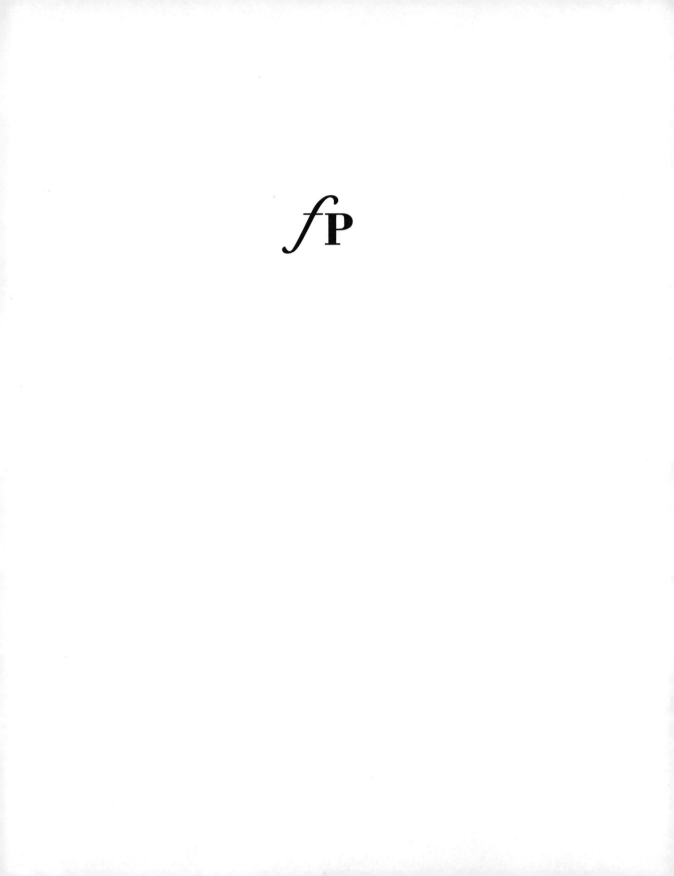

ALSO BY MICHAEL F. ROIZEN AND MEHMET C. OZ

YOU: Staying Young

YOU: On a Diet

YOU: The Smart Patient

YOU: The Owner's Manual

ALSO BY MICHAEL F. ROIZEN

The RealAge Workout:
Maximum Health, Minimum Work

The RealAge Makeover:
Take Years off Your Looks and Add Them to Your Life

Cooking the RealAge Way:
Turn Back Your Biological Clock with More than 80 Delicious and Easy Recipes

The RealAge Diet: Make Yourself Younger with What You Eat

RealAge: Are You as Young as You Can Be?

ALSO BY MEHMET C. OZ

Healing from the Heart:
A Leading Surgeon Combines Eastern and Western Traditions
to Create the Medicine of the Future

YOU

Being BEAUTIFUL

The Owner's Manual to Inner and Outer Beauty

MICHAEL F. ROIZEN, M.D.
and MEHMET C. OZ, M.D.

with Ted Spiker, Craig Wynett, Lisa Oz, and Arthur W. Perry, M.D.

Illustrations by Gary Hallgren

FREE PRESS

NEW YORK   LONDON   TORONTO   SYDNEY

*f*P

Free Press
A Division of Simon & Schuster, Inc.
1230 Avenue of the Americas
New York, NY 10020

First Free Press hardcover edition November 2008

FREE PRESS and colophon are trademarks of Simon & Schuster, Inc.

For information about special discounts for bulk purchases,
please contact Simon & Schuster Special Sales at
1-800-456-6798 or business@simonandschuster.com

Designed by Ruth Lee-Mui

Manufactured in the United States of America

1   3   5   7   9   10   8   6   4   2

Library of Congress Cataloging-in-Publication Data

Roizen, Michael F.
You, being beautiful : the owner's manual to inner and outer beauty /
by Michael F. Roizen and Mehmet C. Oz ; with Ted Spiker ;
illustrations by Gary Hallgren.
     p.   cm.
1. Health.   2. Beauty, Personal.   I. Oz, Mehmet C.   II. Title.
          RA776.096   2008
     613—dc22   2008024414

ISBN-13: 978-1-4165-7234-3
ISBN-10:   1-4165-7234-1

NOTE TO READERS

This publication contains the opinions and ideas of its authors. It is intended to provide helpful and informative material on the subjects addressed in the publication. It is sold with the understanding that the authors and publisher are not engaged in rendering medical, health, or any kind of personal professional services in the book. The reader should consult his or her medical, health, or other competent professional before adopting any of the suggestions in this book or drawing inferences from it.

In addition, this book sometimes recommends particular products or websites for your reference. Drs. Oz and Roizen are not affiliated in any way with such products or entities (with the exception of the Real Age website). In some instances, other coauthors or contributors may be affiliated with a referenced product or website, but recommendations were made independent of such affiliation. In all instances, bear in mind that there are many products or websites other than those recommended here that may work for you or provide useful information to you.

The authors and publisher specifically disclaim all responsibility for any liability, loss, or risk, personal or otherwise, which is incurred as a consequence, directly or indirectly, of the use and application of any of the contents of this book.

To all who radiate outer beauty
because they treasure inner beauty

CONTENTS

Introduction   1

Your YOU-Q: Measure Your Inner and Outer Beauty   8

Part I: Looking Beautiful   21

1. In the Flesh: Make Your Skin Glow   31

2. Head of Class: How to Save Your Hair   65

3. Oral Victories: Your Mouth and Teeth Are a Portal to Your Inside—
   and Say a Lot About Your Outside   87

4. Digital Revolution: Shape Up Your Hands and Feet   107

5. Great Shape: How to Get the Body You've Always Wanted   129

Part II: Feeling Beautiful   151

6. Energized and Revitalized: Power Up Your Body by
   Resetting Your System   155

7. That's Gotta Hurt: How to Manage Your Major Aches and Pains   175

8. Get in the Mood: What You Can Do to Straighten Out Your Mind   223

9. The Worry War: Solve Your Most Troubling Job and Money Issues   255

Part III: Being Beautiful   279

10. That Lovin' Feeling: Improve Your Relationships with the
People Close to You   283

11. That's the Spirit: How to Find True Happiness   311

The Be-YOU-tiful Plan: Live the Ultimate Beautiful Day
(and Improve Your YOU-Q)   337

YOU Tools: More Strategies for Helping You Become Even More
Beautiful   349

Appendix: Healing with Steel   393
Finding the Right Plastic Surgery for You

Acknowledgments   401

Index   407

YOU Tools

The Ideal Wash   56

Body Art   61

Hair Care   83

Foot Play Foreplay   126

Fashion Statements   149

Orthopedic Injuries   205

Breathe-Free Program   246

Finding Your Personality   252

Green Living   333

The Band Workout   351

The Yoga Workout   361

The Perfect Gym Bag   375

Health Utensils (Your Medicine Cabinet, Home Hygiene, Infection Protection)   377

Your Eyes   383

The Biophysical Battery: Energy Blood Tests   387

INTRODUCTION

For those of you who think beauty is about mirrors, makeup, and how many pudding packs you have to sacrifice to fit into your skinny jeans, then pull up a chair, postpone your top-of-the-hour Botox appointment, and hear this.

Beauty isn't some vapid and superficial pursuit that exists solely to sell products, wag tongues, and produce drool. Beauty is actually precisely perceived, purposeful, and rooted more in hard science than in abstract and random opinion. From the time we started prancing around the world with our body-hair parkas and leafy lingerie, evolution has pushed us to be more beautiful. And that's why beauty serves as the foundation for our feelings, our happiness, and our existence. In fact, beauty doesn't reflect our vanity as much as it does our humanity.

Beauty—dear appearance-obsessed friend—*is* health.

We already know that beauty is always on your mind, because it's on everyone's minds. You can't help but think about it or suppress it—consciously or not—every time you step in the shower or in front of the mirror. It drives many of the decisions you make about exercise and eating, and it determines how you choose between the black dress and the white pants.

This kind of traditional beauty—the outer kind—really isn't just about looking good. Outer beauty serves as a proxy of how healthy you are; it's the message you send to others about your health.* Way back when—before we could decode your genome, use fertility tests to see when you're ovulating, and order MRIs to see

---

* Not convinced yet? Look at traditional images of ugliness—pus, blood, gore, Freddy Krueger—and they almost always correlate with something that's *unhealthy*.

1

what was going on with your liver—people used beauty as the serious assessment of the potential health of a partner. Beauty was the best way to figure it out (and in a tenth of a second, mind you). Now, if you take the concept of beauty a few steps deeper, you realize that inner beauty—the idea of feeling good and being happy—also has tremendous health implications in every aspect of your life.

But for so long, we've had it all wrong. We've thought of beauty as nonessential and superficial. Just look at our most popular beauty-based clichés:

- Beauty is in the eye of the beholder. Translation: Just as we all have different taste buds, we all have different beauty buds, as well. Some like blond; some like brown. Some like their men to wear boxers; others prefer leopard-print G-strings.
- Don't judge a book by its cover. Translation: Don't make assumptions or judgments about people just because they have big boobs, no hair, or a belt that's longer than a circus tightrope.
- Beauty is only skin deep. Translation: Stop linking outer beauty with the inner kind. They're as separate as mashed potatoes and maple syrup.

The logic behind all these myths argues that external beauty is unimportant, most likely misleading, and at best relevant only until more useful information becomes available. But we have three words for these three clichés: wrong, wrong, wrong. Scientific study after study shows that these popular principles are more myth than reality.

In fact, research shows that human beings have evolved universal standards of beauty, both within and across cultures. Research also shows that attractive people are judged more positively than unattractive people—even when there's other information available about them. The data show that more attractive people are judged to be better liked, more competent, and more exciting (all by about a two-to-one margin). Research also indicates that external beauty is linked to personality and behavior.*

---

* There are also some interesting historical implications about beauty. In the Middle Ages, pockmarks on the body meant you had already survived smallpox and would be more desirable (since you would be

Though there are biological and social influences on beauty, it does seem that being deemed attractive creates a kind of self-fulfilling prophecy that reinforces and internalizes certain behaviors and self-concepts. And guess what? Most of these crucial factors are ones you can change for the better.

In *YOU: Being Beautiful,* we're going to share with you the biology of beauty, as well as what you can do to be your most beautiful self by making choices and taking actions that will help you look the way you want, and most important, feel and be the way you want.

We're going to clarify what beauty really is—and give you the tools to become healthier and happier by paying a little more attention to it. How? We're going to chop up beauty into three distinct pieces—pieces that will give you a perspective that may change the way others view you and, ultimately, *the way you view the world.* These three hunks serve as the structural outline for this book.

Part 1:

LOOKING BEAUTIFUL: You don't have to be a screen star to know that outer beauty matters. Simply, appearance is the proxy—the instant message to others—for youth, fertility, and health. In this section, we'll explore some of the ways that you can improve your looks when it comes to such things as your skin, your hair, and your body shape. Most of all, these things are important because how you look partly helps determine how you feel.

---

less likely to be killed by the world's biggest plague). And so those people became more sought after—more beautiful. And, in times of little food (like the 15th century and the Great Depression), plump figures were more desirable, because they conveyed that there was enough wealth to provide food for the young.

Part 2:

FEELING BEAUTIFUL: There's no doubt in our minds that looking like diamonds doesn't mean squat if you feel like a wooden nickel. You can have the best hair, skin, and butt this side of Kalamazoo, but if you lack energy or your knees creak or you're sadder than a leashed kitty, then all the outward magnetism you may have will be obscured—and fade fast. Here we'll take a look at the big things that can keep you from feeling beautiful—things like fatigue and chronic pain and destructive attitudes—so you can help turn the blues into, well, hot pinks or purples.

Part 3:

BEING BEAUTIFUL: Though you may assume that we'd be imposing morality in a section about "being beautiful," we're not really talking about behaviors here. We're not here to tell you what's right and wrong but to explain how to take your life one step deeper—to find a more authentic and happier you in your life and relationships—and how to use different strategies to do so.

The beauty of these three kinds of beauty is that they're all tied together: Looking as good as you like helps you feel good about yourself, which serves as the foundation for developing that sense of authenticity and deeper purpose that so many of us crave as we search for meaning in our lives. Plus, being authentic and happier makes you physically more attractive.

Now, let's get one thing straight so you can relax a bit. You wouldn't be here unless your ancestors were beautiful. You need to accept the fact that we're all beautiful; sexual selection guaranteed it, because your ancestors mated with the most beautiful partners. We all have beautiful elements in us; we're going to talk about ways that we can expose and maximize them.

The beauty industry is one of the biggest money-takers around (it sells us *a lot*). We have cosmetics companies and cosmetic surgeons. We have super-models with their own magazine covers, commercials, and reality shows. We're obsessed with fashion and our weight. We fret over inopportune pimples in inopportune places. We exercise our bodies, we scrub our faces, we wax off gnarly hair, we buy expensive underwear to push our breasts up and suck our stomachs in. And maybe you're right. We're all emphasizing the wrong things.

Here we argue that beauty is also much more than outer appearances alone. As we'll explore through the middle and the end of the book, beauty is also about how you feel and how you define your life. These three interlocking elements—look, feel, be—work together to form what we believe is the ultimate goal in all of our lives: *to feel good about yourself because you have strong self-esteem and a healthy, energetic existence that allows you to appreciate the subtle beauty of day-to-day life, and because you know your purpose in life—and to show off that purpose by helping others do the same.*

YOU: Being Beautiful is really about the fact that we're all hardwired with automatic thoughts and perceptions about beauty. That means that many of these ideas have evolved over thousands of years to form a foundation for human behavior, emphasizing that it's especially hard to overcome some of the automatic drives.

To that end, beauty is very serious business—as in survival-of-the-species serious. When we think about survival of the species (living long enough to pass your genes on to the next generation), it's natural to emphasize the survival part of the equation. But when it comes down to a choice between surviving and breeding, breeding often wins. (Think of male grizzlies fighting to the death for a mate.) Considering the stakes, you'd better be sure that the object of your affection (that man with those magnificent abs) is worthy of the effort to attract him. But how can you know for sure? Thankfully, just like the metal detector–toting treasure hunter who leaves luck and serendipity to the amateurs, you come fully equipped with your own professional-grade beauty detectors.

When we spot a particularly attractive person, somewhere deep in our reptilian brains, a beauty alarm goes off. It tells us when we've struck gold, and it does so automatically and subconsciously. Just like a reflex, it's automatic, impossible to stop, and Annie Oakley accurate. Your beauty detectors have the mathematical precision of a Swiss watch, and this precision comes in the form of some very specific numbers that you'll learn about in this book, including something called the Fibonacci sequence. You'll also learn that's the reason why we make so many decisions with our emotions and not our logic; those decisions play a major role in how beautiful and healthy we feel.

To teach you about these things, we're going to use some of the same techniques you may be familiar with if you've followed us along this wonderful journey about YOU. We'll offer YOU Tests to allow you to assess your various states of beauty. We'll explain (both verbally and visually) all of the biology that makes up the systems we talk about; once you know the *why*, you're more likely to take action with a *what*. We'll offer plenty of YOU Tips and YOU Tools that you can use to look and feel better than you ever have before. Right after this introduction, we'll test your YOU-Q—a measurement of how well you're doing in your overall pursuit of authenticity and happiness, since there's quite possibly a large difference between the current you and the potential you (it's hard to be happy if that difference is big). And we'll end up with the ultimate beautiful day—24 hours of simple changes that can help you get where you can.

Along the way, you'll be challenged, shocked, and surprised—and your perceptions about inner and outer beauty may very well implode right in front of your freshly exfoliated face. You'll learn why shampoo may not be all that necessary, why and how the perfect smile can be measured down to the millimeter, how a secret to effective foreplay centers around your ten toes, why female orgasms are crucial to the continuation of the species, how tennis balls can mend an aching back, why a simple change in language fosters or stops addictions, and why our definition of spirituality is like nothing you've ever heard before. We'll cover lots of topics in these three parts of beauty—including all the health implications and easy-to-follow solutions that can help you get the most out of life. (In our humble opinions, it doesn't get more beautiful than that.)

As you dive into this book, you'll come across essential information about the seemingly inconsequential things in life (hello, pores!), and you'll come across mind-blowing inspiration about the absolutely consequential things in life (how to find true meaning and purpose). While we'll hit you with the nuts and bolts of outer beauty, we also hope to inspire you to make changes about how you feel on the inside. Throughout, we'll try to challenge your assumptions about what true beauty is.

Along the way, you'll surely look in the mirror—both literally and metaphorically. You'll get new perspectives on body shapes, on fingernails, on tongues, on depression, on knee pain, on energy levels, on sexuality, on prayer, on so many things in your life that you can strengthen to live healthier and happier. It may be hard to imagine that hangnails and deities belong in the same book. But as we hope you come to appreciate, beauty isn't about the parts. It's about how those parts work together to form the whole. The whole YOU.

YOUR YOU-Q

Measure Your Inner and Outer Beauty

In this book, we're going to give you lots of advice about things you can do to look, feel, and be more beautiful. Some of them you should absolutely do, because they contribute to your overall health. Others? They may not be so clear-cut, because, unlike flip-flops and baby cribs, they're not a one-size-fits-all proposition. What works for you may be absolutely wrong for someone else.

To that end, we've developed the ultimate YOU-Q Test—a quick exercise that will help you identify the things that can help you become happier and more satisfied with yourself. And your life. The key to all of it: finding what we call *authentic beauty.* True beauty comes when you engage with your fellow man in a healthy fashion. That's real authenticity and what will make you happier.

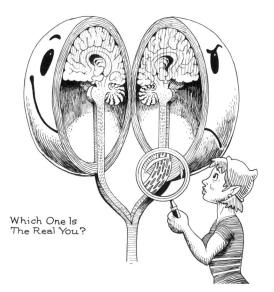

Which One Is The Real You?

Authentic beauty comes from closing the gap between the Current YOU and the Potential YOU.

Current YOU (who you are right now): This includes your physical appearance (bunions and all) and all of the characteristics and quirks that make you, you.

Potential YOU (the person you would like to be, remembering that that may not be the perfect person): Current YOU with some adjustments—perhaps a bit thinner, a little more empathetic, a better cello player, maybe even a redhead.

When the gap between Current YOU and Potential YOU is wider than a 12-lane interstate, you're going to feel less beautiful, less satisfied, and less confident. Close the gap, and bingo, you're hitting the bull's-eye on the target of authentic beauty.

No IQ test or SAT or insect-looking inkblot can help you identify the size of your gap. This YOU-Q Test will. The YOU-Q tests the nature and size of your gaps in four major areas—and gives you plenty of issues to ponder. But don't think of this

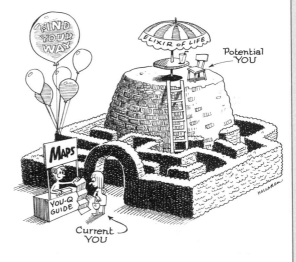

as a final exam. Think of it as more of a practice test that you can retake and retake and retake until you come as close to perfection as possible.

As you read the book, your test results will help you understand where to focus your attention in order to bring Current YOU and Potential YOU into better alignment to find true happiness. To help you along the way, you're going to record your scores on the YOU-Q report sheet at the end of the chapter. OK, sharpen your No. 2 pencils and let's begin.

Note: All the questions in this test are based on validated studies, i.e., real docs spent years proving that these are the appropriate questions to ask to get accurate answers to help you understand yourself. We even enlisted the help of world expert psychologist Dr. Art Markman from the University of Texas to ensure accuracy.

Part I: Looking Beautiful

Think about the appearance you present to the outside world—your face and body. Using the figure below, answer these two questions (be honest, bucko, nobody's looking but you):

1. Circle the image that most closely corresponds to the body type you have *right now.*
2. Circle the image that represents what you think would be the *ideal* body type for you. This body type should be the one that you want, not the one that you think others might want for you.

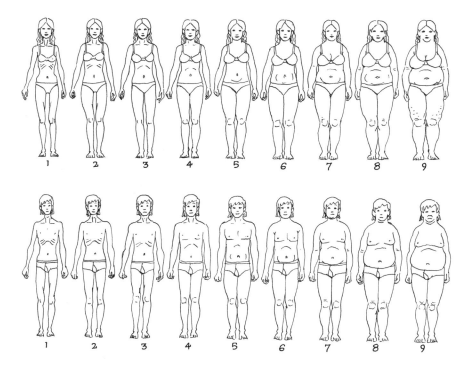

For this part of scoring your test, look at the difference between your responses to questions 1 and 2. Just count how many bodies are between the ones you picked; don't worry about the direction.

If the difference between your answers is:

6 or 7 bodies: We have some work to do. So put **0** in the Body Score box on page 11.

5 bodies: Give yourself **3** body score points in the box at the end of this section.

4 bodies: Give yourself **6** body score points in the box at the end of this section.

3 bodies: Give yourself **9** body score points in the Body Score box below.

2 bodies: Give yourself **12** body score points in the Body Score box below.

1 body: Give yourself **15** body score points in the Body Score box below.

0 body: Give yourself **18** body score points in the Body Score box below.

Picked the same body for both: Congratulations! Give yourself **21** body score points in the Body Score box.

Answer these four questions about your face and skin:

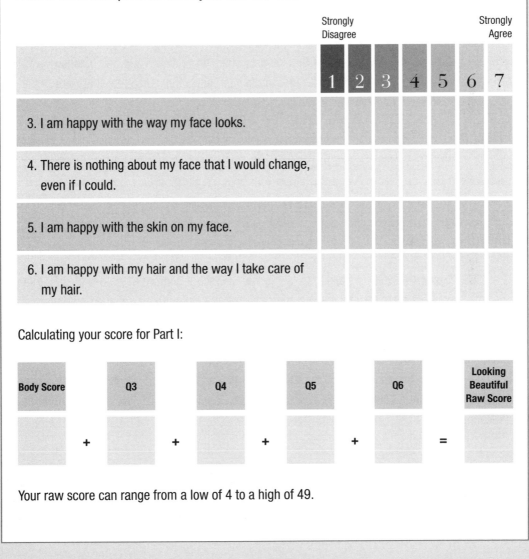

	Strongly Disagree						Strongly Agree
	1	2	3	4	5	6	7
3. I am happy with the way my face looks.							
4. There is nothing about my face that I would change, even if I could.							
5. I am happy with the skin on my face.							
6. I am happy with my hair and the way I take care of my hair.							

Calculating your score for Part I:

Body Score		Q3		Q4		Q5		Q6		Looking Beautiful Raw Score
	+		+		+		+		=	

Your raw score can range from a low of 4 to a high of 49.

Your Looking Beautiful Raw Score

The scales in this section reveal about how happy you are with your overall appearance, focusing on your face and body. Find the range for your score on the Looking Beautiful test analysis below. After you read what scores in that range mean, write down the number of YOU-Q points you get for this score in the YOU-Q worksheet at the end of the section.

If Your Raw Score Is

4–18

There's a lot about your appearance that bothers you. You probably feel bad whenever you look in the mirror. It will take a lot of work to change your appearance, but there are many things you can do to improve your body, face, hair, and skin.

19–30

You don't feel like putting a paper bag over your head, but you also aren't thrilled with the way you look. It may be that you want to change your body, or perhaps your face or your hair. We have a lot of suggestions that will help you improve the way you look, so it won't be long before this score starts to go up.

31–39

Just because you may enjoy walking by a window to catch a glimpse of your reflection, that doesn't mean that there aren't a few changes you'd like to make. There are always things you can do to help maintain the beautiful you and to protect it from bad habits, the sun, and age.

40–49

Frankly, we're surprised you had time to fill out this survey between modeling gigs. All we can say to you is, stay out of the sun, wear your seat belt, keep your feet on the ground, and keep reaching for the stars.

Part II: Feeling Beautiful

The questions in this section focus on how you feel physically.

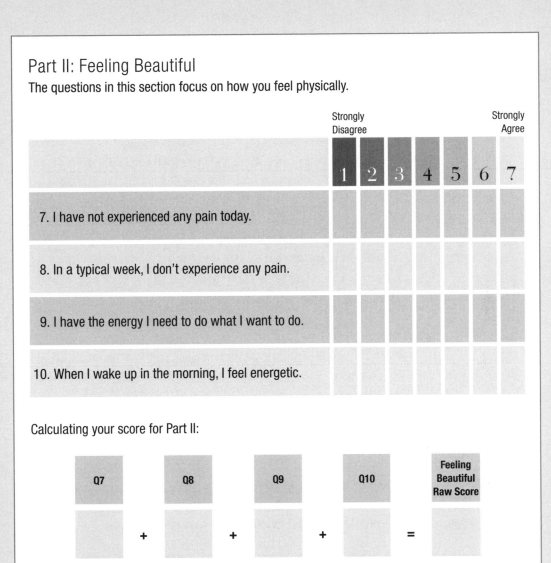

	Strongly Disagree						Strongly Agree
	1	2	3	4	5	6	7
7. I have not experienced any pain today.							
8. In a typical week, I don't experience any pain.							
9. I have the energy I need to do what I want to do.							
10. When I wake up in the morning, I feel energetic.							

Calculating your score for Part II:

Q7 + Q8 + Q9 + Q10 = Feeling Beautiful Raw Score

Your raw score can range from a low of 4 to a high of 28.

Your Feeling Beautiful Raw Score

How you feel is a combination of whether you are in pain and how much energy you have. If you are in pain, it's hard to feel beautiful. If you're dragging all day, it's pretty darn hard also to be a beauty.

If Your Raw Score Is

4–14

If you score in this range, you may have some kind of chronic pain like arthritis that makes you feel like one tired and hurtin' pup. Pain may be keeping you from exercising as much as you would like, which may also affect your energy level. The chapters in Part II will be particularly important to you.

15–21

There are days when you feel as though your get-up-and-go got up and went. On those days, you're just happy to get through the day (certainly not a recipe for beauty). We'll have a lot to say about how you can feel better and increase your energy level.

22–28

Most of the time you feel pretty good. You get out of bed, you have a full day. Not much keeps you from doing what you want to do. Keep it up. And check out the tips in Part II to help you keep feeling good and running strong.

Part III: Being Beautiful

Answer these questions (honestly).

11. Check the *one statement* below that best describes your average happiness.

IN GENERAL, HOW HAPPY OR UNHAPPY DO YOU USUALLY FEEL?	Select *Only* One
Extremely happy (feeling ecstatic, joyous, fantastic)!	(11 pts.)
Very happy (feeling really good, elated)!	(10 pts.)
Pretty happy (spirits high, feeling good).	(9 pts.)
Mildly happy (feeling fairly good and somewhat cheerful).	(8 pts.)
Slightly happy (just a bit above neutral).	(7 pts.)

Neutral (not particularly happy or unhappy).	(6 pts.)
Slightly unhappy (just a bit below neutral).	(5 pts.)
Mildly unhappy (just a little low).	(4 pts.)
Pretty unhappy (somewhat "blue," spirits down).	(3 pts.)
Very unhappy (depressed, spirits very low).	(2 pts.)
Extremely unhappy (utterly depressed, completely down).	(1 pt.)

Now answer these six questions on a scale from 1–7.

	Strongly Disagree						Strongly Agree
	1	2	3	4	5	6	7
12. I am satisfied with my life.							
13. If I could live my life over, I would change almost nothing.							
14. I am very comfortable with myself.							
15. I perform well at many things.							
16. I find inner strength from my prayers, meditations, or quieting my mind.							
17. I believe that on some level my life is intimately connected to all of humankind.							

Calculating your score for Part III:

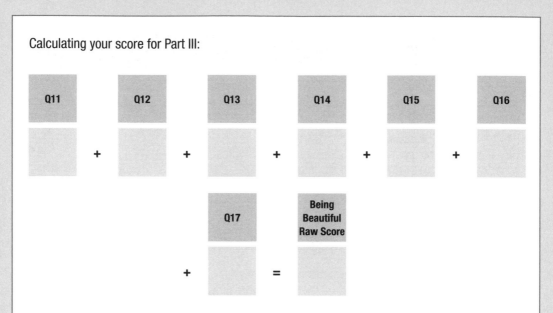

Your raw score can range from a low of 7 to a high of 53.

Your Being Beautiful Raw Score

Life satisfaction is just what it sounds like. How happy are you right now, and how pleased are you with the way your life has turned out so far? Self-esteem is a good marker of how good you feel about your ability to get things done in the world and your influence on other people. By boosting your self-esteem, you are able to be more effective in the world and more beautiful in the broadest sense of the word. Finally, two of the questions ask about the role of spirituality in your life. There is good evidence that having a solid spiritual foundation increases your life satisfaction. We'll have more to say about spirituality in chapter 11.

If Your Raw Score Is

7–19

You're not that happy with life right now. And you're down on yourself quite a bit. There may even be other people who are down on you. You might want to talk to a therapist or counselor (if you aren't doing so already). Depression affects many people over the course of their lives, and it can really stand in the way of your ability to be beautiful.

20–31

There are still days when you wake up and think you could be happier and that you could be doing a better job of living up to your potential. We have a lot of advice to offer. Inner and outer beauty will help increase your life satisfaction, self-esteem, and spiritual health.

32–42

Overall, you feel pretty good about life and your place in the universe. There are days when you can be hard on yourself, but our goal is to help you experience fewer of the bad days and more of the good ones.

43–53

Life feels pretty great to you most days. You probably have a lot of inner and outer beauty already. At the same time, there are a lot of insights in this book that we believe will help you in your continuing quest to make yourself a better person.

Part IV: Understanding YOU

From the list of 60 descriptive words below, pick 5 characteristics that most accurately describe the Current YOU. We know that many of the words could describe YOU, but your challenge is to whittle the number down to the top 5. Next pick 5 words that describe the Potential YOU. Remember, many of the things you would ideally like to be may be things that are already part of the Current YOU. That is, you may be living out some of your ideal characteristics right now.

Since our greatest strengths are often things that are invisible to us, you may want to get some feedback from other people about your strengths. Copy this page and share it with loved ones and coworkers. If they're the same people, perhaps you can forward this document to Human Resources instead.

Smart	Knowledgeable	Honest	Excellent writer
Funny	Empathetic	Great parent	Excellent cook
Caring	Gentle	Musical	In excellent shape
Strict	Capable	Watchful	Entertaining
High achiever at work	Great friend	Artistic	Excellent host/hostess
Confident	Inventive	Organized	Powerful
Humble	Reliable	Outgoing	Excellent caretaker
Rational	Conventional	Personable	Giver (of time or money)
Authentic	Unconventional	Dependent	Neat
Holder of high standards	Breadwinner	Good-looking	Politically active
Easygoing	Moral	Rich	Sexy
Passionate	Supportive	Athletic	Very sexually active
Stylish	Wise	Famous	Loyal
Unflappable	Independent	Leader	Monogamous
Content	Inspiring	Married/Partnered	Spontaneous

Calculating your score for Part IV:

See how many words overlapped between the lists you created for the Current YOU and the Potential YOU. For each word you have in common, take 6 points.

0 overlapping words: Give yourself **0** points.

1 overlapping word: Give yourself **6** points.

2 overlapping words: Give yourself **12** points.

3 overlapping words: Give yourself **18** points.

4 overlapping words: Give yourself **24** points.

5 overlapping words: Give yourself **30** points.

Your raw score can range from a low of 0 to a high of 30.

Your Understanding YOU Raw Score

In this section, you described aspects of who you are that can be changed, and your answers will help focus your efforts.

If Your Raw Score Is

0

Get going, tiger. There's clearly a lot that you would like to be that is not quite the same as who you are.

1–18

You've started to achieve your ideals, but there's still lots more work to go. Part III will help work out a game plan for change.

19–30

You're well on your way. Keep it up. Remember, you don't necessarily want Current YOU and Potential YOU to be identical (you always want to be striving for something!).

Your Final YOU-Q Score

Add your raw scores from each part to determine your YOU-Q Score:

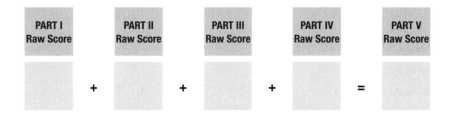

PART I Raw Score		PART II Raw Score		PART III Raw Score		PART IV Raw Score		PART V Raw Score
	+		+		+		=	

The YOU-Q ranges from 15 to 160

Add up your YOU-Q points and start spreading the news. The closer the score is to 160, the more your Current YOU and Potential YOU match. This match between Current YOU and Potential YOU really does tell you a lot about yourself. It tells you how good you feel about who you are. It also gives you a sense of how well you've been able to make changes in yourself in the past and how well you've addressed challenges in your life.

Just to give you an idea about your score, a score of around 160 is nearly impossible to achieve, and you shouldn't think of that as a goal. Just as you probably don't know anybody with an IQ of 160, you probably don't know anybody with a YOU-Q of 160. If your YOU-Q is 100 or above, then you are pretty typical of people who take this test. Finally, don't pay a lot of attention to small differences between scores. If you got a 105 and your best friend got a 110, that is essentially the same score. It does appear that having a younger Real Age than biological age helps you achieve a higher score—and more happiness. (Take the Real Age test at www .realage.com.)

To validate the YOU-Q, we gave the survey to 1,174 women and 533 men who had taken it on the RealAge website. The average YOU-Q score for the women was 95 and for men was 99, so both genders have about the same happiness score. This average stays the same across our lifespan, but individuals can increase and decrease their score as they age. If your YOU-Q is way above 100, congratulations! You're already well on the path to beauty. If it is well below 100, then you have got some work ahead of you. Luckily, your YOU-Q differs from your IQ, because your YOU-Q is easy to change. So no matter what your YOU-Q, you'll find plenty of great advice in the pages to come that will help that score go up.

As you make changes in your body, your health, and your inner self, you will also experience changes in your life satisfaction and self-esteem. All of these factors will increase your YOU-Q. Periodically come back and take the YOU-Q again, and watch the YOU-Q grow—just as you do.

Part I

Looking Beautiful

Glowing Skin

Luscious Hair

Marvelous Mouth

Nice Digits

Sexy Shape

Quick, think of a place that doesn't have a mirror. Pretty hard, right? Bathrooms, of course, have them. So do cars, department stores, gyms, supermarkets, hotel lobbies, bars, subway cars, purses, bedroom walls, and bedroom ceilings. In fact, you'd almost have to be living in solitary confinement or a single-seat submarine not to have the opportunity to judge your own appearance through your reflection.*

Besides constantly being judged by your own gaze, your face and body often serve as the target for other people's eyes (and perhaps whistles). While it may seem unfair to be under such constant visual scrutiny, the fact remains that beautiful people have more advantages than unattractive folks. Sounds harsh, we know, but just consider the evidence:

- Mental acuity, interpersonal skills, and moral goodness are all associated with physically beautiful people.
- Beautiful people are believed by others to have happier marriages and more rewarding jobs. And they're more likely to be hired, have a higher salary, and be promoted sooner.
- Better-looking people are more likely to marry sooner, as well as to marry people who have more money and higher social status.
- More attractive babies have even been shown to be rewarded with greater overt maternal affection.

* Only two animals in the world, humans and great apes, are able to recognize themselves in the mirror. To recognize yourself in a mirror means you must have a self-concept, a mental image of yourself on which to base the match. Which, of course, raises the question of where the mental image came from. Are we constructing our sense of self by virtually superimposing other people's faces on top of our own and somehow sensing the differences? Maybe this is why our self-assessment of our own beauty predictably goes down if we are asked to rate ourselves just after spending time with a substantially more attractive individual.

In this part of the book we'll be examining the elements that primarily determine whether or not you're perceived as beautiful or not—things like skin, hair, and body shape. But before we start any specific discussion of various wrinkles and jiggles, we'd like you to take a step back and look at the bigger picture.

Though we'll have plenty to say about the body's anatomical wonders, the most important body part of all when it comes to beauty isn't a luscious lip or hardened glute. It's your brain.

Now, we're not suggesting that the pituitary gland and hypothalamus are party-stopping body parts the way a silky mane or a plywood-flat waist may be.* What we are suggesting is that beauty is always on your mind. In fact, your brain *needs* beauty.

Your brain—under intense demand to process an infinite amount of information at any given moment—must make choices about whom to trust, whom to mate with, and whom to run from. It does this by dispensing with unnecessary stimuli—and drawing conclusions from a select few pieces of info. So we're not programmed to not worry about whether a strand of hair is out of place but are programmed to note the subtleties of facial expressions, whether the slight curve in a lip is conveying anger, sadness, or fear. That process, really, is the foundation of perception—how you perceive and contextualize the facts and faces all around you.† Beauty is not as much a physical property of the person, as the end product of a complex mental process that translates millions of meaningless dots of light on the back of our retinas into 3-D shapes, objects, and faces. Embedded in the software of the mind is a set of rules that are used to decode these raw "bytes" of visual information. Think of these "bytes" as the letters in the alphabet. The perceptual rules are like grammar; they determine how the parts are combined to create a whole.

What's most interesting is that these observations are automatic—a beauty reflex, if you will. Most of us, especially when we're young, have a strong sex

* Unless, of course, a pretty pituitary is your thing.
† In fact, you have a separate part of your brain just to process faces (the fusiform gyrus).

drive—a drive so strong, in fact, that it often overshadows all of our other natural drives. But nobody instructed us to be sexually attracted to others. We didn't have to learn about hourglass figures or chiseled jaws. It was instinctive—a genetically programmed behavior.

These instinctive behaviors aren't conscious acts. They're spontaneous, irrepressible, and predictable. They're performed without evident reason, but rather with stimulation. Your beauty detectors, like Doppler radar, are able to scan the environment in real time for signs of an attractive mate and forecast a conclusion about that environment. Your assessments are fast and accurate. For example, you can observe a human face for a fraction of a second and accurately rate its beauty—and what it's trying to communicate to you, through expressions, nuances, and all kinds of nonverbal signals. Similarly, your appearance affects the first impressions that others have of you. And that first one can be a lasting one.

So how do we make those snap judgments? It all starts with a group of numbers called the Fibonacci sequence. That sequence is 0, 1, 1, 2, 3, 5, 8, 13, and so on. Each new number is the sum of the two before it, and the ratio of each number to the one before it approximates the value of phi, or 1.618.* OK, so you may be asking what in the world a group of numbers has to do with the fact that you prefer just a little bit of nicely groomed chest hair. Well, phi is the basis for what's called the divine proportion or the golden ratio: the ratio of lengths from one element to another is 1.618 to 1 (see Figure A.1). This golden ratio is found throughout nature, from leaves to seed arrangements to conch shells, and it also figures prominently in a list of man's greatest accomplishments, like the Great Pyramids, the Parthenon, Michelangelo's *David,* and Leonardo's *Mona Lisa.* The omnipresence of phi throughout our world creates a sense of balance, harmony, and beauty in the designs we see naturally and artificially.

Phi is also a driving force in human attraction—men and women around the globe prefer a mate whose face is symmetrical and follows this ratio. (More than

---

*The way scientists came up with this number is through trying to predict reproductive patterns in animals. If you take a male and female rabbit (1 and 1), put them in a cage and reproduce, you'd have 3 (the next number in the sequence). Now with three in the cage (1 male and 2 female), you'd end up with 5 total in a few weeks, and so on (see Figure A.1).

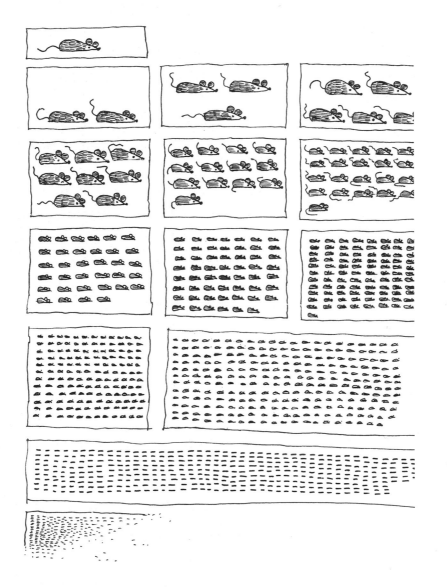

Figure A.1 Oh, Rats! The reproductive patterns of animals gave us the formula for beauty. Each generation of life—whether flower petals or lips—reproduce with a predictable ratio. As the proportion of offspring produced increases, the ratio of one block divided by the one before it serves as the foundation for things we perceive as beautiful. So, ⁵/₃ is about ⁸/₅ is about ¹³/₈, or about 1.6—the golden ratio.

Safari Secrets:
Lessons from the animal kingdom

The reason we all look a little different may not be obvious today, but there's an evolutionary basis for our genetic differences. At first glance, zebra stripes seem like a bull's-eye for predators. In fact they're the wild's greatest camouflage system because predatory animals, which see only in black and white, can't see zebras standing in the tall grass. Also, zebras blend in with the heat waves coming off the ground, which look alternating black and white against the sand, so they're especially confusing to the pestering tsetse flies—an example of how an animal's looks respond to external pressures.

2,000 years ago, Pythagoras developed a formula for the perfect female face, which included such stats as this one: The ratio of the width of the mouth to the width of the nose should be—*tada!*—1.618 to 1.) In this part, you'll see more examples of this on the human body. Now, we're not suggesting that you move your eyeballs closer together or farther apart if they don't meet these statistical standards, but we are suggesting that there are many easier options that can make the ratio closer.

Our point: Humans do have universal (and subconscious) standards of beauty—underscoring its importance and the fact that your brain really does make reflexive decisions about people based on appearance that affect every aspect of your life.

There's a reason why we have to use this reflex—it would take way too much time to assess others if we didn't have it. Consider this:

Just about every situation we confront in life provides infinitely more inputs than we're able to process productively. A classic example of this idea is chess. While the game is reasonably well defined and contained, after just ten moves there are literally billions of possibilities to consider for a next move. Assuming we could evaluate these options at a rate of about one per second, it would take about 9,000 years for us to consider *all* the possibilities. Not only would this make for a really long chess match, it underscores the brain's need to keep it simple.

Because of the immense computational complexity and impracticality of processing all the inputs a particular situation presents, the cognitive system has developed a number of mechanisms that limit the number of possibilities that are considered. How? For one, the eye takes in a limited amount of high-quality information (through a part of the eye called the fovea), which is supplemented with lower-quality info as needed. As your eye moves to process the info, it takes in only a fraction of what's in your horizon. In a constant state of vibration, the eye repeatedly refreshes what it sees (like refreshing web pages). These movements help your brain decide what it is you're looking at (and without the movements, we'd actually lose our vision because the rods and cones in our eyes respond only to certain changes). So you take some shortcuts and make leaps about what you see; you *need* cues like beauty and waist-to-hip ratio—things with scientific and universal standards—to make judgments about people. You can't contemplate 9,000 different nuances in someone's face in a timely fashion. You keep it simple.

For example, the most information-dense visible area in nature is the human face, so we process a small area of the face and extend our conclusions to the entire surface. The right changes (even if they're small) can make a huge impact on how you're perceived. Much of "seeing" someone you know is memory, since we don't reanalyze an entire face each time.* The richest connection of nerve and muscle density in the body is actually around the larynx (voice box), and the face is second—underscoring how important it is that you read subtle messages through speech *and* body language. Some argue that growth of the frontal lobe of the brain happened because of these rich connections and our ability to sense and transmit so much information beyond what most animals can.

Your face communicates whether you're happy, sad, mad, disgusted, surprised, or ready and willing to do the two o'clock tango. Similarly, you receive information about other people through their eyes, their mouth, even their skin. The whole notion of beauty revolves primarily around nature's hockey masks—either you've got a well-designed one or you don't. Now, the question is: How do we define well-designed?

The theory is that the more symmetrical a face is, the healthier it is. As you can see in Figure A.2, that symmetry is divided into several planes, including horizontally, vertically, around the eyes, around the nose, and so on. The formula

---

* It takes one-tenth of a second to recognize someone.

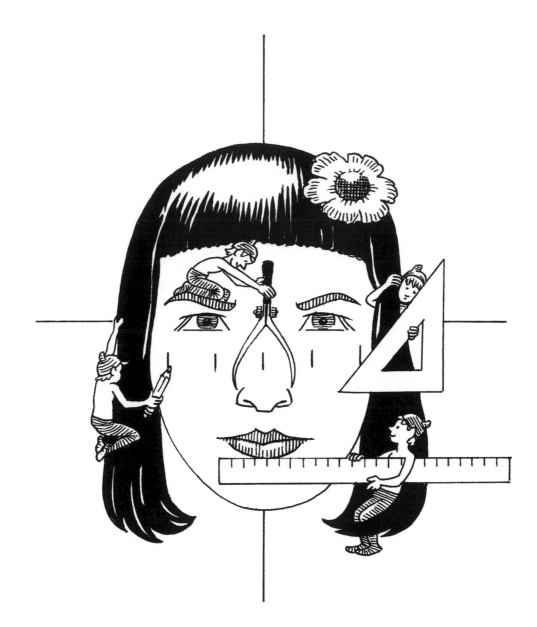

Figure A.2 Divine Ruler Using the golden ratio of 1.6, we judge the beauty of other people's faces (and other body parts). We use that ratio—subconsciously and reflexively—to decode whether someone's eyes, face, and body are, in fact, beautiful.

for beauty is that precise golden ratio (go ahead and pull out a ruler and a calculator on your next date). The same ratio holds for the width of the cheekbones to the width of the mouth. Scientists also believe that symmetry is equated with a strong immune system—indicating that more robust genes make a person more attractive.

Of course, that's the element of beauty that you typically can't control. You have what you were born with. But that doesn't mean that you can't make changes—changes to enhance your beauty and, along with it, the way you feel about yourself.

That begs a few very interesting questions about our own beauty. What do you see when you look in the mirror? How do you think others see you? How much of your self-image has been determined not by who you are but by who others think you are? How much has your sense of the *outer* you influenced the *inner* you? To some degree your appearance influences how well you do in love, at work, and in life, but most of us feel we don't measure up. So the question is, should you just accept yourself as you are? Or should you try to improve your appearance? How far should you go? What should you try to improve? Will it make you happier or feel more satisfied with yourself? And which comes first? Does being satisfied with your appearance lead to a higher self-concept, or does having a high self-concept create a greater sense of happiness?

In the first five chapters of this book, we'll be showing you tips and tricks that will help your skin glow, your hair shine, and your body shrink. They're things that we believe will not only make you look better to the rest of the world but also help you feel a lot better in your inner world.

In the Flesh

Make Your Skin Glow

YOU Test: Tale of the Tape

To take your facial fingerprint, pull out a roll of Scotch tape. Make sure your face is clean (without makeup, sunscreen, moisturizer, or peanut butter for at least two hours). Place a piece of tape vertically on the middle of your forehead from your scalp to the area between your eyebrows. Move it to the outside corners of your eyes, across the apple of each cheek, and above your lip. Press gently in each spot, leave it for a few seconds, and carefully remove. Check the tape for lines and flakiness.

If your tape is completely smooth: You have the skin of a typical 30-year-old.

If you have flaky or dead cells but no lines: You have the skin of a typical 40-year-old.

If you have flaky cells and small lines: You have the skin of a typical 50-year-old.

The world glows all around us. There's the celestial kind of glow—the stars, the moon, the sun. And there's the artificial kind—the night-light inside the baby's room and the neon lights outside the nightclub. But the most wonderful glow we can think of is the living, breathing kind—the kind that comes in the form of human skin.

We all know or have seen people who radiate—who have the kind of smooth, shiny, healthy, glowing skin that could light up Times Square. But you know what? We all have that potential. The problem is that many of us treat our skin like wrapping paper; it starts out looking pretty enough, but eventually we're going to find a way to tear it up.

Now, this glow we're talking about isn't just the result of good genes. It's also the result of making good choices to protect, heal, and clean your skin. We all have the ability to make those decisions. European cars "glow" more than American cars because the manufacturers use smaller drops of color that reflect more light than they refract. Your skin works the same way: If you ruin your reflection through a buildup of oil or dead skin, you lose the glow (and your full beauty potential).

Of course, it goes without saying that pornographic and beauty-product entrepreneurs aren't the only people who know the value of skin. We all know the risks of exposing our bare skin to the sun, snake fangs, and camera phones. And we also know that the way our skin looks goes a long way toward determining how we

FACTOID

We love exercise. But exercise for the face? That's an idea whose time has not come. Exercising the facial muscles is a sure way to *increase* your wrinkles. The facial muscles pull on the skin to give you facial expressions. And the repetitive movements of the skin, over the years, combined with the normal thinning of the collagen and elastin of the dermis, will eventually crack the skin, causing wrinkling. Botox is the reverse of exercise; it paralyzes muscles and lessens wrinkles.

feel about ourselves. If we don't look beautiful, we don't feel it. And if we feel beautiful inside, we reflect it in our skin. So if you have smooth skin that radiates, then you feel and look younger—and probably are younger on the inside, an important aspect of your overall well-being and health. But if you feel depressed and reclusive, you may have more wrinkles than a shar-pei or become spotted, dotted, and blemished. And that's one of the reasons why you should read this chapter. Ultimately, your skin communicates messages about your youthfulness, your vibrancy, and your health. Face it: Skin sells.

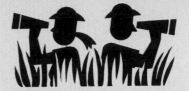

Safari Secrets:
Lessons from the animal kingdom

The reason why there are butterfly collectors and not moth collectors? The colors of moths are determined by scales that are shed, so they don't keep their colors in the box, only in life—just like humans. The colors of a butterfly's wings are never lost.

Your Skin: Let's Flesh a Few Things Out

Funny, whenever we say something's skin deep, we mean that it has about as much depth as a puddle. But that's hardly the case with skin—it's an amazing and complex organ that extends much deeper than the part we can actually see and touch. Your skin is the biggest and heaviest organ of your body, making up 15 percent of your body weight and covering 12 to 20 square feet. The composition: 70 percent water, 25 percent protein, and less than 5 percent fats. The obvious role of skin is to protect and to package. It protects our blood, organs, and bones from what's outside, and it also packages our body neatly together so we're not blobby organisms that leave trails of blood and bits of tissue everywhere we go.

And skin does more than serve as our anatomical casing. Skin also helps us with healing. How? Touching in that loving way reduces levels of the stress chemical cortisol and increases levels of the feel-good chemical oxytocin. And touching in that special way (massaging and caressing, not the touch of a slugger's right hand) also stimulates the vagus nerve, which runs up to the brain to improve the health of our whole body.

So here's how your skin works. While serving as an obvious barrier to the millions of chemicals and germs that want to invade your body, it also has a big sensory function. Deep in the skin, follicles grow hairs that can sense before your skin is actually touched. Eyelashes, for example, prompt the eyelid (through great nerve connections) to involuntarily close to protect the eye before you even know you're in danger and to quickly flick off bugs before they bite.

Besides sprouting up hairs that sense things, your skin lubricates itself with oils we call sebum produced by sebaceous glands and also absorbs certain medications and hormones. But it can also absorb things, such as toxins, that you don't necessarily want. And ultraviolet light can turn your own skin against itself by creating those much-talked-about damaging free radicals, not to mention changing your DNA (and usually not for the better).

Like many structures in your body (including your blood vessels), your skin has several components (see Figure 1.1).

Epidermis: Serving as the body's primary barrier against the outside world, the epidermis is less than a millimeter thick. Your skin is your raincoat, keeping your insides dry and letting you swim without swelling. Your epidermis is so well designed that only the right-size molecules can get through. The cool thing about your skin is that it renews itself every six to eight weeks. How? Dead cells from the epidermis continually slough off and are replaced by new ones from below (that's one major way you get dust in your home—the sloughing off of skin). Your epidermis largely determines how fresh your skin looks—as well as how well it works in terms of absorbing and retaining moisture.

Dermis: The thickest of your skin layers, the dermis is what actually holds you together.* It's your leather. The dermis is made up of cells called fibroblasts,

---

* What, you thought it was duct tape?

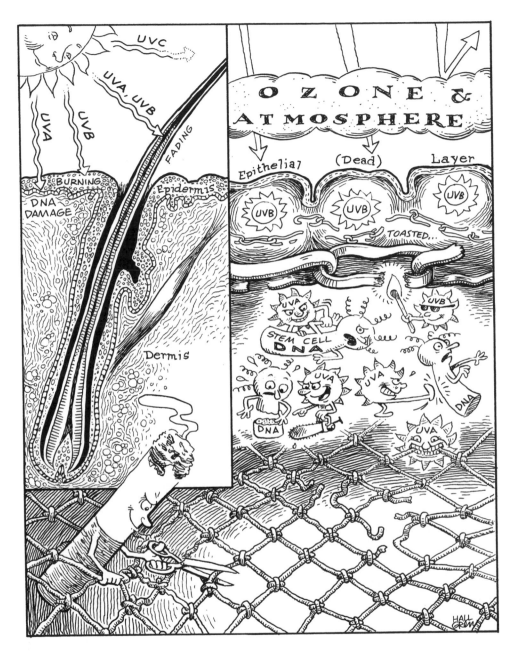

Figure 1.1 Flesh Beating UV radiation damages the skin by weakening elastic collagen fibers and by preventing stem cells from rejuvenating the injured area. It also causes free radicals to damage the DNA, which can lead to cancer. UV-C is blocked by ozone, UV-B penetrates the epidermis, and UV-A goes even deeper to the dermis.

which make collagen and elastin, proteins that give the dermis its strength and allow it to be stretched. Dotting the dermis are hair follicles, sweat glands, and sebaceous glands, which produce the oily sebum that lubricates your skin and hair. This sebum is really a mixed blessing; while it helps keep bacteria under control, it also attracts insects. Finally, the dermis contains tiny blood vessels (to nourish the skin) and lymph nodes (to protect it from toxins).

Subcutaneous tissue: This innermost layer is made up primarily of fat and acts as a shock absorber and heat insulator for your body (many mammals, by the way, don't have this because their fur does the same job).

The Skinny: How Your Skin Works

Your skin can do more than get you arrested. It's able to do many things—some good and some we'd rather live without.

FACTOID

If stretch marks make your skin look like a highway atlas, the answer isn't to try to cover them up with creams or makeup. They actually could be a road map to something more serious that's going on inside your body. First, you need to make sure that your adrenal gland isn't making too many steroids (that could be a sign of Cushing's disease). If the marks are less than a year old and still have a purplish hue, you can have them lasered to lighten them, but other than that, only surgery can remove them.

IT SWEATS: In a way, our skin acts as our third kidney, detoxifying our bodies. When we exert ourselves, not only do we sweat to cool our bodies, we also increase blood flow, which releases toxins. Though it may not be so great on silk blouses and stair climbers, sweating is something you need to do regularly—not just because of the cardiovascular and fat-frying benefits of exercise, but also because of its body-cleansing function.

IT TANS AND BURNS: Exposure to sun causes an immediate release of stored melanin and stimulates the cells designed to protect you from too much sun, the melanocytes, to produce a protective pigment, melanin. But that process takes several days, by which time you have left the beach

Stop the Burning

Some burns are preventable (sideburns and sunburns), some burns are accidental (darn curling iron!), and some burns are downright dumb (leave the fireworks to the pros, smart guy). No matter what the cause, you can take steps to soothe the pain—and prevent scarring or further damage. First, you'll want to cool the burn with water or ice as soon as you can to reduce the prostaglandin response and limit the damage. Clean the area with water and a simple soap such as Ivory, Neutrogena, Dove, or Cetaphil to remove dirt and bacteria, and don't pop any blisters that form. For the small blisters, apply a sterile moisturizer like bacitracin or Neosporin twice a day and leave them intact. They serve as the ideal sterile biologic dressing over the nascent skin that is quickly growing to cover the injured area. Scarring is always worse if the growth of this new skin is hindered. Cover blisters with a fine gauze like Vaseline gauze or Adaptic. The small blisters will dry up and flake off within two weeks.

Note: If the burn is on your hands, face, or genitals (we won't ask) and is bigger than a nickel, it's a good idea to let a doc look at it. She may want to treat it with an antibiotic cream called Silvadene that kills bacteria and keeps the wound moist.

with Santa-suit-colored flesh. The sun, unbuffered by melanin, is your skin's cancer-causing deep fryer.

IT WRINKLES: We all know that wrinkles generally don't look all that good—not in dress shirts and not on your skin. In fact, one main indicator of body aging is wrinkles, especially vertical lines above the lips and between the eyes (each of these stereotypically means different things; cigarette smoking and inflammation in your blood vessels cause lip wrinkles, while vertical lines between eyes reflect stress). How do we get wrinkles? In a couple of ways, actually. Since skin is attached to the muscle beneath it, your skin creases when your muscles move. Over time, that creates a well-worn groove. It's actually like a stress fracture—the repeated bending of skin over the underlying muscle creates inflammation and the collagen gets squeezed together. Young skin stretches and recoils over the muscle, but thinned, old skin loses this ability. And, like an overbent piece of cardboard, it eventually cracks. As we get older, the connections between the skin and underlying connective tissue stretch out, which can cause sagging of the skin. When that happens, gravity pulls down, and the sagging contributes to the formation of wrinkles (see Figure 1.2).

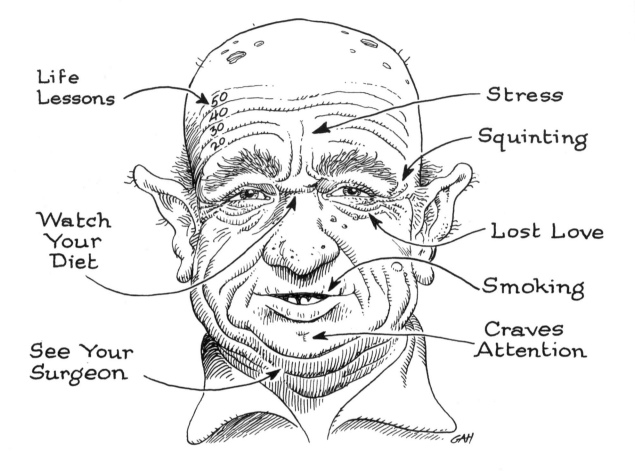

Life Lessons

Stress

Squinting

Watch Your Diet

Lost Love

Smoking

See Your Surgeon

Craves Attention

Figure 1.2 Fine Lines Many things can cause wrinkling, including cigarette smoking and sun exposure. Ultimately, it's caused by thinned, damaged collagen and a loss of elastin fibers (think of it as a kind of stress fracture). When skin loses its elasticity, gravity pulls down on it, and the sagging causes even more wrinkles.

How Skin Ages

When it comes to skin, most of us can spot the good kind a mile away. That's because we can instantly identify all the characteristics of healthy and beautiful skin—it's well hydrated, tight and elastic, not overly oily, has clean pores, and all that. But here's the big myth about skin—that you can stop your skin from aging. No matter what products you use or procedures you undergo, you can't stop time from pulling, tugging, and tearing at your skin. What you can do, however, is slow it down considerably and encourage all of those things that make your skin appear and be healthier.

Skin aging can happen in the matrix between cells, within the dermis, or on the surface. Here's how:

- **In the matrix:** Skin aging happens when your collagen becomes damaged and loses its tight weave, and your elastin loses its zing. The fibroblasts (and their DNA) that produce both collagen and elastin are prone to damage from UV radiation, and as they falter, that DNA, which makes collagen and elastin, makes less and/or defective collagen or elastin. Also, glycosaminoglycans (say that three times fast) are large sugarlike molecules that plump up a bit and fill the skin when they bind with water. As you get older, they become more like an old sponge and don't suck up water as efficiently. The decrease in water content means that the skin becomes like a bad keynote speaker—dull and dry. And those old glycosaminoglycans can link up with proteins and cause yellowing (or browning) of your skin (that's called glycation, and though it happens to all of us, it's especially visible in diabetics).
- **On the surface:** Your skin secretes fat (the technical term is lipids). Fatty acids called ceramides help protect an outer layer of your skin called the stratum corneum, so that you have better skin hydration and are less susceptible to irritation. Think of these fatty acids as a coating on you, like the slimy coating fish have on them; they serve as

an extra buffer layer between you and the outside world. Ceramide concentrations decrease with aging and with washing with fat emulsifiers like soap and alcohol—our mantra isn't "use just water" if you touch people and dirty objects, but using just water helps save those ceramides to help you.

Thinner, duller, less vibrant is what you can expect from your skin as you age, but you can control how fast those changes occur in your skin.

In your 40s, your skin becomes thinner and more translucent so capillaries show through. And those capillaries increase in number as a response to years of inflammation from sun damage. Signs of photoaging—such as wrinkles, age spots, and uneven pigmentation—may show up, especially if your parents or you weren't diligent about sun protection during childhood and in your 20s and 30s. Your skin will produce less oil naturally in your 40s, leading to increased dryness. Cell turnover also is slower, which can cause skin to appear dull.

In your typical 50s, you may experience a deepening of facial lines and wrinkles due to the loss of subcutaneous fat, moisture loss, and accumulated sun damage. As skin elasticity declines, skin may start to sag, especially around the jawline and eye area. If you are postmenopausal, the related drop in estrogen can make your skin thinner, dryer, and more easily irritated. Hydrating moisturizers will decrease water loss but can lead to unnecessary dependence on them (you'll feel as though you always need them). Vitamin A and E creams increase the water

FACTOID

Most of the day, gravity pulls your skin down (contributing to facial sagging and wrinkles). When you sleep faceup, gravity exerts a light stretching effect on your skin; when you sleep face pressed to the pillow, you'll look puffier in the morning and develop sleep lines. There are other reasons for puffiness upon waking. Allergy to dust mites or dust mite poop is common, as are allergies to feather pillows and laundry detergent. These all cause repeated nighttime eyelid swelling. You can prevent leakage of mite poop protein or mites by covering your pillow with a 1-micron case that feels like a pillowcase or a latex cover that feels a bit plasticky; both work to decrease mite allergies and the subsequent puffiness.

Soap It Up

How does soap work? It emulsifies oils—that is, it makes oily substances float away in water. Soaps are all derived from fats—the type of fat used determines the qualities of the soap. In its simplest form, soap is fat mixed with lye. Modern soaps add a chemistry set to the mix, but the simplest soaps are really the best, since every added chemical increases the likelihood of skin irritation, called dermatitis, or allergic reactions to fragrances or preservatives (in the subtle form of puffy eyes or red hands).

We like solid soaps because they can be made with a minimum of ingredients. Liquids often add many chemicals and preservatives. The simplest type of soap is made of saponified olive oil, with a small amount of an essential oil such as lavender or peppermint to give it a nice fragrance. Examples of simple, low-chemical bar soaps are Kiss My Face Pure Olive Oil Soap and Plantlife Aromatherapy Soaps. To prevent the spread of bacteria between users, treat the soap bar as you would treat a toothbrush—don't share.

For liquid soaps, we like Neutrogena and Cetaphil. Check the ingredients—fewer is generally better. You might try See the Dawn Purity facial cleanser, which contains glycerin, aloe vera, and lavender flower–scented water, or Garden of Eve Facial Cleansing Nectar, which contains glycerin, safflower oil, wax, sunflower oil, and water.

content of the skin. Regular exfoliation is a good start, decreasing the thickness of the dry, rough epidermis (more details later).

If you are typical and natural, in your 60s, 70s, 80s, and 90s, cell turnover and skin healing are even slower, and your skin may be very dry, as well. Mature skin may need special care, starting with hydrating moisturizers and regular exfoliation to encourage cell turnover.

Your Skin: What Else Can Go Wrong

As the primary part of your body exposed to external threats, your skin is not only your body's greatest protector* but also extremely vulnerable to the outside world.

Of course, we're most concerned with cancerous growths. Keep an eye out for

---

* Unless, that is, you employ a personal bodyguard.

Keep Off

One of the tricks to using skin products is not only finding the ingredients that will help you but also avoiding the ones that may damage or irritate your skin. Some ingredients you should think about avoiding:

Imidazolidinyl urea and diazolidinyl urea. They're used as preservatives to prevent bacterial growth (not fungi), but they're also a relatively common cause of contact dermatitis.

Fragrances. They may smell good, but these little molecules are responsible for allergic reactions in as many as 14 percent of people. Most skin-care products don't really need added fragrances, but some, like soap, simply smell like the fats they were made from without added fragrance.

Sodium lauryl sulfate. It's common in shampoos and cleaners to create suds and is relatively safe, but longer contact time can cause irritation and dryness, because the detergent strips the skin of lipids.

Mineral oil. Used as a base in some products, it may interfere with perspiration.

MEA, TEA. They're common pH stabilizers, but when they're exposed to air, they form potentially irritating substances called nitrosamines. And they have a tendency to clog pores and create blackheads.

Toluene. This chemical solvent, which the EPA designates as hazardous waste, is found in fingernail polish. Toluene can cause headaches, irritated eyes, and memory loss. The website nottoopretty.com lists perfumes and cosmetics that contain toxic chemicals like toluene. They're not going to kill you, but if you don't feel good, it's worth experimenting to see if beauty products could be the source of your general blahness.

DMAE. This common "instant face-lift" ingredient in wrinkle creams actually does its work by causing cell damage and swelling. Sure, the wrinkles will go away temporarily (they also will if you're slapped in the face), but that doesn't mean it's good for you.

precancerous growths by self-exam with the help of a partner (have your spouse or a close friend look at all the areas you can't see and photograph your total skin surface), and have anything new or different evaluated by a dermatologist. You can even use your cell phone camera to record pictures that your dermatologist can use to compare yearly changes. Put a dime next to any growths that you photograph to provide an estimate of size. By the way, in case you think you're safe just because you stay out of the sun, realize that skin-damaging ozone levels increase in the afternoon, which can affect skin whether it's sunny or not. That un-

YOU Test

What's Your Type?

All that time in front of the mirror, in the shower, and at the nude beach has likely given you some pretty good insight into what type of skin you have. But there's more to skin intelligence than just knowing whether you're happier exposing it or concealing it. Take this test to determine your skin type.

1. Does your skin look dull or flake like a snow globe?
2. Does your skin look like a bathroom floor with a shiny, slippery texture?
3. Does your skin feel itchy and taut like sausage casing?
4. Do you have pores that are enlarged like craters, or clogged pores, or acne?
5. Does your skin react to cosmetics containing alcohol, synthetics, fragrances, and artificial colors?
6. Does your skin appear consistently moist, vibrant, and plumper than a squishy cantaloupe?
7. Does your forehead, nose, or chin appear oilier than a fast-food kitchen, while the skin around your cheeks, eyes, and mouth is normal or dry?

If you answered yes to 1 or 3, you have DRY skin.
If you answered yes to 2 or 4, you have OILY skin.
If you answered yes to 5, you have SENSITIVE skin.
If you answered yes to 6, you have NORMAL skin.
If you answered yes to 7, you have COMBINATION skin.

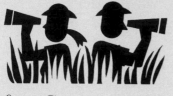

Safari Secrets:
Lessons from the animal kingdom

UV radiation comes in many forms, and we can see only a small spectrum. Other animals see things that we don't (and vice versa), which explains why they are attracted to apparently dull objects or have strange colors themselves. Some animals, including birds, reptiles, and insects such as bees, can see into the near ultraviolet. Many fruits, flowers, and seeds stand out more strongly from the background in ultraviolet wavelengths than in human color vision. Scorpions glow or take on a yellow to green color under UV illumination. Many birds have patterns in their plumage that are invisible at usual wavelengths but observable in ultraviolet, and the urine of some animals is much easier to spot with ultraviolet.

derscores the point that you need to try to keep your skin healthy even if you have the best sun-protecting habits.

Following are some other health issues that have beauty implications. These are irritating conditions that can influence your appearance and self-confidence.

ACNE AND ROSACEA: While people often like to think that things like chocolate are responsible for pimples, there's no proof that what pops up on your dessert plate influences what pops up on your nose the night before a big presentation. What we do know is that 80 percent of U.S. teens and 40 percent of U.S. adults complain of pimples. But in Papua, New Guinea, the figure is nearly 0 percent, so it's a fair guess that something is going on with our lifestyle. One culprit is inadequate intake of omega-3 fatty acids (as opposed to saturated or trans fats or omega-6 fats from corn and soybean oils). Get adequate amounts of these good fats by consuming walnuts, avocados, freshly ground flaxseed, canola oil, fish oils, or DHA supplements from algae. Another culprit? Stress. In studies of college kids during exams, researchers found them to have many more bouts of acne while under pressure. Paradoxically, the steroid medication triamcinolone can be injected to calm a severe form of pimples called cystic acne, but there's a cost—it also thins the skin, often leaving a depression months later. And don't squeeze—you'll damage the skin by increasing inflammation and risk spreading the infection. Instead, wash your face with a coarse washcloth and mild soap to break open any pimples. Salicylic acid, benzoyl peroxide, azelaic acid, and vitamin A creams or gels are all simple and effective methods for reducing acne. You can also try an ancient Chinese remedy—seabuchthorn oil, which has been used for a few millennia in China for a variety of medicinal benefits. More recently, the rich fatty acid mixture has been used topically as a natural treatment for acne and rosacea. Try the soap form.

For rosacea—a form of adult acne that's a fairly common problem—certain antibiotics tend to work not only because they kill bacteria but because of their anti-inflammatory effect. Our recommendation: Ask your doc if an ointment that combines antibiotics and a low-potency steroid cream such as hydrocortisone is right for you. Lasers that target the visible capillaries can have a dramatic immediate effect, and daily topical vitamin C and twice daily topical niacin more subtly reduce the redness in about a month.

ECZEMA: If your skin's looking as if you just did the hubba-hubba in a bed of mashed strawberries, it might be a case of the common skin condition eczema. This is a type of allergic reaction, and it's easily treated with inexpensive skin moisturizers. It's especially common during the winter, when the dry air causes little breaks in the skin, letting in chemicals that rake over your skin, particularly your hands. Treat your skin like an athlete working out in the heat—keep it hydrated. After your daily shower (don't dry yourself first), immediately apply Vaseline or cream (Eucerin, Keri, Nivea) so the moisture is locked in—and the rash-irritating dryness is kept out. If you have stubborn eczema, you might use a moisturizer with lactic acid or a steroid or a prescription drug called tacrolimus. If all else fails, have an allergist get to the bottom of your

FACTOID

African Americans and people with dark skin have natural SPF 16 UV protection, although dark skin blocks Vitamin D3 production even more. So darker-skinned people require 10 to 20 times the sun exposure length (which equates to about two hours of exposure) of lighter-skinned people to build up the same amount of vitamin D. While all humans have the same number of melanocytes (which produce melanin and determine skin color), those melanocytes produce different amounts of melanin. People who moved to northern climates needed more UVB rays to make vitamin D, so they produce less melanin. And over time that has gotten ingrained into the genome so northerners typically have less dark skin.

The skin around the eyes is only ½ millimeter thick compared to 2 millimeters elsewhere on average. As the day progresses, the body accumulates fluid (that's why your ankles might swell as well), and this engorges the veins beneath the eyes and makes them bulge and appear blue through the thin skin. The muscles around the eye also tire as the evening progresses, so they begin to sag. Dark circles can be due to melanin pigment—you can have those peeled away or use pigment reducers for many months. For translucency of skin, when muscles or blood vessels under the skin become visible, only makeup will really work. For shadowing from fat, you'll need an eyelid lift. Finally, if there are larger blood vessels, you can have them zapped with electrocautery. Sleep helps, too.

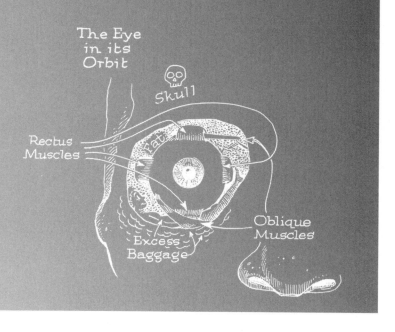

The Eye in its Orbit

Skull

Rectus Muscles

Fat

Excess Baggage

Oblique Muscles

problem—in many cases the culprit is the metal nickel or one of the preservatives or fragrances in skin care products.

PSORIASIS: Signaled by dry, flaking skin, psoriasis is an autoimmune ailment that affects the life cycle of skin cells. Remember how we talked about new cells replacing older cells that slough off and how that process usually takes less than two months?* Well, in people with psoriasis, that process takes only a few weeks. Immune cells go out and attack healthy skin cells by mistake, as if they're trying to heal a wound. The result: Cells build up fast and form thick scales that are dry, patchy, itchy, and sometimes painful. In essence, your body is fighting a chronic civil war and your skin is caught in the middle.

While there's no cure for the disease, people can get some relief from the pain

* No? Then turn back to page 34. We'll wait.

and discomfort. Topical agents and light therapy (exposing yourself to small amounts of UV light) that slow skin replication can help. And powerful agents such as Humira or Remicade that are used to prevent joint destruction and arthritis from autoimmune attack on cartilage seem to slow remodeling enough to make the skin and nails (see chapter 4) much better almost instantly. Also, mindfulness meditation and resistance exercises may help to calm the autoimmune process when it is not so severe as to cause joint damage.

ALLERGIES: People with sensitive skin (about 10 percent of the population) should avoid some of the fragrances, antioxidants, stabilizers, preservatives, and coloring agents that are found in skin care products and cosmetics. Sometimes less is more. While a skin cream might have one or two active ingredients, they all have a dozen or more inactive ingredients—that is, they are supposed to be inactive in making your skin healthy. But those inactive ingredients could be active against you and your skin.

Whatever the case, you can take steps not only to decrease the chances of getting these and other skin conditions, but also to improve the look and vibrancy of your skin, no matter what your age.

YOU Tips!

With just about anything—computers, cars, kids—you've got two choices: You can prevent a problem before it happens, or you can try to repair one if it does. Your skin's no different.* Though many of us have skin that's sustained a demolition derby's worth of damage, that doesn't mean you can't treat those issues. And if you still have young, tight, healthy skin, you can also take steps to ensure it stays that way. The challenge is fighting through all the different products that purport to slather on the lotion of youth. We'll help you separate the skin savers from the money wasters. And also check out our YOU Tool in a few pages on the perfect skin-cleaning steps. The simplest concept for skin care is to feed your skin with nutrients at night, when there is no UV light, and to protect it from UV and toxins during the day.

CHECK LABELS. Going to the beauty counter is like going to the supermarket—there are millions of products, and many times you have no idea which ones are healthy and which ones aren't. Some offer double robbery: They both weigh down your skin and lighten your pocketbook. Look for products that list an "active ingredient" and a particular concentration. Vitamins and supplements in skin lotions, creams, and potions usually have to be in the 1 to 10 percent range to really do something for or to your skin. The formulations also need to be pH balanced, and the active ingredient must be able to penetrate the skin (vitamin A works at a much lower concentration). Your best bet is to try reputable brands, but even some of those use ingredients that could enter the skin only in a science fiction movie. So the bottom line is that you have to read the label and use only the scientifically proven ingredients that are discussed in this chapter. Remember that cosmetic products are just that—cosmetic. Products that make therapeutic claims must be scientifically proven to be safe and effective and are regulated as drugs by the FDA.

CREAM IT ON. There are hundreds of skin-care ingredients, including many with fancy names and expensive price tags. But there is very little science to most of them and no science to many of them. The list of ingredients that really can make a difference in the skin is small. The big ingredients (and their closely related derivatives) to know:

- Vitamin A (retinoids)
- Vitamin B3 (niacin or nicotinamide)
- Vitamin B5 (pantothenic acid, panthenol)

*Except for the fact that it doesn't come with a hard drive, transmission, or a sassy tongue.

- Vitamin C
- Viamin E
- Alpha-hydroxy acids
- Ubiquinone or coenzyme Q10 (small-molecule antioxidant)
- Ferulic acid (small-molecule antioxidant)

These eight are examples of skin-care ingredients you can cream on with solid scientific backing.

It probably makes sense to steer clear of hexapeptides and collagen. However, smaller peptides are okay. Dr. Perry's NightSkin (vitamins A and C, glycolic acid, licorice extract, an herbal skin lightener) and Dr. Perry's DaySkin (zinc oxide–titanium dioxide sunblock, Vitamins B3, B5, and E) are examples of skin creams with a scientific basis. (Of course, we saw the science and recruited him to work with us.)

KNOW YOUR VITAMINS. You know you need to ingest them, but vitamins are also important as topical agents. These are three of our favorites for good skin health.

Vitamin A. Winning our vote for the most valuable skin care nutrient to be applied to the skin—not in a vitamin pill—is vitamin A. Without vitamin A (a "retinoid"), your skin, hair, and nails will be dry and you will be sickly. Vitamin A is found as retinoic acid (Retin-A), retinol (retinaldehyde), or retinyl propionate. Be careful of these if you're potentially pregnant. All of these forms work, because your body can transform one into another. Retinoic acid decreases acne by knocking out bacteria and decreasing the thickness of the dead layer of skin and oils that plug pores—and this decreases visible pore size. Topical vitamin A increases the stretchy elastin fibers, the hearty structural collagen, and the natural moisturizer hyaluronic acid in the skin. It lessens the dark pigmentation in the skin and is the first-line drug for acne, rosacea, and seborrheic dermatitis. Retinoids are really the only thing you can put on your skin that can repair sun damage, giving you smoother, less wrinkled skin. Most important, retinoids decrease things called actinic keratoses that can become skin cancer. These drugs might even be able to help stretch marks. Light destroys vitamin A. Because of this, you'll be wasting your money if you put it on your skin in the morning. Use it at night, when it can do the most good.

Vitamin C. Vitamin C is one of your skin's main water-based antioxidants, although in your skin, vitamin E, because it is lipid soluble, gets the top honor. But you can buttress the vitamin C levels in your skin by 40 times by rubbing in at least a 10 percent concentration of L-ascorbic acid. In your skin and in your orange juice, vitamin C rapidly breaks down with exposure to UV light and oxygen (so remember to close the refrigerator door—and did that light really go out?). So use the vitamin C at night, when it can stimulate your collagen and elastic and help build up your skin. The vitamin C will last a long time in your skin or until it is inactivated by UV light.

Vitamin C protects against sunburn and sun-induced wrinkling. It knocks out those free radicals and inflammation after UV exposure, and it can decrease the rosy look of rosacea. Vitamin C also helps with those brown age spots. If you use it along with vitamin A, you'll get a better effect than with either alone.

Vitamin E. The major lipid-soluble antioxidant in your skin hitches a ride to the stratum corneum, the dead upper layer of skin, with your natural oils, called sebum. Topical vitamin E needs to be in the form of DL-alpha-tocopherol to make a positive difference to your skin. Many skin creams contain a much more user-friendly form, called tocopherol acetate, but this doesn't do the magic of alpha-tocopherol. In fact, tocopherol acetate may actually hurt your skin. Vitamin C, by the way, needs vitamin E like Bonnie needs Clyde. Vitamin C is water soluble and an effective scavenger of free radicals in the water-soluble parts of the skin, while vitamin E works on the lipid-soluble portion. But if all you have is vitamin C, the lipid part of the cell ages. The real vitamin E stuff (DL-alpha-tocopherol) enhances the effects of sunscreen, stops the immune system from getting blitzed, and slows wrinkle production. Because UV light degrades vitamin E (just as it does vitamin C), it should be applied along with sunblock and/or at night.

Other antioxidants. Different plants make different sunblocks to protect themselves from the blistering UV light. And each of these usually dark-colored antioxidants can give the skin their benefits. The problem is that many antioxidants have red, blue, or green pigments, unappealing in skin creams. And while these antioxidants may make sense and even may be proven in animals, very few studies have been done to show that they really work in humans. New antioxidants include ferulic acid, idebenone, ubiquinone (coenzyme Q10), alpha lipoic acid, and resveratrol and are already making their way into our friendly neighborhood counters.

EAT FOR SKIN. Perhaps the only food some people associate with skin is a little whipped cream on Saturday night (more on sex in Chapter 10), but a lot of foods or ingredients in foods can help protect it.

- **Eggs (yolks, unfortunately), legumes, avocados, soybeans, and nuts:** All of these contain biotin, an essential chemical for fat and carbohydrate metabolism. A lack of biotin (caused by taking too many antibiotics or an inadequate diet) can lead to dry skin or dermatitis of the face or scalp. (A deficiency can also cause your hair and nails to become brittle and frail.)
- **Salmon:** It contains astaxanthin, the carotenoid that gives salmon its pink color, which improves skin's elasticity, and the good fat DHA-omega-3, which also makes your skin and hair look younger and healthier.
- **Green tea:** Contains polyphenols that have free oxygen radical scavengers. These protect against photo damage and thicken the epidermis. It can be taken orally or topically. And it may help sunburn.

- **Pomegranates:** In addition to thickening the epidermis and prolonging fibroblast life to produce more collagen and elastin, they contain phytonutrients that seem to accelerate wound healing.
- **Tomatoes:** The nutrients in these reduce the chance that you will get a sunburn, so bulk up on tomatoes (with a little lipid such as a few walnuts beforehand—so the active ingredients are absorbed) before your annual summer vacation. It may be because of the lycopene they contain, but we really do not know the active ingredients for this effect, so enjoy the tomatoes rather than just a lycopene supplement.

ASK FOR A HAND. There are many benefits to massage—relaxation, the release of muscle tension, the chance to chat with strong-handed Sven. There's also another: aromatherapy. Many people think aromatherapy has to do with smelling, but it's really about allowing your body to absorb oils that can have a profound effect on your health. There's an ongoing debate whether massage with aromas is superior to standard massage, but some evidence suggests you may experience more short-term benefits from a massage with scents. The scent with the most data supporting it: lemon. We recommend you use the scent in a variety of ways:

- Spray it on a pillow a couple of hours before bed.
- Take a foot bath with lemon in it. Some studies show that a foot bath with lemon as opposed to a foot bath without lemon helps promote relaxation.
- Have (or give) a massage with lemon oil, or add it to your bathwater.
- Rub your body with lemon oil to promote sleep and soothe skin burns.

Some other aromas and oils we suggest:

- Tea tree oil for topical infection in some of our "dirtier" areas, such as the feet, armpits, or groin, or even the pilonidal cyst area just above the crack between the buttock cheeks in hairy people.
- Rosemary, which can help improve mental alertness and function by reducing the effect of stress so you can focus.
- Peppermint and lavender (we suspect these work, but we're still waiting for good scientific studies to find out).

PUT THE FIRE OUT. Quickly treat burns from both sun and flames with ice water, as mentioned earlier, to slow down the rush of inflammatory cells that create blistering and further the collateral damage of the burn. Sap from the aloe leaf can also be very soothing. Most important, prevent infections in the damaged area (bacteria love dead and burned skin), since infection will worsen the scar. Staying out of the sun for six months after surgery will minimize the risk of brown pigmentation in the scar as it tries to protect itself from UV radiation. By the way, if a new burn hurts, that's good. It means you didn't fry the full thickness of the skin. A deep burn through the dermis kills the nerves so you don't actually feel it. But an old wound that starts hurting is your body's message for you to see a doctor.

SLEEP AND EXERCISE. They stimulate growth hormone, which promotes fibroblast health and allows more production of collagen and elastin to keep your skin taut. They also accelerate the production of epidermis. See more about exercise and our new band workout on page 351.

OIL UP. We love olive oil, and whenever we find another use for this natural wonder, we get excited. Olive oil should find its way into makeup and skin creams, since it has been shown to decrease UVB damage to the skin. Extra-virgin olive oil seems to work better. (Like almost anything, olive oil can be a skin irritant in some people.) To make an olive oil bath, add $1/4$ cup olive oil along with a few drops of lavender or peppermint oil to the bathwater. In the winter or in low humidity, olive oil is the most natural of the moisturizers. Massage it into your skin, particularly the elbows, face, feet, and legs. Olive oil can also be used to moisturize the scalp and hair, the nails, and the lips.

CHECK IT. Treat your skin like a science experiment. Look at it. Inspect the pore size with a magnifying glass. See how much skin you can slough off with sandpaper (kidding on that one). Do it regularly—one of the ways to really assess skin health is to look at your skin often, to compare changes in things like pore size, oil, flakes, and wrinkles.

DON'T TRAP DIRT. Your skin needs to breathe for heat exchange and to get rid of toxins from the sebaceous glands. But your skin can't breathe if it's suffocated by a pancake-thick layer of makeup. While we're not in a position to tell you to flush your cosmetics, we do believe that many women can be brainwashed to believe that makeup is absolutely necessary to improve their appearance. Healthy skin is nature's ultimate cosmetic.

DROP THE FAT. High blood fat levels won't just clog your arteries—they'll clog your skin. Out-of-control levels of cholesterol and triglycerides can wreak havoc on your appearance. A hailstorm of yellow bumps, called xanthomas, results from high triglyceride levels. Scavenger cells clean up the fatty debris beneath the surface of the skin. Diets low in saturated and trans fats, blood sugar control, and LDL cholesterol–lowering and HDL cholesterol–raising medications are essential steps. Once blood fats are lowered, xanthomas can resolve, but this may take years. Adding niacin (300 mg or more twice a day—see your doc on these) and 162 mg of aspirin a day (with half a glass of warm water before and after to minimize stomach damage) will help reduce arterial inflammation and reduce the risk of wrinkles as well as erectile dysfunction.

CHECK FOR CO-Q10. Coenzyme Q10 helps prevent damage to lipids on the surface of the skin. It's good to see Co-Q10 as an ingredient in skin products that you're going to buy. But studies have shown that many products listing Co-Q10 as an ingredient either do not contain Co-Q10 or have less of it than advertised (a lot less—like 90 percent less). Check www.consumerlab.com or look for the USP-verified symbol on the bottle to ensure you are getting the ingredients for which you are paying. After 2011, the FDA will be monitoring to ensure that what is on the label is what is in the bottle, but you should start earlier than that.

LAY OFF THE BOOZE. Alcohol dehydrates the skin and increases the leakiness of capillaries, so more water moves from the bloodstream into soft tissues. Combined with the horizontal position during sleep, this results in facial puffiness, stretched skin, and faster wrinkle formation. While we're knocking vices, cigarettes not only damage your arteries to contribute to the formation of wrinkles, but they're also responsible for vertical lines above the lips. That's partly because cigarettes deplete levels of a gas called nitric oxide from the inner lining cells of your small arteries (and large ones, too). That short-lived gas helps gives skin some of its flexibility, so cigarettes and saturated fats take away your skin's flexibility and contribute to wrinkles. Combine that with decades of puckering your lips around those cancer sticks and you've got prune lips. So when you quit, you often look younger as the nitric oxide returns and the vertical lines decrease.

ENLIST THE PROS. Some say wrinkles look distinguished. Some say they make you look older than a French cathedral. If you fall into the category where you want wrinkles on your skin as much as you want them on your wedding dress, then you have several professional options, besides the do-it-yourself tactics we've outlined above.

Injectible fillers. These plump up the tissue to eliminate wrinkles. Collagen injections are being replaced by hyaluronic acid because it lasts longer and your body can attack your own collagen if you use a lot of that cow stuff—not a good situation. Hyaluronic acid physically plumps up the dermis, making wrinkles virtually disappear. How long these fillers last depends on their thickness and the exact chemicals they are made from. The thinner ones (for fine lines) hurt less but have a shorter duration, while the thicker ones (for big wrinkles) that act more like caulk are inserted deeper and last longer. On average, they last between six and twenty-four months.

Paralyzing agents such as Botox. Originally approved to eliminate excessive twitching of the eye muscles, Botox weakens muscles, smoothing the skin and diminishing wrinkles. A very low dose of

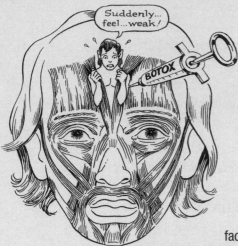

botulism toxin is inserted directly into a muscle and deadens its nerves for an average of four months. It's most often and best used for creases between or around the eyes and the forehead. Daring surgeons inject it around the mouth, sometimes creating the ultra-beautiful effect of drooling. Yes, people have died from Botox, but the doses that were used were at least ten times the cosmetic dose. Around the eyes, go ahead and talk to your doc about Botox if you don't want to scowl.

TRY A PATTY FACIAL. Stimulating the lymph drainage of your face can cleanse toxins and reduce facial swelling. Best of all, it only takes one minute in the shower. With the water caressing your face, gently sweep your hands from your chin down to your neck. This rubs the large nymph nodes (which always swell when your throat hurts) and stimulates the large ducts to drain waste fluid from the face. Then move up as you pat your fingers from the middle of your face outward toward your ears. Start below the lips and move up to beneath the nose, then the bridge of the nose, under the eyes, and finally the forehead.

ERASE THE MARKS. Here's what you can do about some of the spots, blemishes, and lines that may make you feel like jumping out of your skin.

What's On Your Skin	What They Are	What You Can Do
Age Spots	Flat, round, brownish spots that look like freckles. Benign age spots aren't dangerous.	If they bother you, see a dermatologist or plastic surgeon who can treat them with bleaching creams, laser therapy, or such procedures as chemical peels. Using sunscreen can prevent the development of more spots. Sun makes them darker so use sunscreen—at least an SPF 30 with three- to four-star UVA protection. Common skin cream ingredients such as vitamin C, vitamin A, glycolic acid, emblica, and licorice extract can lighten brown spots when used for months (more in Chapter 4), and so can niacin.

What's On Your Skin	What They Are	What You Can Do
Stretch Marks	These scarlike marks appear when the skin stretches beyond its elastic capability and the underlying connective tissue tears.	They tend to diminish over time after the early redness subsides, but there's no known nonsurgical treatment to eliminate the marks. Treatments such as laser therapy or Retin-A are not effective in diminishing the appearance of scars.
Varicose Veins	When valves preventing backflow of blood returning to the heart become weakened (often because of pregnancy or weight gain), blood pools in the veins of the legs, causing them to bulge.	You can reduce some of the symptoms (like pain and swelling) by elevating your legs to promote blood drainage to the heart and avoiding standing for long periods of time. Wearing compression stockings while standing can stall their development. Various kinds of surgery can also address varicose veins—either by removing them or by closing them off.

YOU Tool: The Ideal Wash

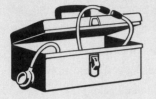

Step 1: WATCH WHAT YOU'RE WASHING

You have an acid mantle (like cellophane) that forms a protective layer on your skin to inhibit the growth of harmful bacteria and fungi. If it loses this acidity, the skin becomes more prone to damage and infection. How do you lose the acidity? By washing your face with ordinary soap. Most of the soaps we use are basic in nature, which counteracts the acidity, so you end up removing the mantle that seals in moisture. Now, we're not trying to encourage that outdoor look or manly smell by not washing. Use pH-balanced soaps and cleansers; if they are gentle enough not to sting your eyes, chances are good they won't harm your skin either. Your pores will look smaller if they're kept free of oils and dirt. Ideally, you should wash your face twice daily, and you don't need to spend more than a few seconds doing it. Excessive rubbing can aggravate eczema and acne. Skip the soaps with colors and fragrances, too. They just add residue and increase the chance of an allergic reaction.

Step 2: ADD ANTI-OXIS

If you read our tip on vitamins, you'll know they can help improve the skin. Here's a quick recap of why antioxidants help. Natural antioxidants inside the membranes of your cells (vitamin E is the most common in the skin) protect you against free oxygen radicals in the membrane and lipid portions of the cell. They're especially important for protecting your skin, because they help thicken your epidermis while the sun quickly depletes levels of vitamin E. Your body will replenish its own vitamin E if you are eating smart, but adding some extra vitamin C (which protects the water-soluble portions of your cells) can help decrease the appearance of wrinkles and improve the formation of collagen and elastin.

Only certain types of vitamin C will penetrate the skin—one called L-ascorbic acid does this particularly well. To work, it must be in a concentration of at least 10 percent and must be kept acidic. So,you can't just rub oranges on your face and expect it to work. L-ascorbic acid is oxidized by the sun, rendering it ineffective, so use it at night.

Topical application of niacinamide (niacin, vitamin B3) and pantothenic acid (vitamin B5) and other antioxidant vitamins (taken orally) are good for the skin. In fact, topical niacin helps prevent injury caused by the sun, and increases the level of certain fats and protein in the skin, which improves its barrier function, and it helps reduce the yellowing of skin that's associated with glycation (the yellowing can disappear between 4 and 12 weeks of use).

Step 3: MOISTEN BEFORE USING

Typically, your skin soaks up moisture to keep itself young and vital, but it loses the ability to do that as you age. Most commercial face creams are oil-based and work by blocking the release of water from the skin. As people grow older, however, they cannot rely on oil-based preparations to block the release of moisture. That's because aged skin loses the ability to attract moisture in the first place and becomes fundamentally dehydrated. But the vitamin A family, commonly called retinoids, can increase the actual water content of the skin without clogging the dead layer of cells. Retin-A contains retinoic acid and requires a prescription. Retinyl propionate, retinyl palmitate, and retinol (retinaldehyde) don't require a prescription, and all are converted by your skin's own enzymes into retinoic acid.

Healthy moisturizers don't disturb the acid mantle of the skin or clog pores. We prefer natural moisturizers, such as squalene (made from olives), avocado oil, walnut butter, or cocoa butter, and ones that are proven to be hypoallergenic. Apply while you're still damp from the shower to seal the moisture in, and remember, it's especially important to moisturize when you're flying, at high altitudes, or in dry climates.

Step 4: EXFOLIATE OFTEN

Which is better for your floor? Sweeping it clean every week or waiting for all the gunk to build up and then doing one big power wash a year? Exactly. You have several choices when deciding to do the same with your face:

- Mop it clean daily or weekly with a light physical exfoliant or a chemical exfoliant. Don't use physical exfoliants that have sharp edges, since they can damage healthy skin below. Apricot seeds are natural and work like an old-fashioned straw broom as opposed to the newfangled chemical beads, which are more symmetrical like a synthetic broom. We favor the latter but won't report you to the authorities if you insist on going the old-fashioned way. Try some on the back of your hand to make sure it's not too harsh.

- Microdermabrasion is industrial-level exfoliation and can be repeated monthly for the best results in typical people. Microdermabrasion uses either aluminum oxide or salt crystals or, even better, embedded diamonds to exfoliate while the oils are sucked right out of those pores. See below for more about microdermabrasion.
- Power-wash it with something stronger, like trichloroacetic acid, which takes off the top layer of skin (it looks so bad for a week that we recommend doing this once yearly around Halloween). This is most useful to lessen that annoying splotchy brown pigmentation. This requires a doc.
- Every few years you can scrape it with a sandblaster or wire brush—that's real dermabrasion and the recovery is not particularly pleasant, so new light lasers are being developed to do this without the downtime. Unfortunately, they're so new we can't recommend one yet.

While they all can be effective, it makes the most sense to us to exfoliate once a week to remove dead skin cells and stimulate growth of new ones. If you wear makeup or are exposed to a lot of dirt, exfoliating nightly is recommended (don't do it at midday, which basically only removes your makeup). Also, for the women here, you produce more oil during your period so you're susceptible to more acne, meaning you should use a lighter peel.

Use a loofah sponge for your body. The loofah mechanically removes the old layer of skin. (Turkish baths require loofahs, and folks don't feel really clean unless they've had a vigorous rubdown.)

If you're going to do it yourself, look for exfoliating products that contain acids compatible with your skin's own natural acidity. Some options:

- Alpha-hydroxy acid (usually listed as glycolic acid) works as an exfoliant by peeling off the top layer of dead skin and hydrating with moisturizer. Alpha-hydroxy acids (skin-rejuvenating fruit acids) have been around for about 20 years and make a marked improvement in skin quality by sloughing dead skin cells off the surface so that more youthful-appearing fresh cells become visible. Fine lines and wrinkles lessen and your skin takes on a fresher-looking tone.
- Glycolic acid (less than 10 percent concentration is safest; docs use higher concentrations), which is derived from sugarcane, traps moisture in skin and releases dead cells. Use it sparingly at first to make sure it doesn't cause skin irritation.
- Hyaluronic acid is a large sugarlike molecule in the extracellular matrix that binds with water and provides volume and fullness for skin, making skin smooth and moist. Hyaluronic acid

can't penetrate the skin, however, so when you put it on your skin, it's really just a moisturizer.

- Apple cider vinegar also works as an exfoliant for the top layer of skin.

Step 5: PICK THE BLOCK

You're supposed to get 20 minutes of sunlight a day—but only when it's at low levels (a good rule to tell: your shadow should be longer than your height). This includes even on a cloudy day, which stops only 20 to 40 percent of UV radiation. Beyond that, you know the drill. You know it, you hear it, you see the ads with the baby's butt on billboards. Wear sunscreen. Like punishment doled out in the principal's office, sun protection is nonnegotiable—because it's the most critical factor in keeping skin healthy. It's best to make sunscreen a part of your daily regimen so you won't get unexpected exposure (or get a sunburn). Use a great moisturizer that you love that also contains an SPF 30 sunscreen and affords the protection you need. If you're going to be outside for sports, use a lotion with SPF 30 (for UVB) and a four-star rating (for UVA) and reapply every two hours.

Our recommendation: Always protect your face and the backs of your hands but allow your body to be exposed to some sun for a few minutes before you add sunscreen. A little redness in the skin signifies that vitamin D is being made. Here's a helpful hint: zinc oxide and titanium dioxide sunscreens protect immediately, and newer versions of these sunscreens form a thin film rather than making you look as if you smeared crayon all over your face. All the rest of the sunscreens—called chemical or organic sunscreens (misnomers if we ever heard one)—take 20 minutes to absorb into your skin before protecting. So get those few minutes of sun and then apply the zinc.

You need to slather all sunscreens on thickly and apply them evenly, making sure not to miss any spots such as the back of the neck, the top of the ears, and any exposed scalp. Most of us don't put on enough sunscreen, and if that's the case with you, then you're getting only half the

FACTOID Within 1,000 years of a population's migration from one climate to another, its descendants have the correct color skin to protect them and maximize nutrients in their environment. If you chart the evolution of skin color of populations living in one area for 500 years, the curve perfectly correlates UV radiation with skin color. The only exception is the Inuit, who have dark skin and hair even though they inhabit northern climates; that's because they eat lots of fatty fish, which provide vitamin D, so they don't need it from the sun. Our ancestors began migrating from northern Africa 250,000 years ago, so there has been lots of time for our skin types to adapt to our climate.

effectiveness (if you're putting on SPF 30, it's more like SPF 15). You really need 1–2 ounces of sunscreen to cover your whole body.

Which product is the best? Look for ones that are hypoallergenic and noncomedogenic, because you don't want to cause other skin damage while trying to protect from sun damage. But don't put a lot of faith in those labels, since all creams can cause pimples and rashes. It's really hit or miss. Also make sure that your sunscreen is water-resistant so it doesn't end up in your eyes while the rest of the players on your team watch you drop the ball in painful anguish. Water resistant also means it will stay on your body past the first droplet of sweat when you are hot. But even if it says "water-resistant," reapply it after swimming. By the way, hats and T-shirts don't provide enough SPF protection. Hats provide an SPF of 10 at the most, and T-shirts only about SPF 5 (but sun-protective clothing with higher SPFs are available).

Ever wonder what the heck the SPF numbers truly mean? An SPF of 1 means that your skin covered in SPF 1 would turn red in about 20 minutes; SPF 2 would require 40 minutes, and so on. The most common reason for sunscreen failure is using inadequate amounts.

Step 6: HAVE A PRO SAVE YOUR FACE

While some cosmetic procedures may seem as unnecessary as gumball machines, there are a lot of advantages to getting regular facials or microdermabrasion. Microdermabrasion is really a facial without all the glitz. It simply exfoliates your skin and sucks the dirt out of your pores. If you can afford it, get a facial or microdermabrasion monthly to clear pores, which can be clogged by makeup. The massage part will also stimulate blood flow. These cleaning procedures must be followed by proper skin care at home twice a day—cleaning, antioxidant protection, hydrating, protecting against the sun, and exfoliating regularly.

YOU Tool: Body Art

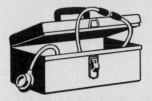

It used to be that people would decorate their bodies with the big three—clothes, makeup, and facial hair. These days, bodily decoration has become infinitely more creative and colorful. With the prevalence of tattoos and piercings on the rise (24 percent of people between the ages of 18 and 50 have tats), it seems that everywhere you turn, you're looking at a skull, rose, or some Asian symbol. Some of us scar our bodies and embed metal under our skin. We're not telling you that you can't look like a Ferengi from *Star Trek,* but if you do choose that alien look, we want you to stay safe.

Professional tattoos are applied with a sewing machine–type needle that drags ink into the mid to upper dermis as it penetrates. Some pigments contain iron oxides and some organic chemicals. Most inks/pigments are from nonsterile bottles, but some companies do make sterile pigments, which cost hundreds of times more than the nonsterile ones (which makes them hard to find). Here's the lowdown on what you need to know if you decide to have yourself inked or pierced.

STAY STERILE. Your artist should wear sterile gloves and a surgical mask, and your skin should be cleaned with an antibacterial solution. We prefer Betadine, but most will just use alcohol. Betadine is better because it lasts longer and kills a wider variety of bugs. But it needs to be applied wet and allowed to dry to really work its wonders. Infections can occur because the barrier of the skin is broken during the procedure. (Tattooing and piercing are the only situations where the skin is intentionally penetrated by nonmedical people.) Because pigment is not sterile, bacteria and viruses can contaminate it, and infections can come to you from parts of the machine that can't be sterilized (even though your artist may think the machine is spotless). HIV and hepatitis B and C can be transmitted through tattoos and take a long time to show up in blood tests, so you won't be able to donate blood for a year after receiving a tattoo. People with tattoos are nine times more likely to contract hepatitis C than people who never get tattoos. Essentially, you're having sex with your tattoo artist and everyone else he's used the pigment on. If you wouldn't have sex with these unknowns, don't get tattooed with that old pigment.

THINK AHEAD. A letter on your cheek? Dots on your fingers? You might want to think twice or even three times about putting a tattoo on an area that is visible in normal clothing. What you do to your privates stays private, but your neck will be visible to every employer and customer for your entire life. Pick spots that can be concealed and are more amenable to future modification, such as upper legs, buttocks, and back. When the skin is thin, it's more difficult and painful to remove or alter.

KEEP IT CLEAN. Treat your tattoo like a wound for the first week or so. Keep it clean by washing it with soap and water twice a day. Coat the area with bacitracin, Neosporin, or Vaseline. You'll know when it's healed; it'll stop hurting. If it still hurts after five days, give your doc a call.

TAKING IT OFF. Maybe you've decided that Yosemite Sam on your forehead doesn't go over all that well at job interviews. If the tattoo is small, you might consider having it cut out—one procedure and it's done. You'll be replacing the tattoo with a scar, however. If it's larger, lasers might be the answer. Different lasers are used for the different colors in your tattoo. The laser heats up the pigment and explodes the cells that contain it. The pigment then disperses and other cells pick it up. Each treatment blurs the tattoo until it is hard to see. But there are many drawbacks to lasering; it takes many painful, expensive treatments and often leaves white scars behind.

For the time being, you've got a problem if you don't like your tattoo because the pigments are permanent, but removable tattoos are around the corner. Within a few years biodegradable pigment sealed into tiny plastic capsules will be used. When the capsules are lasered, they break open, and the biodegradable tattoo disappears.

CHECK THE PIERCING TOOLS. Piercing instruments must be sterilized in autoclaves—medical-type machines that kill every little germ that can cause infections. The instruments shouldn't be boiled, placed in hot glass beads, or dipped in some strange chemical. The piercing instrument should be wrapped in a bag with an indicator that tells you the proper temperature was reached to kill bacteria and viruses. And that's not enough. The autoclave must be tested every week with live bacteria to make sure it's really working.

Like a tattooer, your piercer should wash his hands and put on sterile gloves, and your skin should be cleaned with Betadine before any piercing. The Betadine should dry on your skin to a beautiful orange. The jewelry should also be sterilized before it is put into your body. Since stones will loosen in an autoclave, we recommend using only metal jewelry right after a piercing. You can bring your jewelry to your family doctor and ask her to sterilize it for you. After the piercing, keep the area clean with hydrogen peroxide on a Q-tip or washcloth. Then coat the area with bacitracin or Neosporin. Skip where they tell you to clean the area with alcohol. That will actually stall healing. It takes weeks to months for the piercing tract to heal. Until that time, don't remove the jewelry for more than a few minutes.

BE SMART. Earlobes are a pretty safe area to pierce; that's why 12-year-olds with an ice cube and a needle can usually pull this one off. We recommend that you draw an ink spot exactly where you want the piercing on one side, then measure the distance up from the bottom of the lobe and back from the cheek. This is the spot the piercing should go on the other side. If they come out crooked, just take the earrings out and wait a month to repierce. Other than the lobes and the belly button, you're increasing your risk of trouble if you stray to other areas. Ear cartilage, for example, has poor blood supply and can't fight germs if they get in. An infection here will leave you looking like a basset hound. In the eyebrow, there's a nerve that supplies sensation to the forehead that might be speared with the piercing. You'll remember the piercing every day because painful scar tissue, called a neuroma, can form here. Other areas such as the nose, labia, and nipples are definite danger zones when it comes to infection and other long-term issues, like breast-feeding. And the tongue? Make sure you have good dental insurance; you'll need it as the piercing destroys your teeth by clanging against your precious enamel and gives your breath that sweet odor of trapped bacteria. Ugh.

Cosmetic Enhancement?

Queen Cleopatra of Egypt set the trend for thousands of years. A little green copper and black kohl around the eyes and some red iron ore on the cheeks and lips and, voilà, Madonna had nothing on her. Since then, most women (and a few men) older than 12 have practiced the fine art of makeup to hide wrinkles, look younger, and attract mates. Early cosmetics were made of toxic metals such as lead, arsenic, and mercury that ate away at the skin if they were used long enough. Safer cosmetics have been in use for the last 200 years. Even so, toxins such as lead keep cropping up in makeup.

While the FDA supervises the cosmetics industry, that control is with a very long leash. Most creams and cosmetics contain many ingredients, and any one of the ingredients can cause contact dermatitis, a type of allergic reaction. Fragrances are the main culprits, but preservatives, chemicals (such as p-phenylenediamine and glyceryl monothioglycolate), UV sunscreens, resins, and nail acrylates cause many allergic reactions. If you suffer an allergic reaction, you may need a dermatologist or an allergist to perform a patch test on you to determine the cause.

Some other dangers to be aware of:

- In the Middle East, Asia, and Africa, kohl is still used as an eyeliner. More than half of these products contain lead. Users have been found to have high body lead levels, which can lead to nerve damage. Lead has also recently been found in lipsticks manufactured in China.

- Powders improve facial color and also absorb oil. They are made of either talc (magnesium silicate) or zinc stearate with added magnesium carbonate (chalk). Since inhaled talc and titanium dioxide cause lung injuries that some scientists think eventually lead to cancer, it's a good idea to avoid powders with them. The industry is beginning to respond by creating "green" cosmetics. Powder made from velvety smooth cornstarch can safely replace the minerals that are toxic to your lungs.

- Because germs can contaminate mascara, preservatives must be used. Mascara is probably the most dangerous of cosmetics, with risks of bacterial and fungal eye infections and allergic reactions to the preservatives, all occurring close to the eye. The dyes can also permanently color the inside of the eyelid.

For a list of specific product recommendations, see www.realage.com, where we have enlisted the help of cosmetics specialist Paula Begoun.

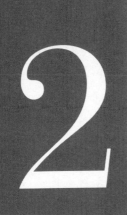

Head of Class

How to Save Your Hair

YOU Test: Mane Squeeze

Grab a group of hairs on your head (aim for about 60—or the amount that would fit through a straw). Starting at the base, gently tug at the hairs, pulling up and out.*

Result: If more than a tenth of the hairs that you clumped together at the beginning come out when you pull, it's a sign that you may be experiencing some accelerated hair loss.

* An even better test for men: Comb your hair for 60 seconds over a towel, then count the hairs deposited there. If you count more than 10 hairs, you're losing hair faster than the average man.

When it comes to appearances, some of us may be predominantly defined by our faces, some by our bodies, and some by our addiction to tattoo ink (nice skull, Grandma!). Many others, of course, are largely judged by their hair. And for good reason. Your hair—on your scalp, face, or back—is your body's fashion statement. While you're born with a natural color, shape, and style of hair, you also have the power to control how good (or bad) it looks, how long (or short) it is, and whether it's black or blond (or blue). With a few snips or tricks, you can tell the world you're wacky (Britney's shave job and Sanjaya's famous faux-hawk). You can say you're sexy (pick your favorite celeb). You can let it grow (Rapunzel) or hack it off (Kojak). You can be the inspiration for millions (thank you, Ms. Aniston) or the proud butt of jokes (sorry, Mr. Trump).

Sure, hair is great for running your fingers through and growing make-a-statement goatees, but hair used to be more purposeful than simply serving as bodily ornamentation. Today, the hair on our scalps protects us against the sun, and our eyelashes act as our first defense against bugs, dust, and other irritating objects. But back when clothes were as scarce as skyscrapers, the hair in our nether regions camouflaged our reproductive parts from generation-threatening spears. And by lining our armpits (we docs call them the axillae) and groins, our dry hair actually acts as a lubricant, allowing our arms and legs to move without chafing. Then and now, our body hair serves as a protector against malaria (see more on body hair on page 75). The anopheles mosquito—a low-flying bug that likes the legs—hates hair, in part because hair warns its victim to start swatting. While their bite is painless, our hair signals their presence before they bite (it's why kids are at greater risk—they have less hair on

Hair Today, Gone Tomorrow

In one of life's injustices, many of us have the frustrating experience of losing hair in the places we want to keep it (the scalp) and growing it in the places where we want to lose it (perhaps the back and shoulders for men and the chin and around the belly button for women). Though there are plenty of remedies that can eliminate unwanted hair, such as Nair and other hair dissolvers, waxing, and shaving, the latest hair zapper is laser therapy. Here's how it works: The brown pigment in the hair soaks up the laser light, acting like a firecracker fuse leading to the follicle 2 millimeters under the skin. The laser's heat travels down through the hair to zap the follicle so it can never grow hair again. It doesn't work with blond, red, or silver hair because there's not enough brown pigment to fry. It takes several treatments to remove lots of hair in one area (it removes about 20 to 40 percent each time). The coolest thing is that the laser works like military weapons, seeking out and frying hairs, even ingrown hairs, diving beneath the surface of the skin (as long as part is above the skin). They can grow, but they can't hide.

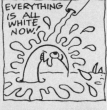

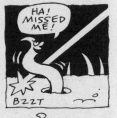

Now, growing a mustache may very well be a rite of passage for teenage boys,* but it can also be one for menopausal women, because of hormonal changes. About 30 percent of women report unwanted hair on the face. The cause? A predominance of male hormone, often caused by polycystic ovarian syndrome or menopause, which accelerates hair growth. This excess hair is generally a harmless condition, but you can treat it a number of ways, including bleaching, plucking, laser therapy, or electrolysis (an electric current damages follicles so hairs don't grow back). Electrolysis (as long as it's done by someone who's trained to do it) can work well for those with unwanted blond or white hair, since lasers aren't as effective for them. If you're going to wax any part of your body, ask to have room-temperature wax, not hot wax; the cooler kind will generally do less damage as the wax rips the hair and follicle from your skin. Wait a year after stopping Accutane or steroids before considering waxing. If you don't, you might be not only hairless but skinless. Another remedy: losing weight. Weight loss (works in women and men to decrease unwanted hair and increase wanted hair) can decrease male hormone levels and slow down the growth of unwanted mustaches.

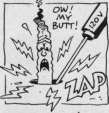

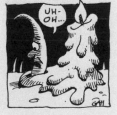

*And '70s sitcom actors.

their legs). That's most likely the original purpose of hair: It served as an early-warning system of bodily threats. We seem to ignore the armor function of our hair today, removing it every chance we get, except on our heads and eyes.

In addition to its utilitarian functions, hair reflects a lot about our self-esteem, taste, gender, age, and attitude. It also plays a major role in how we're attracted to and attractive to other people (more on this in chapter 10). It can even be a source of conflict. While men tend to prefer women with long hair (ever see a painting of Eve with a buzz cut?), women, especially as they age, seem to prefer wearing shorter hair. More important, our hair tells us a ton about our overall health status, as the growth or loss of hair can signal other malfunctions going on *inside* our bodies. Whatever the case, we all know why in the United States alone we spend $50 billion a year* on hair care: because we care about our hair.

We care about cleaning it. We care about beautifying it. We care about keeping it in some places and losing it in others. Just as skin can shine and glow, so can your locks—as long as you use the right tactics to maintain your mane.

Your Hair: Losing It and Abusing It

In today's world, we don't treat our hair all that well. In fact, if your hair knew what was going on, it would be pulling its hair out.

To show you how, let's talk about the structure of hair—how it grows, how it

---

* That's roughly equivalent to the gross national products of Iceland, Costa Rica, and Bolivia combined.

Gone Today, Hair Tomorrow?

If you lose a little grass in the yard, you just plant some new sod and let it grow. Seems like the perfect remedy, right? Well, that's why many men have turned to hair replacement surgery as a way to deal with their male-pattern baldness. We have to say that we don't think bald men need to hide their heads under hats or hairpieces. But many men do, and that's why some have turned to this procedure in which hair is harvested from the back of the head and inserted in the front. These procedures have declined in popularity—not because the surgeries can't be well done (they can be quite good if performed by a specialist, although nowadays many unqualified docs are getting in on the act). It's because of genetics. After 20 years or so, the newly transplanted hair can thin as well—leaving very visible scarring. Isn't a smooth, shiny scalp more attractive than one that looks like a connect-the-dots workbook?

can end up in your shower drain, and how it can end up looking about as lively and healthy as sun-scorched grass. The average person's head has up to 150,000 hair follicles (the adult body has 5 million). That number is constant over a lifetime; it's hereditary, so only thickness, condition, and whether you lose the actual strands that come from those follicles can change. Each one of those strands grows about six inches a year—women between the ages of 16 and 24 pump it out the fastest.

FACTOID It's a myth that wearing a hat causes baldness. As long as the hat is not tight enough to restrict circulation (therefore cutting off circulation to the follicles), a hat will not cause hair loss.

While it may seem that your hair is as far removed from your internal organs as your clothes or jewelry, each strand of hair has its own blood supply. Because of that, hair is greatly influenced by health and diet. Hair is also under the delicate control of hormones, which is why men have beards and hair on their chests and male-pattern baldness on their heads, and women don't.*

As you can see in Figure 2.1, your hair is made up of distinct structures: the follicle and the shaft. A tunnel-like segment in the epidermis portion of your skin, the follicle resides under the surface of the skin and extends down into the

* Usually.

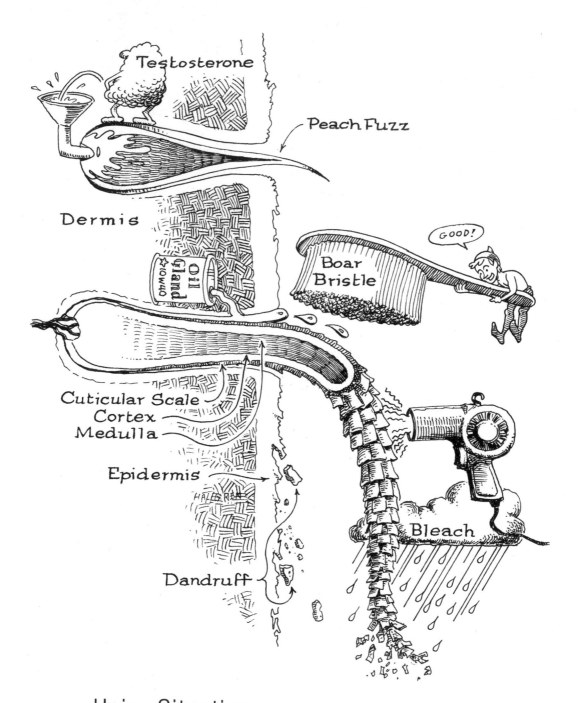

Figure 2.1 **Hairy Situation** While a hair follicle begins deep below the skin, what we do to the outside of hair can be criminal. Excess heat and other harsh treatments can make hair look frazzled, not dazzled.

dermis. The base of the follicle contains little blood vessels that nourish the cells. The living part is the bulb at the base, while the shaft—the part of the hair that we see above the skin—is dead.

That hair shaft is made up of a protein called keratin. The inner layer (the medulla) and the middle layer (the cortex) make up the majority of the shaft. Like the nail's structure, the hair's cuticle, which looks like a tile roof under the microscope, serves as the outer, protective layer that covers the medulla and cortex.

Now, to keep your hair shiny, it needs oil. Surrounding your hairs are tiny muscles that give you goose bumps, standing your hairs on end when you're cold or during a scary movie. These muscles also squeeze the glands that lube up your hair, which produce sebum—your own natural vitamin E–rich hair and skin conditioner.

Safari Secrets:
Lessons from the animal kingdom

Monkeys of certain species have patches of hair on their heads very similar to humans'; they develop during puberty and are found only among the males. In evolutionist language this is called epigamic hair, which means that it is a sign of sexual dominance. The lion's mane is an example of epigamic hair, because it's used as a scare technique during sexual fighting.

How Hair Is Lost

When it comes to hairy situations, many of us can live with a bad haircut or a little graying or the occasional day when our hair looks like a haystack. But the most frustrating problem for many people—men especially—is what's perceived to be the start of the downhill slide to death, or at least the impetus for wanting that Corvette: hair loss.

While we tend to say that baldness comes from the mother's side, an individual's genes *from both parents* influence that person's predisposition to male- or female-pattern baldness. Of

FACTOID

On average, you lose 50 to 200 hairs a day. Any guess as to when we have the most hair follicles? Bzzzz, try again. It's when we're in week 22 as a fetus; that's the largest number we'll ever have, since we don't generate new follicles as we age.

Underwear Under Hair

As you may have noticed, pubic hair is quite different from hair on the head. Short, coarse, and curly, public hair never gets a chance to grow long because it has a short growth period. Within six months, the follicle dies and the hair falls out. Pubic hair—which acts as a buffer to reduce chafing and maybe to hide our genitals—provides a large surface area to disperse the naturally smelly sweat. Many animals use the odor of sweat from the groin and underarms (pheromones—see chapter 10 on sex and attraction) to attract the opposite gender. Today, it more often keeps people on the other side of the elevator.

course, hair loss is far more visible in men (80 percent of whom experience some degree of baldness), but nearly 40 percent of women lose substantial amounts of hair after menopause, as well (women tend to thin out all over, rather than develop the signature spots that men do), making it a major appearance issue for both genders.

To learn how you lose hair, you first have to understand how it grows. Hair goes through its own growth cycle that's unrelated to seasons or hormones or anything else. It's a random biological process that's dictated largely by your genetic disposition. The two main phases:

Anagen (active): Cells in the root are dividing quickly and pushing the hair out. It averages two to three years.

Telogen (resting): This phase lasts for about 100 days on the scalp. Consider it hair hibernation—the follicle is completely at rest.

Doctors don't know why certain hair follicles are programmed to have a shorter growth period than others. One suspected factor for age-related male-pattern baldness is a person's level of androgens—the "male" hormones that are actually produced by both men and women. Take a look at Figure 2.2. For many years, people believed that a predominance of testosterone was the root cause of baldness, but it's not quite that simple. We do know that we lose hair especially

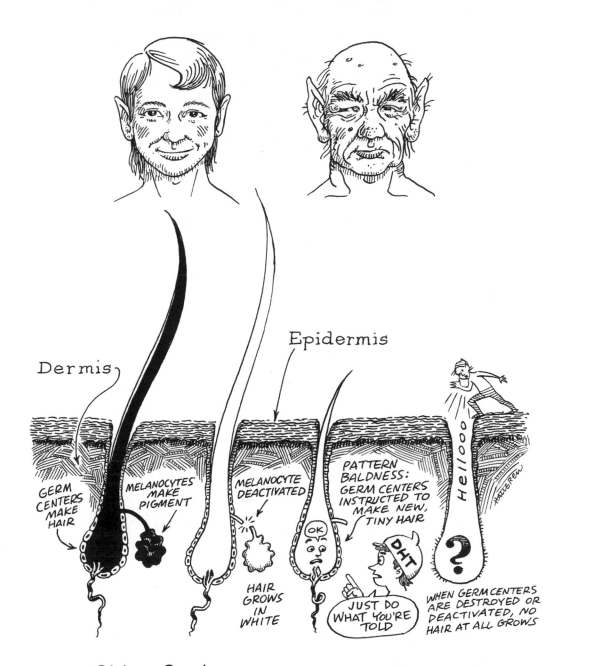

Figure 2.2 Shiny Scalp The reason we go bald isn't because of our mother's father. It's because of DHT (a product of testosterone), which first makes hair turn thin and fuzzy and then makes it fall out from our head to the shower drain. The distinguished graying around the temples (and elsewhere) occurs as we lose melanocytes.

The Future of Hair Loss Treatments

Anybody who's lost a lot of hair probably knows why the race to find a cure for baldness is a competitive one—there are a lot of willing customers ready to try and buy. Many different therapies are being tested as we speak, including gene therapy (in which genes involved in hair growth would be delivered directly to the follicle) and chemicals that increase hair's growth cycle. One of the more interesting ones involves cloning—a process in which scientists would clone your hair so you could donate to yourself all the hair you'd ever need or want.

fast if it is exposed to dihydrotestosterone (DHT, which comes from metabolism of testosterone). It's believed that the exposure of follicles to levels of testosterone that are normal for adult males causes the hair follicles to go into a resting state. This DHT is formed in the testes, prostate, adrenals, and hair follicles themselves through an enzyme called 5-alpha reductase. The enzyme raises the levels of DHT, and that's why there's a link between higher levels of this enzyme and areas of baldness. DHT changes healthy follicles to follicles that grow thin dwarf hairs—hairs that resemble peach fuzz. Essentially, DHT shrinks hair follicles, making it impossible for healthy hair to survive. Drug companies have targeted this process by making antibaldness medication that inhibits 5-alpha reductase, the enzyme that makes DHT. (Some of the infrequent side effects of these meds include impotence, decreased libido, and breast enlargement.)

Now, age-related baldness isn't the only reason why clumps of hair start falling from the head like raindrops from the sky. Other causes, especially for women, include low iron levels and anemia (low blood count), recent anesthesia for surgery (it's the stress of the surgery and the pressure on one area of the head, not the anesthesia), menopause or being postpartum, autoimmune diseases such as lupus, thyroid disease, and polycystic ovarian disease (PCOS).

Rapid hair loss is often a strong sign that you

FACTOID

People who constantly pull their hair out aren't overcrazed parents; they're more likely suffering from a form of obsessive-compulsive disorder. This habit—called trichotillomania—keeps happening because the puller is always searching for the perfect "pull" (so they keep on pulling when it's not). The treatment: Follow the addiction principles on page 246, or just make it harder to do, by wearing gloves at night or keeping a rubber band handy so you can play with that rather than fiddling with your follicles.

Hairloom

We all know people have varying degrees of body hair: Some men have chests and backs that double as winter coats, while others have torsos that are slicker than an ice patch. That begs the question of why we even have body hair in the first place. Of course, for early humans, hair kept them warm, protected them from cuts and scrapes, provided camouflage, and even served as a nice handhold for the young. The reason why we lost a lot of body hair over time isn't because we invented heaters and parkas. More likely, our ancestors started having to hunt in hot, tropical areas—and bare skin adds to the efficiency of our cooling system. The reason why we kept the tuft at the top? Many experts agree that it had to do with a mating ritual that went a little something like this: The male with the most impressive hair—or he who could make it look that way—frightened away his rivals, got his girl, and fathered the next generation. Hence, head hair played a major role in obtaining a partner and successfully producing offspring.

ought to have a battery of tests to evaluate your nutrition, health, and hormone levels. And that makes an important point: Hair loss isn't just an appearance issue; it can be a sign that something wacky is going on elsewhere in your body. Inflammation in the scalp, from an overdose of sun or from seborrheic dermatitis, can speed up hair loss. More often than not, it's a hormone issue—especially one involving your thyroid gland. In women especially, it's common to experience a decline in thyroid hormone (that's called hypothyroidism), where some of your bodily systems slow down. Scalp hair loss or facial hair growth is a sign that you should have your hormone levels checked. We recommend having your thyroid-stimulating hormone checked every other year if you're losing hair, or, for all others, once at age 20, then at age 35, and every

FACTOID The hair you have in your ears comes to life only as you age. As one of the pleasures of growing older, this hair protects you from insects that find the ear canal interesting. Also, like sheep, you recruit dormant follicles so you can grow more hair to keep yourself warm in the winter.

other year after age 50 (TSH is the trigger from the brain that tells your thyroid gland to make thyroid hormone). If your level of thyroid hormone is low or if it's normal but you are experiencing thyroid-related symptoms, you can be (and usually need to be) treated with a synthetic (sometimes bioidentical) hormone. You'll need to be rechecked six weeks later to see if the supplemented dose is enough.

For a man, a decline in the need to shave signals a decrease in testosterone (for a woman, it's the same clue if she needs to shave her legs less often).

How Hair Is Destroyed

Our hair occasionally needs lubrication the way other parts of our bodies do.* But with hair, the things many of us do to help it are actually hurting it. Most of us treat shampoo as if it's toothpaste for our head—we've got to use it every day. But that doesn't have to be the case. Some people find that their hair has just as much body and shine without shampooing every day (and they like the fact that they can take a break from putting additional chemicals on their head). On the other hand, if shampooing is a Zen experience for you, its calming benefits may well do more for you than its hair-stripping effects, so we can't argue with daily shampoos (you can also use conditioner alone). See below for our specific recommendations for hair washing.

FACTOID

Big hair is a competitive enterprise from the highlands of New Guinea to the shopping malls of the United States. In the highlands of New Guinea, tribesmen think that the ghosts of ancestors lodge in the hair and that baldness is a sign that the ancestors have abandoned a man. When they court women, tribesmen build large wigs made of hair mixed with clay and then sewn onto a frame of cane, hardened with dipped wax, painted, and adorned with vines, beetles, side ringlets, and fur.

Now, here's some information that's going to make your hair stand up. Artificial coloring on your head—whether you're bleaching it or coloring it—is the equivalent of artificial coloring in food: It may make it look as pretty as can be, but it's not always the healthiest thing you can do to your head. There is some suspicion that permanent black hair dye can cause leukemia and lymphomas and some chemicals that are no longer used caused bladder cancer. So the purple Mohawk you're considering? It's probably fine for your health (temporary hair dyes are safer than permanent dyes), though probably not for your

* We're talking about your joints, funny girl.

next job interview. Bleaching, on the other hand, will really run up your hair bill as you try to salvage permanent damage.

Here's why: The pigment of your hair comes from the inner two layers. When you bleach your hair, you damage the shingles that create the covering of the hair shaft. The dye, which slips through the gaps in the outer layers, swells to give your hair a different color. But the prior or current damage the bleach caused allows the dye to slowly slip out of the hair, so you end up losing the full body of the hair faster than if you just left it alone.

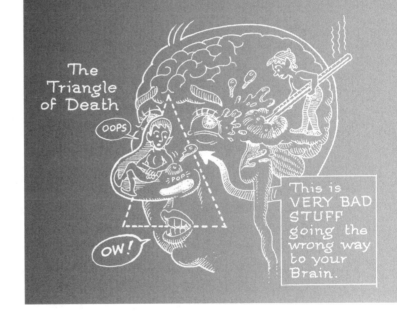

The Triangle of Death

OOPS

OW!

This is VERY BAD STUFF going the wrong way to your Brain.

YOU Tips!

Most people tend to think that the only things you can do to protect your hair are to give it a good wash and watch out for clipper-toting frat boys. The reality is that there are many things you can do to make sure you make the most of what hair you have and save the hair you want to keep.

PRACTICE GOOD HAIR HYGIENE. Most of what we do to hair is hairicidal: We blast it with hot air, bleach it, and then dye it. High hair-dryer heat (and that from curling irons) causes the water under the cuticles (the outermost layer of the hair) to form bubbles that stress and break the hair. The tiles that cover the hair dislodge, and your hair handles water like an unroofed house. You'll get those dreaded split ends and your collie's hair will outshine yours. It's best to blot hair dry with a towel and then use low heat if you use a dryer. Your hair is actually most vulnerable when it's wet, and you should treat your hair almost as you would a silk blouse—don't iron it or heat it up to extremes. Also, it's smart to use a brush with smooth or rounded teeth or bristles, which will massage the hair and scalp without damaging them. And you know that we're going to quote Billy Joel when it comes to bleaching, dying, and adding hot-pink highlights: We like you just the way you are. Still, we also know that changing hair color can be an appearance advantage if it makes you feel better and healthier. Here's an example of what we call biological budgeting—traditionally, you may have needed the cleanliness of your hair (for mating purposes), but you also run the risk of taking it to the extreme by overcleaning or overcoloring, which can damage your hair in the process.

EXAMINE YOUR SHAMPOO. Not that we've got webcams in your bathroom, but we pretty much know your in-the-shower routine: Rinse yourself, shampoo your hair, rinse your hair, add conditioner, wash body, shave legs (or face), rinse, dry off. Sounds great, but it's not ideal for you in at least one way. There isn't one "right" answer to the question of how often to wash your hair. Your physical activities, your use of styling products, and your hair type will usually determine how often you wash your hair. If washing every day makes your hair too dry, try every other day or every third day. Or you may have very oily hair that needs washing more than once a day. If you condition when you shampoo, it could be that you need to shampoo daily but need to adjust the level of conditioning. However, if you have dandruff, it is advisable to wash your hair daily. More frequent washing has been shown to reduce the food source (sebaceous lipids) for the organism—*Malassezia*—that causes dandruff. Less frequent removal of these lipids by shampooing leads to overgrowth of *Malassezia* and increased dandruff. Conditioners, on the other hand, do seal in moisture, so they can be helpful. Apply conditioner daily and don't bother washing it out if you don't want to. Ideally, use an all-natural pH-balanced shampoo that's gentle; remember, just because it's *natural* doesn't mean it's always the best (cyanide is natural). We love shampoos from these makers: Aubrey Organics, Quinessence, So Organic, Avalon Organics, and Organic Excellence.

STAY PURE. Drinking water isn't the only water that should be free of toxins. You should also shower and especially bathe with toxin-free H_2O. Instead of squirting yourself with Evian, remove chlorine by adding a charcoal filter to your shower or bath. Chlorine—which isn't just in swimming pools but also in tap water—dries out the hair (as well as the skin). It's especially important if you take ten-minute showers or baths rather than a quick rinse. The problem isn't the straight chlorine but what it turns into—stronger toxins called trichloromethanes.

CHECK YOUR DIET. We're not recommending you scrub your scalp with salmon (though the thought has crossed our minds), but the omega-3 fatty acids found in fish, distilled fish oils, or DHA supplements from algae are the primary nutritional component that makes hair shinier. Other recommended foods: walnuts, flaxseed, avocados, sardines, eggs, milk (skim), and green tea. There's also a connection between balding and eating animal fat—particularly red meat—because high-fat diets lead to more DHT production and more damage to hair follicles. Instead, make caffeine your vice, which has been shown over time and through a series of reactions to *decrease* DHT levels. Get yours via green tea, which also has been shown to help slow baldness by slowing down DHT production. There's not much in the way of hard science that shows a direct link between these foods and pedestrian-stopping hair, but anyone who has pets knows that the better you feed your pets, the better their coats look: They feel softer, and their sheen is brighter.

CHECK HORMONE LEVELS. If you experience sudden hair loss or lose hair in clumps, it may be a sign of a hormone imbalance or condition. It's worth seeing a doctor to get a blood test that will measure your thyroid-stimulating and thyroid hormone levels. You'll have better results trying to treat the cause if it is thyroid disease (and practically any other disease), rather than the symptom.

SLOW BALDING. If you want to treat male-pattern baldness, you can try the medications minoxidil (Rogaine) and finasteride (Propecia). Minoxidil works by increasing the anagen growth phase and enlarging the hair follicle, while finasteride inhibits the conversion of testosterone to DHT (by blocking that enzyme we mentioned earlier), which causes hair loss. Research shows that two-thirds of men who use finasteride slow down hair loss. And the earlier this drug is used after noticing hair loss, the more effective it will be. But this drug has that pesky little side effect of occasionally (rarely, actually) leading to decreased sexual desire and difficulty in achieving an erection. Interestingly, minoxidil was originally used to treat blood pressure, but researchers noted that it had a strange side effect: It grew hair on the backs of hands, cheeks, and fingers, and that's how it was developed as a hair-loss treatment. When it comes to other products or procedures that claim to grow hair—everything from the HairMax LaserComb to Scalp Med—you should be wary of a wallet transplant. Yours to theirs. No potions or lotions other than minoxidil and finasteride have been shown to predictably increase hair growth or prevent its destruction.

ADD REINFORCEMENTS. These are the vitamins and supplements that have been most favorably linked with good hair health.

Vitamins. The most important vitamins for hair loss are the B group (B6, biotin, and folate for slowing loss and pantothenic acid and niacin for promoting hair growth). You can get B vitamins through diet, as well, by eating such foods as beans, peas, carrots, cauliflower, soybeans, bran, nuts, and eggs. See www.realage.com for our vitamin dosing recommendations.

Supplements. The extract of the berries of the saw palmetto shrub and the oil in avocados may slow hair loss and promote hair growth by preventing follicle-killing DHT from binding to receptor sites at the hair follicles. These supplements are controversial, however, and there are few studies that show their effectiveness. There is also some evidence that the amino acid L-lysine (at 500 to 1,000 mg) can help hair grow thicker (it hasn't been tested in humans, but the coats of sheep grew thicker after being given L-lysine). And expect a new generation of shampoos containing pepper. Pepper has recently been shown in animals to knock out that evil enzyme that leads to hair loss.

KNOW HOW TO DYE. Surely you've read about links between hair dye and lymphoma. After a somewhat checkered history, hair dyeing today is considered safe and effective. Some dye ingredients that were a potential health concern in the past were removed many decades ago and are no longer used in the United States, although some ingredients may still represent a concern in other countries (like lead-containing products, which may represent a neurological risk). It will take several more decades to know if hair dyes currently in use have subtle side effects. Because of extensive lobbying in the 1930s, hair dye manufacturers have to put warnings on the labels only for skin and eye irritation. But in the late 1970s, the FDA proposed a warning linked to products that used two coal tar ingredients—4-methoxy-m-phenylenediamine (4-MMPD) or its sulfate cousin (it never was implemented). Professional colorists can decrease your exposure to potential toxins, but if you're going to dye your hair yourself (though we think you look just fine), follow this advice:

- Don't leave the dye on your head any longer than necessary. Rinse your scalp thoroughly with water after use.

- Wear gloves when applying hair dye (nitrile gloves are the best when dealing with chemicals), and carefully follow the directions.
- Never be a home chemist and mix different hair dye products—you never know what you might create!

DEFROST THE FLAKES. The only flakes we tend to enjoy are the ones that cancel school and the ones we put in our cereal bowl. If white ones are falling from our head, we want no part of them. Dandruff results from inflammation of the scalp as well as from a fungus called *Malassezia furfur,* formerly called *Pityrosporum ovale* (stellar work by the ad agency that changed that name). The fungus loves the dark, warm jungle you call your hair.

The way to treat it: frequent washing with a medicated shampoo that helps control the scaling. This works by stopping your immune system from overreacting so your scalp doesn't itch and you

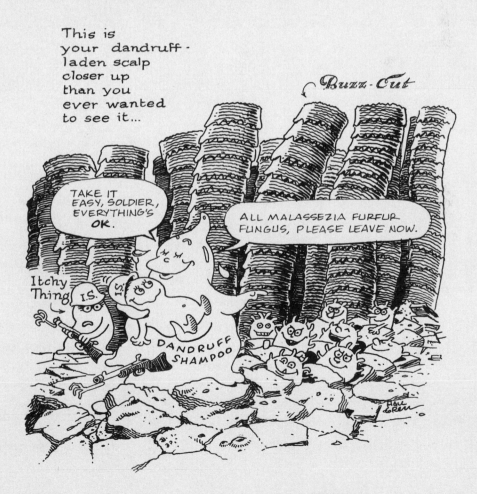

This is your dandruff-laden scalp closer up than you ever wanted to see it...

Buzz-Cut

TAKE IT EASY, SOLDIER, EVERYTHING'S OK.

ALL MALASSEZIA FURFUR FUNGUS, PLEASE LEAVE NOW.

Itchy Thing

I.S.

I.S.

DANDRUFF SHAMPOO

don't scratch off the epidermis. Look for antimicrobial and antifungal shampoos that contain ingredients such as tar, selenium sulfide, zinc pyrithione, ketoconazole, or ciclopirox. Don't use these if you're pregnant, nursing, or trying to conceive. Home remedies, herbals, and nontraditional medicines can have side effects, particularly when combined with traditional medicines and even foods. You should check with your doc and pharmacist about these and all medicines, especially if you're pregnant or nursing. One solution: Green tea applied to your scalp. Green tea contains a polyphenol (called EGCG) that's been shown to help. Unfortunately, green tea doesn't work when it's mixed with other chemicals, so shampoos with EGCG might not offer long-term answers. Just make a strong cup of green tea and apply it directly to your scalp. Cool it first—you do not want to burn the fungus if your scalp is attached. Like so many herbal remedies, however, the studies just haven't been done showing that tea shampoos make a difference. (If psoriasis is the source of scalp flaking, you'll want to limit washing so you don't dry the scalp out further.)

YOU Tool: Hair Care

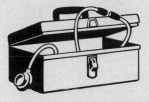

It's no secret that your hair—be it on your head, chin, or back—goes a long way toward determining how you feel and how you're perceived by the outside world. So that warrants some further discussion on making the most of your hair and minimizing damage to it. We'll leave the goatee braids to you and concentrate on helping you make those strands on your scalp shine through.

PERFECT HAIR MAINTENANCE
Step 1: SHAMPOO

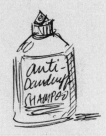

Before getting into the shower, gently brush or finger-comb your hair to loosen up tangles and residue. When washing your hair, treat it as if it were fine silk—delicately. Leave hair hanging down and gently massage in shampoo starting at the roots and working down. Never pile shampoo on top of your head.

Step 2: CONDITION
Conditioner creates shine and preserves hair health by giving it smoothness and protecting against damage. For volume, condition only the middle and ends of your hair, where it's most susceptible to damage. For shine, condition the entire strand. Do it every time you use shampoo and more often if you want.

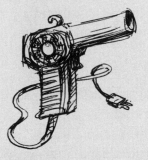

Step 3: DRY
Don't rub your hair with a towel or twist it tightly into a turban. Wet hair is delicate and breaks easily. Pat it gently and squeeze it with your towel or use a superabsorbent towel sold at salons. A wide-toothed comb is the best way to detangle and distribute styling products when hair is wet. And keep any dryers at low-heat settings.

SOLVING THE MANE PROBLEMS
Issue: Damage
Many people damage their hair during the maintenance and styling process—often without even knowing it. Here are the major damagers:

Excessive combing. Over time, excessive combing and brushing, especially of wet hair, can cause the delicate cuticle scales to lift and, in extreme cases, peel away. Forget those 100 strokes a night. The idea was to move oil from scalp into hair to give it shine. But if you comb aggressively when hair is wet, it will be damaged.

The wrong tools. Using the wrong combs and brushes (a wide-toothed comb is best), especially on fragile, chemically treated hair, can remove the cuticle layer in large portions, creating porous and dull hair strands.

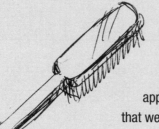

Back-combing and teasing. Back-combing and teasing are extremely harmful, since they tug in the opposite direction of the cuticle scales, which can eventually rip them off, leaving the inner cortex exposed.

Heated appliances. When too hot or used on wet hair, heated appliances can actually cause hair to boil, creating permanent welts that weaken and dull the hair shaft and set the stage for breakage. Never use ceramic appliances on wet hair. If possible, do not blow-dry hair.

Issue: Split Ends

A split end develops when the hair's cuticle layer is severely weathered or missing, causing the exposed shaft to fray like a piece of yarn. Wind can cause hair to tangle and make it hard to comb, which can eventually lead to split ends.

Solution: Give your hair a dose of protection and intense moisture by using conditioner daily. Regular trims help, too.

Issue: Lackluster Locks

Daily environmental wear and tear and a buildup of styling products both contribute to hair's looking dry and dull.

Solution: A mild shampoo will remove residue. But be careful you don't overdo it and strip the hair of all its natural oils. A deep conditioning (conditioner on for 10 minutes) will give you softness as well as shine.

FACTOID

Many drugs may cause hair loss, including acne drugs like Accutane, blood thinners like Coumadin, antidepressants like Paxil and Prozac, some blood pressure drugs, and antifungals, as well as hormonal drugs. If you're possibly experiencing bothersome hair loss as a side effect of medication, check with your pharmacist and/or doc about alternatives.

Issue: Oily Hair

When hair follicles release an excessive amount of the natural protein sebum, hair can look flat, oily, and greasy.

Solution: An oily scalp needs consistent care. When you shampoo, massage into the roots and down the hair shaft. Another habit that may increase the appearance of oily hair is frequent grooming. Combing, brushing, and running your fingers through your hair aid in the movement of sebum from the scalp down the hair shaft, so try to handle your hair as little as possible.

Issue: Lackluster Hair Color

No matter how permanent your chemical hair color claims to be, all dyes will fade with time. The sun, air, and harsh shampoos all contribute to a lackluster shade.

Solution: When coloring, use a semipermanent rather than a permanent hair color system. Semipermanents are far gentler than permanent dyes and are designed to fade over time, allowing you to replenish your color sooner without causing as much damage. Use shampoos and conditioners designed for the maintenance of hair color.

FACTOID

Women's hair is considered so sexually provocative that in many cultures it is concealed after marriage for fear of inciting uncontrollable desires. In the first century, a married Roman woman could be divorced for uncovering her head. To this day, Muslim women and Orthodox Jewish women, once married, cover their hair with a kerchief or scarf or wear a wig.

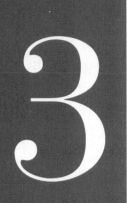

3 Oral Victories

Your Mouth and Teeth Are a Portal to Your Inside—and Say a Lot About Your Outside

YOU Test: The Real Tooth

Look in the mirror. After taking a moment to admire and primp, open wide. Take a close look at your teeth. Yes, beyond the popcorn remnants. And the taffy. Are the tops of your bottom incisor teeth and bottoms of your top teeth flat or somewhat jagged?

If they're flat, that indicates that you could be a teeth grinder—putting you at greater risk for wearing down, breaking, or splitting your teeth and leading to gum and mouth problems as you age, not to mention your looking like a jack-o'-lantern.

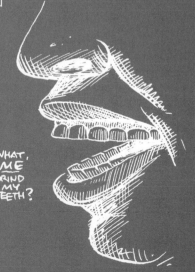

WHAT, ME GRIND MY TEETH?

If our ancestors could see us now. They used their teeth for two things and two things only: one, to shred their fire-cooked meat and feast like the hungry warriors they were. And two, as a last line of personal defense, biting off attackers' ears and noses. Us? Oh, let's see. We use our teeth for such vital tasks as whittling toenails, tearing open cellophane wrappers, and carrying bags when you have kids in both arms.

It's not that we don't appreciate our own meat cutters. It's just that the invention of such things as knives and fruit smoothies has shifted our priorities. Our teeth and mouths aren't quite as essential for survival as they used to be, yet they're still critical to our happiness. The mouth serves as our entrance portal for food and our exit shaft for words, songs, laughter, gas, and salmonella. That's not even mentioning the fringe functions: Mouths allow us to kiss babies, taste falling snow, bite in self-defense, and earn elite status as a sexual dynamo. For your purposes here, however, it's important to note that your mouth is more than a mere functional tool; it's a key indicator of your vitality, your beauty, and even your ability to get a good job and spouse.

Your teeth, in addition to helping with a wide range of tasks and with chewing, are also a very clear marker of your health. If your gums are inflamed, your teeth are falling out, or your teeth are getting ground like fresh pepper from wear and tear, those problems can affect and reflect the health and beauty of your entire body.

As part of your smile, your teeth serve as one of your main markers for beauty. Together, your teeth and mouth act as a stage: You want that stage to be bright, white, and well lit. Though there's no direct correlation, the common perception is that our oral appearance is linked to our cerebral powers. How? We equate snow-white teeth with high-powered brains. Just add a set of Bubba teeth to your mouth. Not only will you scare off neighborhood kids, your perceived IQ will immediately drop 20 points (and your real IQ will fade, too, due to gum inflammation).

Your Mouth: Beauty Markers

On the surface, it would seem that mouths are as nondescript as file cabinets—they all look about the same. But if you think about it a bit more, you'll realize that mouths are much more like fingerprints or eyes—on the surface they are similar, but the difference is in the details. Think of how mouths convey emotions—a smile at a lover's gaze, a frown at a lover's propensity to adore remote controls, a gasp, bewilderment, anger, or the inner happiness that you can't hide. And that's not even taking into consideration that lips come in all shapes and sizes. There are thin ones and plump, full, juicy ones. So it should be no wonder that your mouth is a messenger in many ways.

Plastic surgeons have pored over thousands of pictures of beautiful men and women to come up with the perfectly proportioned mouth (tough work, but someone's got to do it), and this is what they've found. Rulers ready?

- The width of the mouth should be roughly 1.6 times the width of the bottom of the nose (what a coincidence—the golden ratio!).
- If you drop lines down from the inner part of the colored part of your eyeballs, your mouth should fit right between those two lines.

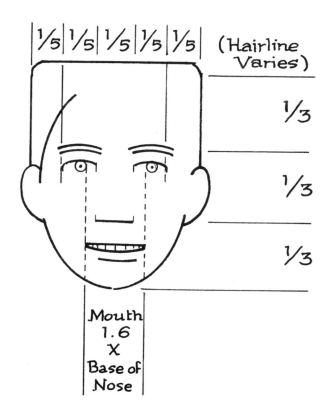

- Your upper incisor (front) teeth should be visible below your upper lip for 1–4 millimeters and your lower teeth should not be visible when your lips are open. As you get older, the upper lip drops and you see less of your upper teeth. At the same time, your lower lip sags, exposing more of your lower teeth. When Shakespeare mentioned older people as "long in the tooth" he was describing this drop. The real reason for being "long in the tooth" is periodontal disease, where the gum recedes and the bone follows. That creates triangles of space between the teeth and exposes their roots.

- Your upper teeth should also overlap the lower teeth by 1 millimeter.

- Your jaw should be level. How can you tell? Take a double-wide Popsicle stick and bite on it. If your jaw is asymmetrical, the stick will tilt.

Stink Mouth

We all know the nasty feeling of holding a conversation with a person whose breath smells like three-week-old leftovers. And we all pray that we're never the source of such stench. Bad breath (or halitosis) comes from lots of places: Some stems from food getting trapped in pockets in the tonsils, some comes from the stomach, and still more originates from the tongue—where the stench from bacteria buildup can clear a room. Some even comes as a side effect of medication (as is the case with Benadryl). One good way to handle bad breath: a tongue scraper, which removes bacteria and takes some of the stink away. Some research shows that the tongue scraper reduces nasty compounds on the tongue by 75 percent (compared to only 45 percent by toothbrush alone). You need only about ten seconds. Just take the scraper and run it over your tongue. If your breath is just relentlessly offensive, talk to your dentist, who might even prescribe a few days of antibiotics. Your dates (and coworkers and subway companions) will thank you.

Now, we're not suggesting that you go in, cut around, and move your facial features a smidge here or smidge there (though there's more on cosmetic procedures in the appendix), but we are suggesting that there are objective standards to beauty (and you automatically calculate those when you look at others—almost instantly, even if you got a C in algebra). And if your mouth's features don't measure up to a perfect score along these scientific standards, there are still plenty of other ways that you can make the most of your mouth. Let's take a closer look at the anatomy of the mouth when it comes to ideal standards of beauty (we'll talk about health implications in a few pages).

FACTOID

Our wisdom teeth were nature's version of a backup system—giving us one last set of teeth that would come out by the age we would've destroyed our molars when we lived in the wild. Why are they called wisdom teeth? Hopefully, we would get them at the age when we were wise enough to take care of them properly, usually by our midteens. But unlike for your relatives 10,000 years ago, hopefully your molars haven't fallen out yet. Because of this, crowding often occurs when wisdom teeth erupt, causing them to come in sideways. Cockeyed teeth can't be cleaned and will destroy adjacent teeth—which is why they're often removed.

Lips: We all know the main things we use lips for, so we'll leave the sexy details to your imagination. (OK, back with us now? Good.) If you'll allow us to go from sultry to scientific

Sore Sport

Surely, there are plenty of places on your body where you love a little tingling, but not right above your lip before a first date, an interview, or your reality show tryout. What starts as a tingle and ends as a full-blown cold sore can be as painful as it is embarrassing. The leading cause: herpes infections, which are transmitted through saliva, kissing, or sharing other people's cups. This is called type 1, not to be confused with the genital variety, called type 2. The best treatment is a short course of virus-killing drugs like acyclovir (Zovirax) or valacyclovir (Valtrex) combined with hydrocortisone cream. By the way, these infections aren't just painful or embarrassing; they seem to relate to an increase in cancers of the mouth. If you know the sore is on its way, you'd do better to start the drug sooner, to try to shorten the nearly two weeks of suffering (they can come back when you have a cold, which is why they're called cold sores). An over-the-counter drug called Abreva seems to superpower your cells to resist this type of herpes infection. Give it a try if you don't have the prescription stuff, and eat a soft, bland diet while you have the sores. If you figure that out on your own, your family won't have to scrape you off the ceiling if you eat pickles.

The other type of mouth sore happens on the inside; they're called aphthous ulcers (otherwise known as canker sores). People with iron, folate, and vitamin B12 deficiencies are more likely to get these sores, and sodium lauryl sulfate (SLS) in toothpaste triggers them. It takes about ten days for these to go away, but hydrocortisone ointment and keeping the sores clean with antibacterial mouthwash can reduce the duration.

for just a moment, there's more to know about your pinkish pucker. In the ideal scenario, the upper lip should be slightly larger than the lower with a gentle curve that peaks at what's called a Cupid's bow. The upper lip is divided symmetrically in two by two vertical lines under your nose called the central philtrum. The color of the lips also reflects what's going on inside, as pale lips reflect anemia (lack of red cells or abnormalities of red cell contents) and blue reflects lack of oxygenation of blood (which can come from many causes). As we all know by now, lips—like faces, fat, and breasts—are a supreme target of the beauty counter and the plastic surgeon's tools, and we'll talk in more detail about these options in our YOU Tips.

Teeth: One thing we know for sure about mouth beauty: If your teeth look more like randomly shaped shards of glass than perfectly aligned chompers, then it's a pretty good bet that those malformed biters can overshadow other beautiful body parts. Research shows that women tend to prefer upper front teeth that are rounded and men like a more square look, but it does seem that most of us prefer the height of the two front teeth to be about 1.6 times the width (phi ratio!). The front six teeth also should follow the golden rule that we discussed earlier—with the larger ones being 1.6 times the size of each successive smaller one.

Smile. Normally, we think of muscles as giving us the power to push, to pull, to heave, and to haul. But of the seven zillion cool things about the human body, here's one of our favorites: The ever-so-subtle muscles in your mouth (and how you use them) determine exactly how you communicate with the world (see Figure 3.1). To do so, your mouth is controlled by a dozen or so muscles that all connect with the circular muscle around your mouth. Amazed that you have that many? That's just a fraction of those around your eyes. Some pucker the lips, some suck in the cheeks, others lift or lower the lips. Just fire a few neurons that instruct your mouth to move a certain way,

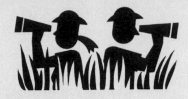

Safari Secrets:
Lessons from the animal kingdom

Elephants replace their teeth five times and then they die. Great white sharks? They spit out new teeth as if they're on a conveyor belt. Both are signs that the animal kingdom knows the true value of our munchers. Without them, you can't survive.

FACTOID Mercury fillings may not have gotten more bad press than conniving government officials, but they certainly have taken their own share of hits. The fact is that there's nothing that shows that mercury in fillings causes any neurological damage, but there are better alternatives than having a mine in your mouth. (Note, however, that if you're pregnant or nursing or plan to be, you should avoid any new mercury fillings because potentially damaging toxins can be released during the procedure that are toxic to incubating infants.) Fillings made of composite resin or ceramic are aesthetically more pleasing and may last longer. Also, there's no need to have a silver filling removed and replaced unless there's leaking, there's decay under the filling, or it has a rough surface that keeps you from being able to floss.

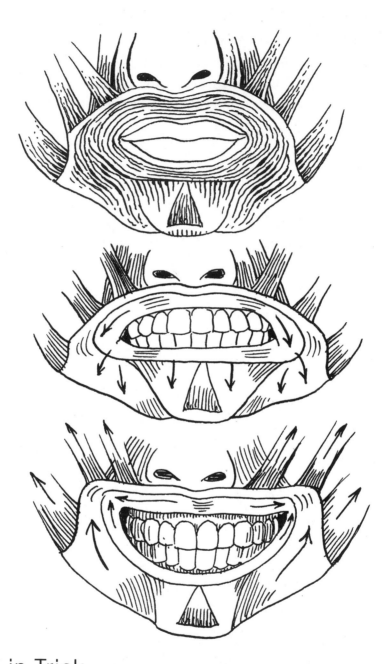

Figure 3.1 Lip Trick Dozens of muscles around your mouth send messages about your thoughts and feelings—without your ever having to utter a word. The subtle cues you communicate through facial expression reveal the secrets you may be thinking.

and depending on which direction those muscles pull, you can convey rage, sadness, happiness, sarcasm, excitement, fear, arousal, confidence, and on and on and on. Even smiles can be categorized by their beauty. The prettier the teeth, the more a person smiles. And the more a person expresses emotion by using the muscles of the face (especially around the eyes and mouth), the younger she looks.

These are the three classic types of smile:

- **The Mona Lisa** (two-thirds of people): The corners of the mouth are pulled up and out, and the upper lip raises to show the upper teeth. The most attractive show all of their top teeth and about 2 millimeters of gums (any more and the smile is classified as "gummy"). Mona Lisa

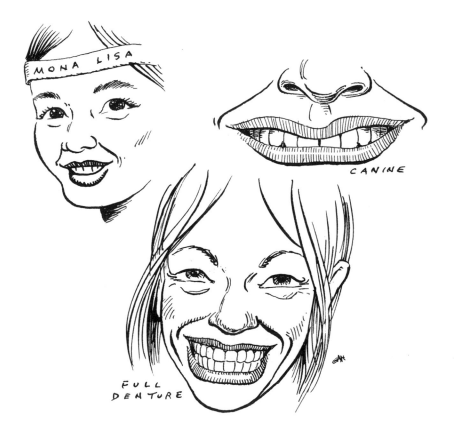

is considered most attractive, with the upper and lower lips moving out half an inch and up at a 40-degree angle.

- **The Canine** (one-third of people): Here a particular muscle (called the levator labii superioris, for you anatomy junkies) is dominant and exposes the canine teeth before the full smile.
- **The Full Denture** (rare): Here all of the upper and lower lips are working overtime to expose the whole dang shebang of teeth.

As you age, you can work to change your smile with facial exercises and by taking care of your teeth. That's important: Your teeth get worn down naturally as you age, and at the same the soft tissue around the mouth descends, leaving you with a Richard Nixon smile—showing all lower teeth and no upper. Teeth are going to move until they touch something that will make them stop. That might be a tongue, dental appliance, or other teeth. As teeth wear down and get shorter, this changes the normal tooth-to-gum ratio and gives the "gummy smile."

Tongue: Besides being your taster, your tongue also helps you swallow and protects you from swallowing poison; you can thank your taste buds for that. Controlled by eight muscles and four nerves, your tongue helps move food and liquids down your esophagus. Of course, few people* think of the tongue as an organ of beauty; normal tongues are moist and pink and have bigger bumps toward the back. It's when you develop problems that things can get a little hairy. Black hairy tongue, for example, occurs when taste buds elongate and change color (due to smoking or antibiot-

* Other than Gene Simmons.

ics). Your tongue can also develop cysts, ulcers, herpes infections, and yeast infections (which are called thrush; milk of magnesia or nystatin can chase the yeast right out of your mouth).

The Tooth About Health

Besides being the tunnel that food and flies enter, your mouth gives you lots of clues about your overall health—especially when it comes to your teeth and their surrounding structures. Some things you can decipher for yourself, but for others, you'll need a dentist and a hygienist to inspect for you. So let's get into our literary dentist's chair and do a quick inspection of the other elements of your mouth. Sit back, cue instrumental rendition of "Kokomo," and we'll take a look inside (see Figure 3.2).

Your jawbone (docs call it the mandible): The only time we ever get to see jaws is in muse-

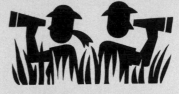

Safari Secrets:
Lessons from the animal kingdom

Elephants displace teeth from the back; they're grinders. But most animals are like us and have a single series of adult teeth, since we need to develop perfect occlusion and would lose this with continual change. Crocodiles have "nails" for teeth, which are designed for grabbing rather than chewing. Our mandibles were fused about 40 million years ago. We lost the independence of selective chewing but gained the ability to spread the force of chewing to the entire jaw. We also have a two-post jaw joint, which allows our mandible to slide forward and then drop down. This enables the masseter muscle to develop increased force during chewing. Carnivores don't have the mechanism since they must grab and tear their food.

ums, and they're usually of the shark or dinosaur variety. But the human jaw is a powerful little clamp of its own—exerting 50 to 250 pounds per square inch of pressure during chewing. It's also extremely efficient: It's the only joint in the body that purposely dislocates itself during a motion, using two points of attachment—one lever point in the back of the jaw and another two inches in front. Every time you chew, your jaw dislocates and relocates, allowing you to crush food so you can swallow and digest. But the muscles that move the jaw can also be a source of pain. If you chew too much or subconsciously clench your jaw during stressful times, your jaw muscles can spasm. Stress-induced

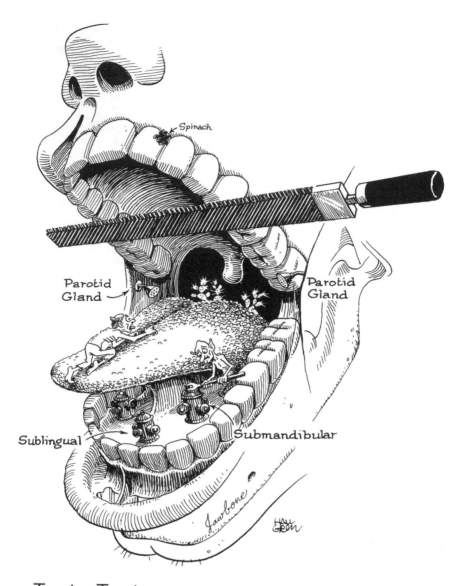

Figure 3.2 Taste Test Much of our perceived beauty comes from deep inside our voice portal: The way our teeth look (not to mention the way our breath smells) influences our relationships with others. Proper flossing, tongue scraping, and other methods of oral hygiene are little things you can do that have major results. Grinding your teeth will flatten them and can cause one heck of a headache. As we age, we make less saliva from our mouth glands, which besides causing us to made weird noises with our tongues can lead to tooth decay.

clenching or grinding can cause slight mis-alignment of the jaw, leading to jaw, neck, or eye pain, as well as jackhammer-like headaches. By the way, if you lose your teeth—be it through decay or an errant baseball—your jawbone will eventually erode away as well (use it or lose it). The main purpose of your jawbone is to support teeth, and a very intricate and complicated set of muscles, ligaments, and skin holds your jaw in place.

Your gums: We all know how well that peas-in-the-teeth look impresses first dates and job interviewers, and it doesn't go over too well with the rest of your body either. Lest you think your gums aren't important: The amount of tissue involved in a severe gum disease case is approximately the same as the surface of the skin on the back of the hand. What would you do if the back of your hand was bloodred and swollen and bled at the slightest touch? You would haul your buns to the doctor. But when the same thing happens in the mouth, you think it's normal. When plaque—that sticky gunk made up of bacteria, saliva, and yesterday's dinner—wedges between your teeth into your gums, it triggers a process of inflammation that leads to periodontal disease (gingivitis is infection of the gums, while periodontitis occurs when the disease progresses to the ligaments and bones around the teeth). Regular flossing and checkups can

FACTOID

You may sleep next to a person who snoozes with a mouth that's open wide enough for a subway to get through. The reason why it's a problem? It's like driving a car without the windshield. When mouth breathers (sleeping or not) are exposed to all that air (caused by a clogged nose), it dries the gum and enamel to create gingivitis and possible bone decay.

FACTOID

You're naturally susceptible to tooth decay if your mother was unhealthy during pregnancy or you had poor childhood health, perhaps because the foundations of the teeth were not created well. Today, major food sources that cause decay include carbonated drinks that dissolve enamel and sugary gums and mints, since these continually bathe our teeth with food bacteria love. Also, avoid sticky foods and candies (such as raisins, unless you religiously brush afterward), which can stick to your teeth (sucking candies are better for the health of your teeth).

rid you of plaque and help save your teeth. Gum disease is linked to many other problems, likely because the same bacteria that can cause periodontal disease can also trigger an immune response that causes inflammation and hardening of the arteries. That plaque that's found near your teeth contains a zoo of bacteria and proteins, sugars, and fat, as well as calcium and phosphorus. This tough stuff sticks to your teeth and causes gingivitis (gingivitis is an even better indicator of heart disease than levels of cholesterol).

Your teeth. Wiggle your jaw around (go ahead, nobody's looking). Your top teeth are fixed to your skull, while your lower jaw has the flexibility to move front to back and side to side. If the top and bottom are misaligned, your upper teeth can't adjust, so you end up wearing down your teeth. How do you know if you're a teeth grinder? One, by taking the flat-teeth test on page 87, and two, because teeth grinders show less tooth when they smile, which makes them look older and less attractive.

While acceptable on dance floors, grinding isn't so great for your mouth. It causes premature aging as the wearing down of the front teeth inhibits the ability of the jaw to work efficiently, causing back teeth to wear down as well. Grinding can also injure your jawbone joint, called the TMJ (temporomandibular joint). If you're a grinder (which can be caused by stress or misalignment), you'll want early detection so your bite can be analyzed and you can be fitted for a night-guard mouth-piece that prevents you from grinding while you sleep. Left untreated, your teeth will eventually break and split from your gums. It depends on the break or the severity of the split if they can be saved or not. If it's not too severe, crowns can cover them. Severely worn teeth may have to be replaced (and that can cost up to $2,000 per tooth).

YOU Tips!

It's one of the most common dreams around: losing your teeth by the bucketful. We're not dream psychologists, so it's not our place to suggest that such dreams are symbolic of your chaotic life (though some people believe that these dreams indicate that you're a grinder). But we do want to help you avoid the nightmare of your teeth falling out in real life. Of course, you know the basics—you gotta brush, you gotta floss, you gotta see a dentist and dental professionals, you gotta avoid barroom brawls. But here are some more details that'll ensure that your new nickname becomes Mighty Mouth.

TAKE TWO. Waiting in traffic, two minutes seems like an eternity. Playing in bed, two minutes feels like a flash. At the sink, two minutes is the time you need to spend brushing your teeth in order to clean them adequately and reduce plaque. Use a soft brush and rub the bristles up toward the gums, so you can get to the actual cusps and gum. Change your toothbrush every two months. Those newfangled ultrasonic brushes amaze many dentists with their plaque-fighting abilities (and some have two-minute timers built in). Many cultures, by the way, believe that massaging your gums with your fingers is helpful in preventing periodontal disease. We actually prefer sonic brushes, since they produce more than 30,000 brushstrokes a minute (compared to about 5,000 of typical electrical ones) and spray into the crevices of teeth to clean beyond where the tips of the bristles actually touch. In other words, they're more effective at dislodging plaque. To use one, follow these instructions:

- Wet the bristles and use a small bit of toothpaste.
- Place the toothbrush bristles against the teeth at a slight angle toward the gumline. Power up.
- Apply light pressure to let the brush do the brushing for you (as with a sensitive coworker, don't push too hard).
- Gently brush the head slowly across the teeth in small back-and-forth motions so the longer bristles reach between your teeth.
- Do the outside top teeth, inside top teeth, outside bottom teeth, and inside bottom teeth each for 30 seconds. Then do the chewing surfaces and anywhere else that may have stains. Feel free to brush your tongue, too, which can help with bad breath.

GET BETWEEN THE CRACKS. Despite the pleading from dentists, from doctors, and from people who notice that ill-placed broccoli floret, 80 percent of us still don't floss. When you don't floss, you're not cleaning 40 percent of the tooth. Dentists consider flossing even more crucial for preventing tooth decay and periodontal disease than brushing. But you've got to know how to do it.

The right way: The floss should barely pass between each tooth and should gently touch the gums. If your floss breaks, try the thicker or waxed stuff, or one made with Gore-Tex material, or have your dentist file down the "contact points" between your teeth.

The wrong way: You can't get into certain openings, so you jam it in between, forcing it into spaces, which then causes gum bleeding and your sink to look like a bowlful of steak juice. Ick.

Now, if you don't floss, at least remember to save up the money to buy the dentures you're eventually going to need (as well as the the coronary artery bypass graft, Viagra, and Botox, since gum disease says a lot about how you look and about the inner health of your arteries).

TOOTHBRUSHING 101

THINK ABOUT YOUR OWN ALIGNMENT.

The only time most of us think about our jaw is when someone's looking to break it. But you can improve your jaw health—and thus reduce tooth problems—by thinking a little bit more about your mouth. Make these adjustments in your alignment until they become habit:

- The only time your teeth should actually be touching each other is when you eat. Otherwise, keep your tongue between your teeth. That will prevent the clenching (and subsequent grinding and aching) that's associated with stress. Your new mandible mantra: Lips together, teeth apart, lips together, teeth apart, lips together, teeth apart, lips together, teeth apart.
- Stand tall. Not only will improved posture improve your back, strengthen your core muscles, and make you look thinner than a flat-screen TV, good posture will naturally correct your jaw alignment. Go ahead and try it. Stand straight and feel what happens to your jaw as it moves back into proper, healthy position.

WHITE UP YOUR LIFE. If your teeth are the approximate hue of hamburger, then surely you've considered the popular cosmetic procedure of whitening. Here's how whitening works: No matter what the delivery method, teeth are whitened by hydrogen peroxide. The oxygen hits the stains and breaks them up; then you wipe them off into oral oblivion. Be careful: It can be irritating to some people. In the dental office, a high-intensity light is used to activate the oxygen, while over-the-counter methods rely more on longer periods of contact time (half an hour for 10 days to two weeks) to deliver the oxygen. For the average person, we recommend the tray method (see below), but there are several options:

In-office whitening: Fastest and strongest effects, up to ten shades lighter, but costs $500 to $1,200.

Brush-ons: Best over-the-counter method. You can see results four shades lighter. Great options are Rembrandt Whitening Wand, BriteSmile To Go pen, and GoSmile Daily, but the first two are reusable, so bacteria can build up; GoSmile is single use, so there are no hygiene issues, but it is more expensive. These get the back teeth better than the strips do.

Strips: You can get four to six shades lighter, but only on the front six teeth.

Tray and gels (in-office or OTC): It's an older technology and has potential for gum irritation, so it's best to do with a doc. At home, the temptation is to abuse it, which can lead to tooth sensitivity.

Whitening toothpastes: An everyday experience, these toothpastes (the best is Ultrabrite in some tests) remove stains from teeth by polishing or chemical removal.

The ideal combo: If you can afford it, use an in-office whitening, then follow up with brush-ons and toothpastes. Studies have shown that repetitive whitening at safe, low concentrations of the active ingredients gives longer-lasting results. Just be sure not to do more than once every two weeks or you'll thin the enamel (home whitening strips don't appear to harm enamel). A simple five-minute fluoride treatment before bleaching will allow the teeth to recover fully in two weeks.

USE TOOLS. It may be tempting to pop beer bottles, tear wrappers, and fix kids' toys by using your teeth. But, really now, is it worth sacrificing your teeth just to save yourself from having to get off the couch and get a bottle opener, knife, or pair of scissors?

EMPLOY ANTISTAINING TECHNIQUES. Certain foods will stain your teeth as surely as a new puppy will stain the carpet. The culprits include red wine, coffee, tea, blueberries, soy sauce, balsamic vinegar, tomato sauce, and grape and cranberry juice. We don't want you to avoid these foods, because of their obvious health benefits, but here's how to combat their staining ways:

- When you eat staining foods, keep a glass of water handy. Swishing and sipping after every couple of bites or slurps will help decrease staining.
- Never skip a bedtime brush, and brush your teeth as soon as possible after a staining meal. Here's where a travel toothbrush comes in handy.
- Some foods can whiten your teeth. Apples, celery, and carrots act as a natural stain remover, while greens such as spinach, broccoli, and lettuce create a film over your teeth that acts as a barrier against staining.

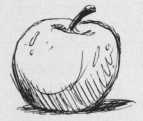

CHECK IT OUT. There are some things you can do yourself to test the health of your mouth: Bleeding, bad breath (you may need a partner to confirm this—they say a skunk doesn't smell his own odor, but then how do we verify this?), an itchy feeling in the gums, a change in gum color, and increased space between the teeth are all signs you should see a dentist. While some people consider dentist visits as optional as a side of mayo, you do need to see a dentist every six months (or every four, if you have gum issues). And that's especially important if you have a family history of gingivitis. Why? Because no matter how much you brush or if you floss with the speed of an expert fiddler, you simply can't dig up and obliterate all the gum-destroying plaque that's deposited between your teeth and near your gums. Dental hygienists have those fun ultrasonic thingos and lovely hooks that do this well. Plus, early detection of gingivitis will make it easier to treat.

WATCH YOUR LIPS. It's not as if lips are high-maintenance items, like skin, hair, or overbearing cousins. But you should protect them with sunblock. If they get damaged by the sun, they'll crinkle and wrinkle and are liable to develop lip cancers, especially on the lower lip. Why? That's where we get more sun exposure. Men and women: You should also use only lip gloss with titanium or zinc oxide sunblock because lip gloss focuses the sun and thus causes more injury. And everyone should make sure their dentists are inspecting their lips for funny marks or nodules as a check against cancer. If you've had an injury to the lip* the small

FACTOID

Don't put Vaseline on your lips. Vaseline is made from the goop that comes from oil wells (petroleum jelly, remember?), so it's something you don't want too close to your mouth because you'll ingest little bits each day. Instead, use cocoa butter or Burt's Bees lip balm to moisten dry lips (they use beeswax—good for bees and OK for you).

*Via hockey stick, dog mouth, overeager date.

blood vessels in the injured areas can dilate and cause blue bulges. Your doc can fix these by making a little nick in the lip and either frying the blood vessel or fishing it out and tying it off.

KEEP PLUMPING IN CHECK. Flick through TV channels long enough, and you're sure to come across someone who has lips as big as dachshunds. Over the last decade, women have put everything except salami into their lips, thinking that bigger is better. What have they used? Silicone, fat, their own skin (dermis), collagen, hyaluronic acid, and even Gore-Tex. But here's our thinking: A little looks good; a lot looks like a horror flick. Keep plastic items out, since they don't seem to do well over time. For more on cosmetic procedures, see the appendix.

4 Digital Revolution

Shape Up Your Hands and Feet

YOU Test: A Nail Space

Place the back of your fingertips against each other, as shown. Look at the space in between them.

Ideally, that space should be triangular or diamond shaped. If the nails are flush together or rounded like the top of a baseball bat, you're experiencing what's called nail clubbing, which could be a sign of bigger health problems, such as lung disease, Crohn's disease, and even hyperthyroidism. It's believed that this clubbing happens from dilation of small arteries in the fingertips.

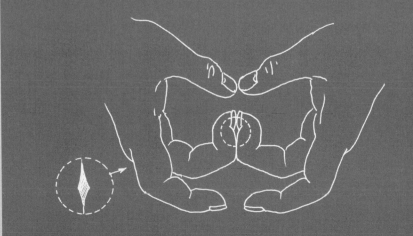

In the pecking order of beautiful body parts, your feet and hands are the source of some pretty diverse opinions. Take feet, for example. Some people pamper their feet (pedicures), and some people idolize feet (foot fetishes). Other people, however, hate feet because of the way they look, smell, and react to tickling fingers.

Of course, ugly digits—whether signified by nasty nails or toes the shape of monkey wrenches—can be a source of embarrassment, sexual avoidance, and frustration. No matter your preference, we should all take a page from the digit lovers of the world and celebrate not only the function of hands and feet but their beauty as well.

Take the foot first. Besides the fact that the structure of the foot makes upright posture possible, the human foot also possesses a natural sexuality. It's one of the body's most sensitive tactile organs. Some cultures believe it's also rich with vibratory and electromagnetic powers that are linked to contact with the earth (one of the reasons why feet are traditionally associated with fertility).

And the hands? They, too, come in all different shapes with all different meanings. There are big, bear-paw hands best suited for manual labor, and thin, dainty hands that are traditionally a sign of aristocracy. The hand is also one of the only body parts that's continually exposed to the outside world—making it a major advertisement of

FACTOID

We all know the joke about how women can tell a lot about men just by looking at their hands. In research that surely was conducted by men, there's absolutely no correlation between finger or foot size and the size of the penis. It's safe to take your hands out of your pockets, bub. But research shows that something called the digit-length ratio (that is, the variance from the second finger to the fourth) can predict such things as IQ, fertility, even the ability to perform in sports. For men, the typical ratio is for the index finger to be 96 percent the size of the ring finger, while women typically have a 1:1 ratio—that is, the two fingers are about the same size. The argument is that this ratio is actually a marker for being exposed to androgens (like testosterone) in utero.

beauty. Plus, there are many examples of how we communicate strong messages through our hands. Gentlemen kiss ladies' hands. Couples hold each other's hands. And strangers and friends greet each other with a shake of the hands to show respect and interact with potential mates.*

We understand that a few blemishes on your hands or feet may be lower on your priority list than wrinkles, dandruff, or missing teeth. But that doesn't mean you should ignore those issues altogether. In fact, unlike some aspects of your appearance where you can't make significant changes, your feet and hands are a few of the places where you can.

You Nailed It: Your Digits

They may come in handy for scratching backs, digging around nostrils, and gouging attackers' eyeballs. But if your nails look like cracked and crumbling sidewalks, they can also crack and crumble your appearance and your confidence (and give you some health headaches along the way). So let's take a look at the things that play a central role in the visual state of your hands and feet.

As you can see in Figure 4.1, your nails are composed of laminated layers of a protein called keratin, which as you know by now is also found in your hair and skin. Each nail has several parts, including:

- **The nail plate:** The visible hard part of the nail.
- **Nail folds:** The skin that frames each of your nail plates on three sides.

* By the way, the reason why we shake with our right hands isn't only because most of us are right-hand dominant. It's partly because shaking with our right was once the signal to foes that we weren't armed. In some cultures, people wipe their tushes with their left hand—shaking with the right, in that case, is simply more hygienic.

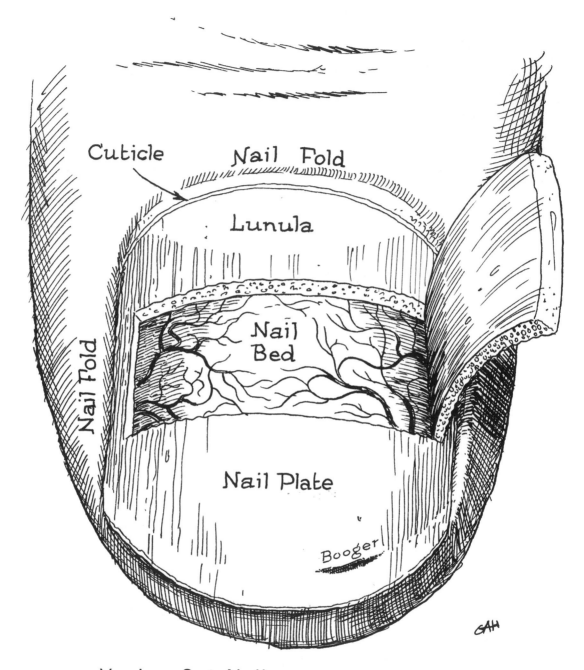

Cuticle

Nail Fold

Lunula

Nail Fold

Nail Bed

Nail Plate

Booger

GAH

Figure 4.1 You've Got Nail Your back-scratchers are made up of several parts. The nail plate is the visible part, but it's locked in by various parts of the skin to keep it in place. Underneath the plate, the nail bed is what actually produces the plate.

- **The nail bed:** The skin beneath the nail plate. The cells at the base of your nail bed are the ones that actually produce the fingernail or toenail plate.
- **The cuticle:** The tissue that overlaps your nail plate at the base of your nail. It protects the new keratin cells that slowly emerge from the nail bed.
- **The lunula:** The whitish, half-moon shape at the base of your nail underneath the plate.

Your nails grow from the area under your cuticle (called the matrix) the same way hairs grow from follicles. As new cells grow, older cells become hard and compacted, basically becoming the keratin, and are eventually pushed out toward your fingertips. Fingernails—which grow faster than toenails and grow faster over the summer than over the winter—grow about a tenth of a millimeter a day, which means that it takes a fingernail about four to six months to fully grow out. As you age, your nail growth slows down, eventually growing half as fast when you're 80 as when you're 10. But, other than Howard Hughes and certain circus actors, who cares about how fast your nails grow? What we're really looking for is not the growth rate but the health of our nails—to make sure they're smooth, without ridges or grooves (although these are often normal variants). Ideally, they're uniform in color and consistency and free of spots or discoloration.

FACTOID

Dietary changes that supposedly strengthen nails don't work. Unless you're deficient in protein—rare among people in the United States—adding protein to your diet won't strengthen your nails. Similarly, all those teenagers in the 1960s were wrong; eating or soaking your nails in gelatin won't help either. There is some evidence that biotin, a water-soluble B vitamin, does help treat brittle nails.

While we trust you know the basics of what looks good (bloody hangnails and gnawed-off nails are indeed gnarly), you should know a little bit about the other things that can make your nails look like the remnants from the bottom of a cereal box.

Finger Looking Good?

Most minor nail injuries heal on their own, but they might be unsightly for a while because the nail is like a kid's science experiment—it takes a heck of a long time to grow. Here, some common nail-related issues.

White spots: These small, semicircular spots result from injury to the base (matrix) of the nail, where nail cells are produced. They'll eventually grow out.

Splinter hemorrhages: A disruption of blood vessels in the nail bed can cause fine, splinter-like vertical lines to appear under the nail plate. Caused by injury and some drugs, splinter hemorrhages resolve spontaneously. However, since an infection in your heart can also cause these, call a doc to make sure, especially if you feel under the weather and have a fever.

Ingrown toenails: Improper nail trimming, tight shoes, or poor posture can cause a corner of the nail to curve downward into the skin. Ingrown nails can be painful and sometimes even lead to infection. To avoid infection, see a doctor rather than attempting to saw away the nail yourself. Your doc will numb the toe and trim the ingrown nail. To prevent the nail from regrowing, an 80 percent phenol solution destroys the nail-growing cells on the side that is growing in. Or you could pay $800 more per nail than the phenol if you want it removed by a laser, which is no more effective.

Finger Cracks: Second only to a toe stub, a pesky hangnail (or a finger crack, technically) wins the award for the smallest, most annoying pain in our lives. How do we get them? When humidity is low, your fingertips and cuticles can crack. Best prevention: Use a moisturizer routinely to keep your skin from drying up. And if you do crack up, try Johnson & Johnson's Liquid Bandage (like Krazy Glue for your skin) to seal the cracks and eliminate the pain within a few seconds.

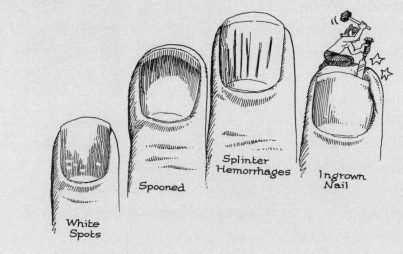

Spooned

Splinter Hemorrhages

Ingrown Nail

White Spots

FUNGAL TOENAILS. Nail fungus—signaled by ugly, thickened, yellow nails—is more common in older adults than in younger ones, because nails grow more slowly and thicken with aging, making them more susceptible to infection. Nail fungus usually begins as a white or yellow spot under the tip of your fingernail or toenail and can be caused by three different fungi. (Toenails are more susceptible to fungal infection because they spend most of their time in dark, damp shoes and socks; fingernails are dry and are exposed to UV light, which kills fungi.)

Fungus is made up of microscopic organisms (see Figure 4.2) that can invade through invisible cuts in your skin, through a small separation between your nail and the nail bed, or after an injury such as dropping a hammer on your toes. As the fungus spreads deeper into the nail, it may cause the nail

to discolor, thicken, and develop crumbling edges that are sometimes as painful as they are ugly. Fungus usually grows when your nails are continually exposed to moist environments, such as sweaty shoes or shower floors (by the way, it's not the same as athlete's foot, which affects the skin; see below).

You (and those around you) can tell if you've developed a nail fungus if your nails are thickened, brittle, distorted, and flat and have turned yellow (without the

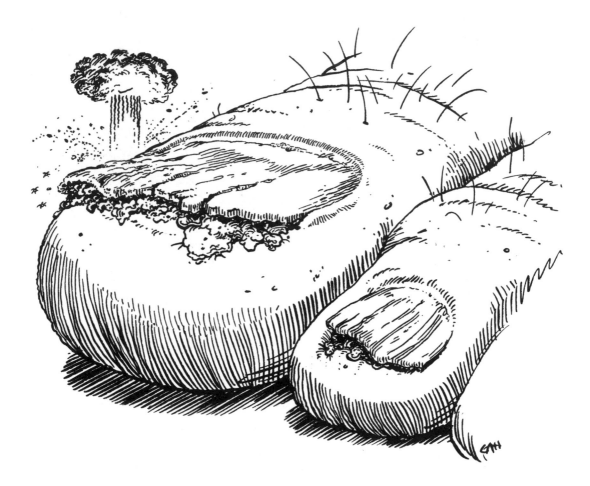

Figure 4.2 Fungus Among Us The cracks and crumbles associated with a nail fungus increase with age. It's especially important to keep your feet dry and get out of your sweaty shoes, since damp, moist areas are a breeding ground for fungi. Luckily, there are medications that can help control the fungus.

benefit of yellow polish), a side effect of debris building up under the nails. While over-the-counter creams, ointments, and expensive pills are available, they may be more effective when combined with some do-it-yourself tactics that we'll outline below. Only the prescription pills with the expensive ingredients work well for fungus. However, the active ingredients can poison your liver, often do not work, and have to be used for many months, which is why so many folks wander around with untreated nail fungus.

Since nail fungus infects the live part of the nail, it can be tough to rid yourself of it. Some people try to cure the ugliness of the fungus (this doesn't treat the fungus itself) by using a Dremel rotary tool with a burr attached. The burr thins the nail and then nail polish is painted on the surface. (If you do this, please wear a mask every time so you don't inhale the fungus and develop a fungus ball in your lung, which is deadly if your immune system is not running on all cylinders.)

The best medical treatment is antifungal drugs taken by mouth, such as ketoconazole or Lamisil. Other drugs that are used include Sporanox, Diflucan, and Penlac.

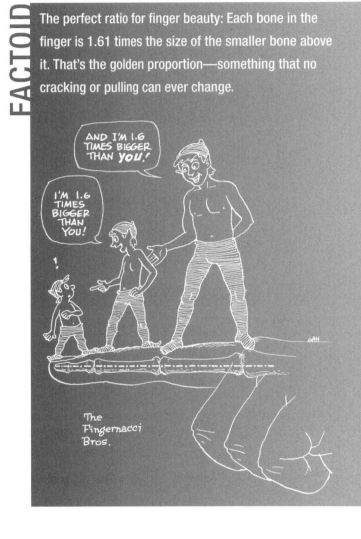

(All of these are potentially toxic, with about 1 in 10,000 patients developing bad liver complications from them, so we recommend avoiding them unless the fungus is really affecting your life.) Remember, these nail fungi never ever cause a problem that is more than superficial (unless you use that Dremel or do a lot of toe sucking), so unless your nails are keeping you from the love of your life, be careful about taking a drug with real risk. (On the other hand, if you get nauseated looking at your nails and are too thin, maybe getting rid of the fungus is worth the effort for you.) These drugs work by letting a new nail grow fungus-free and replacing the old one. You must be patient with them, since fingernails grow in over a six-month period and toenails can take a year. And they appear to work for the typical person less than 30 percent of the time.

PSORIATIC NAILS. Patients with the "skin condition"* psoriasis often develop problems with their nails. Since psoriatic nails look like fungal infections, your doctor will take a snip (a biopsy) to be sure. Generally, psoriatic nails look flakier and are softer than those with fungal infections, like shingles coming off your roof, with pinpoint bleeding. Even a biopsy isn't perfect; under the microscope, psoriasis is misdiagnosed as fungus a third of the time—another reason to get a second opinion on everything. Unfortunately, treatment of psoriatic nails can be as tough as, er, nails. Sometimes the nail has to be removed, but docs will also try light therapy, or topical, oral, and even injected steroids. New drugs such as Humira or Remicade may help heal both nail and skin problems from psoriasis.

INJURED NAILS. A hammer, car door, or angry cat at the wrong place and the wrong time can leave your nail looking like a Jackson Pollock original. While new interns at hospitals salivate at the thought of searing your nail with a hot paper clip to drain the blood, the better solution is to have a more experienced doc pop the nail off, drain the blood, and put a few dissolving stitches in the nail so that it doesn't grow back looking like a kaleidoscope. After repair, the nail will be glued or taped back on to direct the growth of the new nail and prevent you from screaming every time your toe hits a stair. In about six months or so, a brand-new nail will be welcomed into the world, pushing out the old one.

Now, we'd be remiss if we didn't mention this very important fact about nails:

* It really isn't just a skin disorder, because it can affect your kidneys, joints, and other organs as well.

Nails are more than just fingertip armor, tootsie protectors, and ornaments; they can also serve as the smoke alarm for more serious health issues. Heart and lung diseases, as well as some infections and immune disorders, may leave traces in your nails. Changes in nails can be the tip-off to send you scurrying to your doctor. So use your digits not for an in-traffic stress reliever but as a gauge of your health. Yellow or green discoloration in your nails may result from a respiratory condition, such as chronic bronchitis, or from swelling of your hands (lymphedema). Indentations that run across your nails, called Beau's lines, appear when growth at the area under your cuticle is interrupted. This might happen because of an injury or severe illness, such as a heart attack.

Foot Notes: We've Got Them Covered

Though most of us keep our feet hidden from the rest of the world, we've all likely seen some flippers that are scarier than Halloween masks. You know—the warts, the blood, the cracks, the overall ugliness that can make sandal sales plummet. The reality is that a lot of people do have huge issues with the way their feet look (the foot problem plantar fasciitis is covered in chapter 7). We even know of some women who have resisted getting into relationships because they were so ashamed of their feet. So, in the spirit of improving beauty and celebrating the joy of wearing flip-flops, let's slip off the shoes and take a look at what you might be hiding in there (see Figure 4.3).

> **Corns:** When your shoe's too tight, the toe and the surrounding tendons stretch, causing the toe joint to dig into the top of the shoe. This causes a corn to develop—it's the foot's way of protecting itself from that rubbing. If you catch it early enough, the toe can be splinted to regain its form, but if not, surgery can help straighten things out. (Corns aren't a health problem, but a doc can trim them, and you can then use a pad to relieve the pressure.)
> **Bunions:** Unless you have very narrow feet, frequent wearing of beautiful, pointy, high-heeled shoes will push your big toe out of alignment, causing a

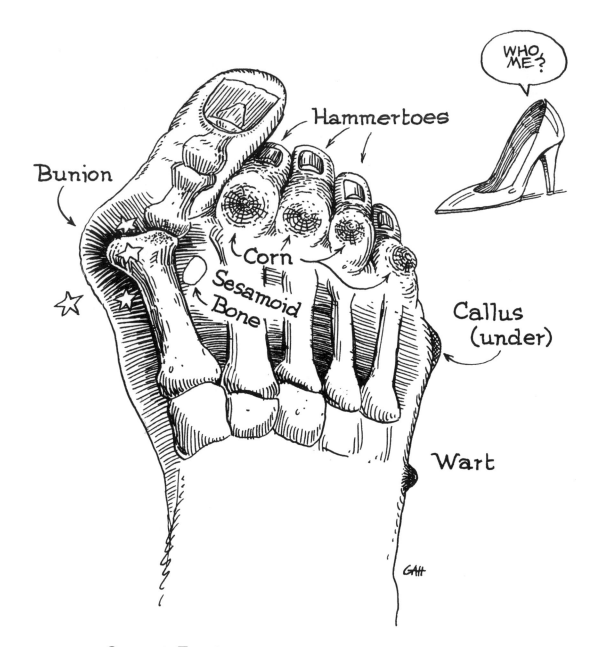

Figure 4.3 Sweet Feet As our primary contact point with the earth, our feet have to stand the wear and tear of everyday living (and our own methods of torture, namely high heels). While podiatrists can help with some of the unsightly marks such as bunions, you can also go a long way in helping out your feet by choosing a proper-fitting shoe that will protect your valuable pups.

partial dislocation of the toe. This creates a bony prominence on the medial aspect of your foot; that bump is a bunion. If you continue to wear tight, pointy shoes, the big toe continues to get pushed out of its joint. This is why bunions are progressive; like a building falling over, they tend to get worse with time. You have two options for treatment: Either you can modify your shoes or a surgeon can modify your foot with an operation that corrects the alignment of the toe. Look for shoes with a toe box that is wide and high; this will stop the irritation over the bump and slow down the progression of the deformity. Unfortunately, these types of shoes are not particularly pretty. The best time to consider surgery is when your pain symptoms are in the moderate category or there's been a significant change in shoe comfort. The good news about a bunionectomy is that once the bunion is corrected properly, it most likely will never come back again. The bad news about a bunion operation is that full recovery to normal shoes can take several months. And there are a lot of shady bunion doctors out there. Make sure yours has loads of experience. If a podiatrist does this, she should have done a surgical residency, and if it's an orthopedic doc, make sure she did a foot and ankle fellowship.

Calluses: If you've spent any time with a shovel or walking barefoot through the neighborhood, you know exactly what a callus is: It's your body's way of protecting you. Calluses are dead, thickened skin that builds up from too much pressure or bearing too much weight (often occurring on the ball of the foot, between your big and second toes). Don't try to slice one down with your triple-blade razor;* it's better to have a doc file it down or to use a toe pad if the callus isn't too serious.

Warts: Caused by a papillomavirus, warts can be treated with acids, liquid nitrogen, or a carbon dioxide laser that kills the cells and causes an inflammatory reaction. You can also suffocate them by placing adhesive tape over the area for a week. One note: If you do have warts, keep your feet to yourself, especially in the bedroom, since you can spread those bad boys to others.

* It'll leave a painful scar—painful for the rest of your life—and your bathroom looking like the local blood bank.

To remove a splinter—whether it's in the form of a rose thorn or shards of wood or glass—lay a piece of duct tape on your skin and lift straight up. If the splinter is exposed, it will lift off with the tape. If the splinter is still there, try snipping the skin with a fingernail clipper (sterilize the clipper by boiling in hot water for ten minutes or at least wash it off with alcohol first). Then use tweezers (we like to call them forceps) to pull out the splinter in the direction it entered. If this fails, a doc can numb the skin and remove it.

What might start out as a game of footsie can lead to genital warts if you take the game too far.

Athlete's foot: You don't have to be a jock to get this. But the name comes from the shared showers that athletes use, since they can share fungus there. The first thing you need to do if you have this ugly, red, and smelly fungal skin infection: Toss the shoes you're wearing, since the fungus can be living there, as well as on your body. You'll want to use a topical antifungal medication such as Lamisil to kill the fungus. And by the way, most health clubs do not use high enough temperature and enough sodium hydroxide (bleach-like treatment) to kill many of these fungi, bacteria, and viruses from a towel's previous user, so you might want to provide your own towels.

Foot shapes are like fingerprints—they're all unique. One thing to check: whether you have a flat foot or high arch, which can be the source of common foot pains and make you more prone to discomfort or even stress fractures (you're less stable when less of your foot hits the ground). How to check: Walk on sand to see what kind of shape your foot makes. Or wet your feet and step on a paper bag. To take a more elaborate test explaining what your foot says about you, see www.realage.com.

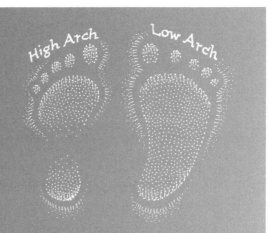

Though you don't have to worry about hand shape in the same way, it is interesting to note that there are different classifications of hand shape: There are (1) leptosome-asthenic, which are long, slender hands characterized by long fingers, (2) athletic, which are rougher, wider hands, but overall is the best balanced, and (3) the picnic, which is classified as short and wide, with conically formed fingers.

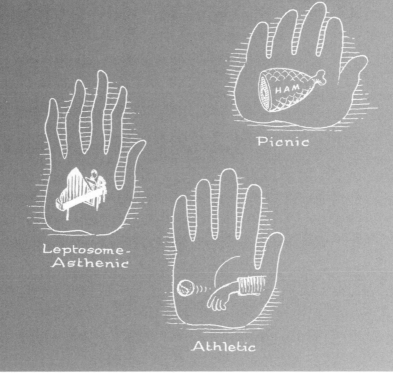

YOU Tips!

These days, we're bombarded with messages that you can make extreme changes to your appearance (as long as you have the money, a surgeon, and a TV camera crew). When it comes to your hands and feet, however, you typically don't need such an extreme approach. In fact, you can see exponential results with just a few simple strategies.

FOCUS ON YOUR FEET. Your toenails are more susceptible to fungus than your fingernails. Keep your nails dry with absorbent socks and wear open-toe shoes when you can. And don't walk barefoot unless the floor is clean enough to lick (lick first, walk second). Fungus hides in the cracks on the shower floor and seeks any opportunity to cause a nail infection. And for common showers—dorms, gyms, and hotel rooms—bring along a little Lysol, Clorox, or even better, a green-friendly bleachlike product to kill those little germs before they find your feet.

NAIL YOURSELF. You should keep your toenails short, dry, and clean by trimming the nails straight across (you can file down the thickened areas). This will help prevent bacteria from collecting under the nail. As opposed to your teeth, where you don't want to see flat surfaces, toenails were designed to be cut flat. You can use a small emery board or file to smooth off the sharp edges. After bathing, make sure you dry your hands and feet (even between your toes) to prevent fungi from being attracted to moist areas. And, by all means, don't create a digital bloodbath by trimming or picking the skin around your nails—it'll give germs access to your skin and nails. And don't cut your cuticle, which can allow infections to develop. Hint: If your toenails are thick and hard to cut, soak them in warm salt water (add one teaspoon of salt for every pint of water) for five to ten minutes. Then apply a cream made with urea (available at drugstores). That should soften them up enough to cut. And use the industrial-strength nail cutters—weak ones can split the nails.

USE HOME REMEDIES. Using tea tree oil and vinegar on a nail can help clear up some infections. But because these compounds can't penetrate deep beneath the nail, they tend not to work when infections are caused by a fungus. One home remedy for nail fungus is to soak the infected areas for five minutes twice a day in 5 grams of Chinese golden larch bark with 2 ounces of vinegar. This treatment requires months of application until the new nail is formed. An alternative, especially if the nail fungus is also associated with a skin condition such as athlete's foot: Soak the area in a mixture that combines a whole clove of garlic and 8 ounces of vinegar for five minutes twice a day. You can keep the mixture for a week. Another one we've found works to clear up infections, though we're not sure how or why: Rub the area with Vicks VapoRub. Generally speaking, the home remedies are worth trying, because you can't be sure if a nail problem is caused by a fungus or bacteria.

PICK YOUR SALON WISELY. While you know you shouldn't abuse your nails by picking, biting, or poking at them with screwdriver-like utensils, you also need to be careful about the people you hire to sculpt them for you. If you get manicures and pedicures, don't have your cuticles removed (it can lead to infection). Choose a reputable salon where the tools are properly sterilized, so that you avoid situations where you risk being contaminated with someone else's fungus or with a viral infection such as hepatitis B or C, HIV, or warts. Ideally, bring your own instruments and sterilize them yourself by boiling them in water for 10 minutes. (Don't use the leftover water for pasta.)

PROTECT YOUR NAILS. Your nails are exposed to lots of threats: bacteria, incisors, circular saws. Here's how to protect them from threats that come from the outside world—and those that come from you.

- Wear cotton-lined rubber gloves when using soap and water for prolonged periods or when using harsh chemicals or cement. Use nitrile gloves if the chemicals will dissolve rubber.
- Trim fingernails and clean under the nails regularly. Use a sharp manicure scissors or clippers and an emery board to smooth nail edges. Filing alone will weaken nails (use a fine-textured file to keep the shape and smooth away snags). Cut flat as we indicated above. Fingernails should be cut straight across and rounded slightly for maximum strength. Never pull off hangnails; doing so almost always results in ripping living tissue—painful at best, and possibly a cause of severe infections.
- Nails need moisture just as skin does. Rub lotion into your nails when moisturizing your hands. Apply a moisturizer each time you wash your hands.

STOP CHEWING. To stop your nail-biting habit, try carrying a squishy ball to squeeze or a rubber band to snap or applying bad-tasting nail polish to keep you from gnawing away. Need something to crunch on to help you get through a stressful time? Celery sticks, my friend, celery sticks.

SQUASH THE SMELL. If your feet smell like spoiled egg salad, the root of the stench is likely a fungus or bacterium. To get rid of it (and have your spouse thank you), spray your entire foot with rubbing alcohol three times a day. Don't wipe it off; let it dry. Before bed, put on a moisturizing cream such as sheep lanolin. After about ten days, the smell should be gone and your mate will return (no guarantees!). If this doesn't work, step up to Betadine. Coat your skin and let the Betadine dry. Then wash it off after half an hour. Do this carefully, since Betadine can dry out your skin.

WRAP IT UP. Sandal-wearing women often develop heel calluses; that's because low humidity causes the heel to dry out and become irritated. A good remedy: a light mixture of Vaseline with salicylic acid. Just grind up two aspirin into 2 tablespoons of Vaseline, rub the heel with it, and wrap the heel in plastic wrap to keep the moisture in. Then you can use a pumice stone to take the dead skin off.

DRY UP. Though sweat is a natural bodily process, about 1 percent of all Americans suffer from hyperhidrosis (loosely translates as "sweats like a tripped-up witness"). This is a condition that affects hands, feet, and armpits because the nerves to those areas relax the arteries and turn on extra sweat glands just beneath the skin and allow excessive moisture to escape. While it's an appearance issue, it's also a function issue—excess sweat makes it more difficult to drive, work, or simply grab a can of beans off the pantry shelf. And that's not even mentioning the anxiety that can come from meeting people, going on job interviews, or needing to change outfits more often than a runway model.

Though we don't favor the average person using antiperspirants (deodorant will do just fine), if you really suffer from the embarrassment of hyperhidrosis, you might want to try a boric acid or tannic acid solution as a first step. If you're still dripping, give 20 percent aluminum chloride a whirl. Put it on at night and wash it off in the morning. If this fails, you can talk to your doctor about using Botox every six to twelve months. It's the pits thinking about shots right there in the pits, but it might be better than a surgical procedure. There's one such procedure that cuts the nerves that cause sweaty hands (fixes the problem in nearly all cases). But that's a pretty big procedure, so you need to sweat an awful lot to justify it. For feet, try soaking your feet in tea, which removes the odor that drives your roommate out the door. In Germany, sage has also traditionally been used to treat excessive sweating and night sweats caused by menopause and tuberculosis. It can be taken as a tea or in capsule form daily and is reported anecdotally to reduce sweating by 50 percent or more. For the groin, a new technique called a sweat-gland suction may be an option. Similar to liposuction, this procedure works by suctioning the sweat glands permanently out of the area. Not many plastic surgeons do this one, however. Other options: Cut down on nicotine and caffeine to reduce the anxiety associated with the condition. Botox injected directly into the area can also help.

HIDE THE SPOT. Age spots are nature's way of tattooing you. But unlike the flaming dolphin you got inked when you turned 18, these tats aren't ones you may want to show off. There are several ways to get them removed. We prefer the TCA chemical spot peel, in which acid is applied to skin and the spots peel away. You can also have them frozen off (cryotherapy), but the freezing can cause blistering and white spots to form. Other options include dermabrasion (sandblasting them off), medications (bleaching creams that gradually fade them), and laser therapy (which destroys the substance that creates the dark pigment). Talk to your doc about what might work best for you. By the way, skin creams with niacin (niacinamide) in over 3 percent concentration applied nightly seem to work in about a month. The age spot is actually glycation of skin (glucose added to the skin protein), and niacin prevents this free radical reaction in your skin to a large degree.

GET THE RIGHT SHOES. If women were intended to have their heels higher than their toes, wouldn't evolution have provided that? One in six people have trouble with their feet from improperly fitted shoes. Heels higher than two inches should be worn only for short periods of time, if at all. High-heeled shoes cause excess pressure on the toes and double the pressure under the bottom of the foot. Cramped toes lead to bunions, corns, calluses, hammertoes, and other deformities. Leave a half inch of space between your toes and the end of the shoe and be able to wiggle those tootsies. Also, don't let the shoes be so big that your feet slip in them. Remember that the purpose of shoes is to protect the feet and keep them comfortable. Athletic shoes are ideal; a compromise is a shoe with a heel lower than one inch with a wide toe box. Fashion has joined comfort in the new generation of sneaker-shoes.

FACTOID

The best way to pick running shoes is to try five different ones and rate them from 1 to 10 on comfort. The most common mistake people make when buying running shoes is that they don't try on enough pairs to really gauge relative comfort. By the way, it's hard for people with long second toes to find shoes. While they're actually considered a sign of intelligence, the bad news is that if you have a long second toe, you're more susceptible to pain under the bone due to high heels or running shoes.

YOU Tool: Foot Play Foreplay

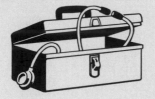 Ask anyone to define foreplay, and you'll likely get different answers from men and women. Women may say foreplay includes things like kind words, romantic gestures, and an offer to wash the dishes. Men? Use your imagination. A wonderful foreplay strategy that shouldn't be used solely as a preamble to sex and that has health benefits way beyond being a sexual stimulus is a foot rub.

A good foot rub works for body and mind because:

- It elevates levels of oxytocin, which are the hormones that make you feel warm and fuzzy (it's the same hormone that a mother's brain secretes when she's breast-feeding).
- It causes arousal, as the foot contains its own set of sexual nerves.
- It stimulates lymphatic drainage. Massage helps drain waste material out of your system.

How to do it:

1. Clean up. To make your partner comfortable, clean his or her feet with a warm washcloth or in a shallow basin of warm water.
2. Use the right lotion—one scented with lavender, which is perceived as an aphrodisiac by both men and women.
3. Do the whole foot. In reflexology (which shares some philosophical roots with acupuncture), the foot is seen as a metaphor for the body. The big toe is seen as the top of the head, and the sensitive area at the base of the toes represents the neck. The inner sole of the foot is the belly, while the outer sole is the spine. If an area is bothering your partner, spend some time there to get the good vibes flowing.*
4. Work your way up. We store a lot of tension in our ankles, so move the foot around passively to help relax the joint. Start with the heel and push up toward the leg; pull it down and work it side to side. On the bottoms of the feet, use firm pressure with your thumbs (too light and it'll be ticklish). Use slow, deep pressure, and work the whole foot and in between toes. Pull each toe for ten seconds. Rub the calves from ankle toward knee. Since the calves and feet are farthest from the heart and fighting gravity, it is challenging for them to move lymphatic

*While you're down there, look in between your partner's toes; that's where some of the deadliest melanomas appear.

waste along. You want to be moving in that direction anyway, and now you have an excuse. Even if your sexual advances have the opposite effect, you can be proud: Professional massage therapists consider sleep or drooling a sign of a job well done.

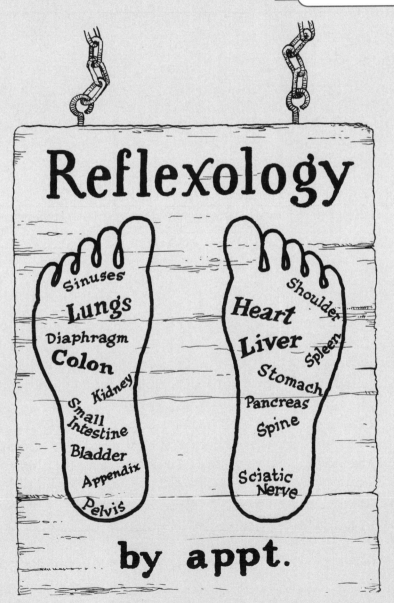

Reflexology

Sinuses
Lungs
Diaphragm
Colon
Kidney
Small Intestine
Bladder
Appendix
Pelvis

Shoulder
Heart
Liver
Spleen
Stomach
Pancreas
Spine
Sciatic Nerve

by appt.

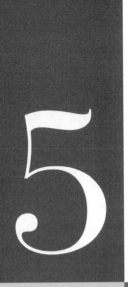

Great Shape

How to Get the Body You've Always Wanted

YOU Test: Waist-to-Hip Ratio

Take a tape measure and measure your waist (at the point of your belly button, while sucking in—you will anyway). Now measure your hips at the largest point around the buttocks. Do this calculation: waist size divided by hip size.

Results: Women: Ideal waist-to-hip ratio is around 0.7, while the ideal for men is around 1.0 (the same size waist and hips).

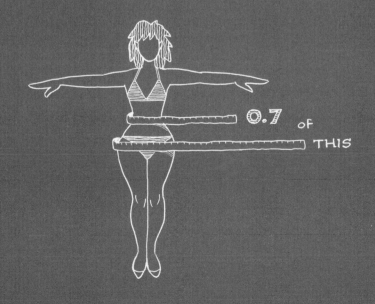

Before you wad up a ball of phlegm and hurl it at these pages, hear us out. We know there are all kinds of "ideal" bodies. We know that our differences in anatomical tastes are part of the beauty of being human. Some like round, some like flat, some like perky, some like steely. You like what you like (on yourself and on others), and whatever makes you happy, well, makes us pretty dang happy, too (as long as your tastes don't include living at an unhealthy waist size and weight). But let's also not be naive enough to think that there aren't some objective standards of beauty—not standards dictated by magazines, celebrities, or the porn industry but standards set by science and evolution.

Prehistoric men and women had to make decisions about how and with whom they were going to mate. They didn't get those messages from the media. There were no ads on rock faces, no fashion shoots with buffalo hides, and no reality shows (*Extreme Makeover: The Neanderthals!*). They had to make the ultimate reproductive decision based on a novel concept: each other.

So what did they do? They made judgments about partners based largely on appearance, because you could improve your reproductive success, the theory goes, if you chose someone deemed to be of high quality. A woman would choose a man with lots of resources and loads of strength to protect a potential family. Women didn't make that decision based on the amount of tree trunks a man could bench-press but on his outward appearance: Muscles signaled strength. Strength signaled he was a veritable reproductive hottie. And that signaled he was a prime candidate to do the boop-dee-boop.*

When it comes to the reproductive value of a woman, well, that was a little harder for a man to judge, because there was no direct outward signal of ovulation and fertility, so man had to use indirect clues such as physical attractiveness to judge the reproductive value of a woman. His main criterion: distribution of body fat. In other words, the waist-to-hip ratio. In still other words, body shape.

* Odds are, early man did not actually use the phrase *boop-dee-boop* or any derivatives thereof.

Every Side Is Her Best Side

An additional evolutionary advantage of why women are shaped like pears: The shape remains constant whether viewed from front, behind, or side. As a matter of fact, the degree of femininity can be easily and accurately assessed by viewing the back of a woman. Some researchers have argued that the front view is more important (under the assumption that breast size signals reproductive value, though it's also been shown that breasts do not always accurately reflect the reproductive capability of a woman). So this might magnify the sexual attractiveness of a woman who has shapely breasts and broad hips set against a narrow waist (the hourglass). In the same vein, the bodily feature that is most altered by pregnancy in a woman is, of course, the waist. So a high waist-to-hip ratio may mimic pregnancy—and thereby make the woman less sexually attractive when she's off limits for men looking to fertilize.

Now, before we get started in our discussion about diet and body shape, we should make a few things perfectly clear. There are vital reasons that some bodies need to be changed—because the people who live in them are at risk of loads of health problems if they don't get in better shape (that's the subject of *YOU: On a Diet*). That said, we also know that the medical definitions of what constitutes being healthy don't necessarily constitute those of being beautiful. Ultimately, we want you to be in better shape for you. For your health, for your mind, for you to feel beautiful. If good things are happening on the outside, then chances are they're happening on the inside, too.

It's also worth mentioning that part of the reason so many of us are obsessed with our weight is because of an emotional phenomenon called body dysmorphic disorder—that is, you're never satisfied with the way your body looks, you're convinced that you're ugly, and you have an unrealistic perception of what your body truly looks like. This disorder may manifest itself in all kinds of ways—obsessing over the mirror, getting addicted to plastic surgery, even exercising hours on end in pursuit of the perfect body. (This disorder is actually a form of obsessive-compulsive disorder.)

The real trick is to put into perspective what our bodies really look like, accept our imperfections, and acknowledge how much work we need to do. Do that, and you'll be better able to take actions to feel and act better as you try to make healthy changes to how your body looks and feels.

There's no question that a hot body is an instinctual sign of health (though true, bad health that docs measure doesn't usually show up unless you're obese). So what we're going to explore in this chapter isn't just for vain people or mirror hogs; body size and shape are important for all of us—in terms of both our looks and our health.

Your Body: What Shape Are You In?

To start, let's discuss how you got the shape you developed as an adult (we're all basically the same shape as kids). It all comes down to sex hormones, which regulate how you use and store fat. The big gender difference comes in the form of the classic apple and pear shapes (called gynoid and android). Testosterone stimulates fat deposits in the belly and inhibits it in the thighs, which is why men are typically apples, and estrogen inhibits fat in the belly and stores it on the ole thighs, which is why women are typically pears. There's also an evolutionary reason for this: Fat deposits on the thighs are almost exclusively used during late pregnancy and when a woman is nursing. In eras when men and women all needed fat storage during times of famine, 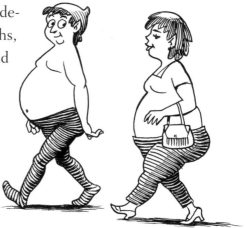 the fat deposits on thighs (as opposed to the belly deposits on men) helped women provide calories not just for themselves but for their offspring as well.

While produce makes a nice metaphor for describing the general shapes of bodies, we also know that there are more subtleties when it comes to how we look. And that's where waist-to-hip ratio comes in. (Remember our test: Waist-to-hip ratio measures the waist at the narrowest portion between the ribs and the iliac crest, measured at the belly button with you sucking in, and the hips at the point of the greatest protrusion of the buttocks.) Men are generally close to 1:1

(same size waist and hips). The ideal figure that science has determined for women is 0.7 (in our terms that's at most a 32.5-inch waist if 46-inch hips).

So you may be asking what the big deal is over a few decimal points. On the surface, there isn't one. Or is there? Studies actually show that waist-to-hip ratio is a very reliable signal of reproductive age, reproductive potential, and potential for disease. The closer your body is to the ideal measurements, the closer it is to ideal for childbearing.

Your Shape: How to Change It

Snowflakes and meat loaves aren't the only things that come in different shapes and sizes. Bodies, of course, do, too. There are the apple, the pear, the hourglass, the telephone pole, the Mack truck, the beanbag chair, you name it. Of course, genetics do play a role in some of our shapes and sizes, but you have the ability to tweak, push, and shove your body's chemistry to eventually change your shape and size. While there's also help that comes in the form of scalpels and fat vacuums (we'll get to that later), you can also make changes the old-fashioned way—with a little bit of chemistry, a little bit of know-how, and a little bit of gumption to get your marshmallowy middle off the couch. So let's take a look at the places where you can have the most effect (see Figure 5.1).

FACTOID
The waist and buttocks are uniquely human features. None of the great apes (orangutan, chimpanzee, and gorilla) has a waist or full buttocks. (Think of that next time you're visiting a zoo.)

Your Brain

SATIETY CENTERS. Think about what motivates us to work, to love, to parent, and to do all the things we need to do from day to day. One of the driving forces for all of our action? Satisfaction. We're constantly in search of experiences and people who leave us feeling fulfilled and, essentially, satisfied. That's not because we're selfish people. It's because satiety is a basic biological drive that originates

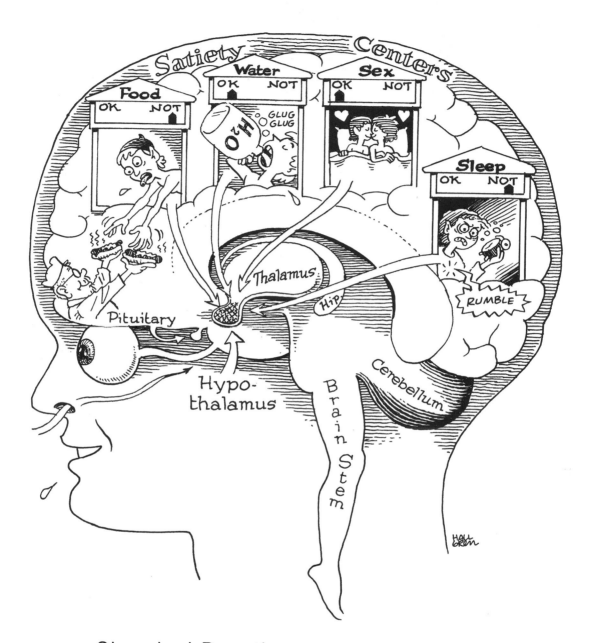

Figure 5.1 Chemical Reaction The reason for overeating may be caused not as much[...] example, reacts because it longs for satisfaction in the areas of hunger, thirst, sleep, and sex. In you[...] flip the switch to make you want to eat more, others help turn off the switch.

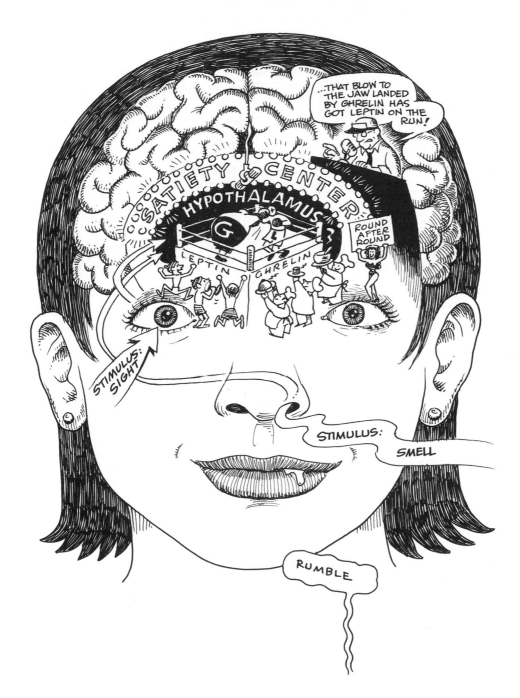

y your love of three-cheese pizza as it is by chemical systems in your brain. The satiety center, for

rain, two chemicals, leptin and ghrelin, duke it out for control over your appetite: While some foods

The Breast Evidence

There's no disputing that a large chunk of society spends a lot of time thinking about (and a lot of attention focusing on) breasts. Hef and Victoria's Secret have made millions off them. Some people have been sued because of them. Others have been mesmerized by them. While there's no scientific evidence showing that size and shape have any correlation with reproductive success, researchers have uncovered interesting info about how breasts are perceived. Turns out that medium-size breasts evoke the most favorable ratings (from both male and female reviewers). And the viewers even went so far as to make psychological assessments about women based on their breast size. Smaller-breasted women were rated as competent, ambitious, intelligent, moral, and modest. Big-boobed women? The exact opposite. What's also interesting is that breast size complements waist-to-hip ratio; it's the total package that influences whether a woman is judged as attractive, feminine, and healthy. Large breasts consistently enhanced the attractiveness ratings of both slender and heavy figures, as long as they had a low waist-to-hip ratio. If a woman had a high waist-to-hip ratio, large breasts appeared to decrease the attractiveness ratings. The one instance where large breasts raised the attractiveness ratings of a high waist-to-hip ratio figure was when she was heavy. This may have occurred because large breasts can make a woman look as if she has a lower waist-to-hip ratio than she actually does. The cause: a perceived shift in her proportions, created by the large bustline.

in the brain. While there are infinite ways to feel satisfied, the four main drives that exist in the brain's satiety center are these: food, water, sex, and sleep. Our brains (and bodies) need those elements to prevent our body chemistry from spinning out of control like a hydroplaning vehicle.

Now, the interesting thing about these drives is that they all rely on one another a bit. When one drive isn't being satisfied, your body makes up for it by relying on others. If you're not getting enough sleep, for example, you compensate for that lack of fulfillment with an out-of-control sausage binge. In fact, that's one of the main reasons why people overeat: They're not getting enough sleep, they're not getting enough sex, and they're not drinking enough water. To compensate, they end up getting way more cream cheese than they can burn off. Though it may seem a little tabloid-esque to say that more romps in the bedroom can help you lose weight, there's some truth to it.* Make sure you get enough water, sleep,

* You're welcome, fellas.

and sex, and you'll not only enjoy the benefits from them individually, but the trickle-down effect is that you will reduce the chances that your satiety center will go schizo.

CANNABINOIDS. If you ever wondered why your college roommates used to get the munchies after they smoked a little of the cheech, look no further than another system of hormones called cannabinoids. These little suckers hinder the ability of insulin to push sugar into your cells. (The receptors are influenced by marijuana, or the cannabis plant, which is why they're called cannabinoids.) So? Well, if your body doesn't sense that it's been fed (via glucose), your brain gets the signal that you're still hungry. People who have a haywire cannabinoid system never get that signal, so they eat and eat, and gain and gain. The most frustrating thing about these receptors is that you could be a person who does everything right (eating, exercising) and still not budge when it comes to the scale or the tape measure. The cannabinoid system has that much influence on your body. Up to 20 percent of obese people probably have a major problem with the cannabinoid system and could one day benefit from drugs. Cannabinoid-receptor-blocking drugs are in development, and we may very well see antiobesity drugs that work via this system. But eliminating omental fat (that's the fat around your waist between your organs, especially hanging off your stomach) through the choices you make reduces the production and amount of cannabinoids that wreak hormonal havoc, so even without drugs, you can help yourself.

FACTOID

People who sleep more lose more weight. Not only does less sleep mean that you have more hours to gobble down Goobers, it also means that you have more hormone stimulants for food. Get more downtime (as long as it's not over nine hours a night) and you'll be better able to downsize.

GHRELIN AND LEPTIN. Think of any classic mano a mano matchup: Ali vs. Frazier. Dog vs. cat. Trump vs. Rosie. In any classic battle pitting one opponent against another, there's a simple equation: One wins, one loses. And the way they fight—via strength or smarts—largely dictates who's victorious. That's essentially

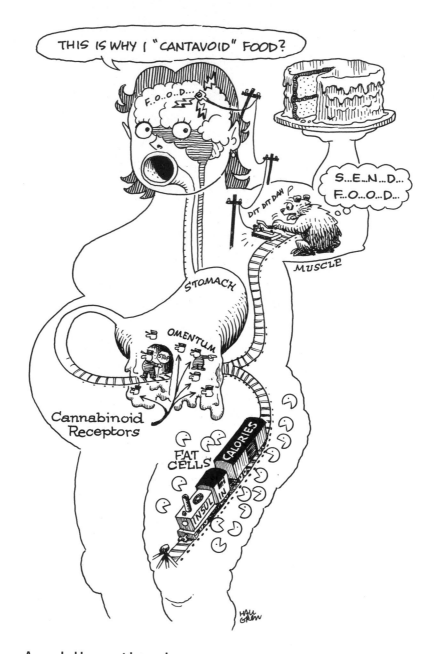

Figure 5.2 Avoiding the Issue We call the cannabinoid system the "can't avoid" system because when it's activated, the fact is, it's awfully hard to avoid the foods you should.

what you need to know about two hormones that are pitted against each other in the supreme battle of hunger versus satisfaction. When the level of leptin is high in your body, that's when you feel satisfied, with little desire to eat. When the level of ghrelin (think gremlin) is high, that's when your body sends emergency signals to the pantry: Hungry. Send food. Now. You don't need to be an endocrinologist to realize that this hormonal battle largely dictates how much, how often, and how smart you eat. Of course, the trick in all this is that there's no little nodule on your body that regulates these hormone levels; you have to do all the regulation internally—primarily through your food choices, by focusing on foods that make leptin levels surge and ghrelin levels plummet.

In this grudge match, leptin works over the long term, so if you

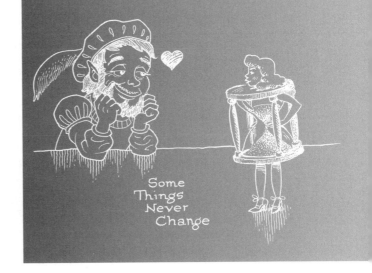

Some Things Never Change

can increase leptin levels, you'll be able to maintain that satisfaction over time (walking and other exercise are good ways to increase leptin). Ghrelin works in the short term, shooting up when your body feels hungry and shooting down when the stomach is full or 70 calories of healthy fat (such as six walnuts) hit your intestinal wall (the intestine comes right after the stomach as one goes from mouth down) or sugar hits your brain, except when your body consumes fructose

Hidden Causes of Weight Gain

You may feel as if you're doing everything right—restricting your calories, exercising your body—yet you keep gaining weight. The issue may be hormonal. Some possibilities:

- Abnormal thyroid levels are one big cause. Hypothyroidism slows down your metabolism so that you can't burn calories the way you used to (more on this in chapter 6, as it relates to your energy levels).
- PCOS, or polycystic ovarian disease, which accounts for a huge amount of unexplained weight gain in 20 percent of women. This is a form of insulin resistance, which wreaks hormonal havoc, which leads to the additional poundage.
- Testosterone levels can fall in older men and postmenopausal women, especially if they have belly fat, which converts testosterone to estrogen. That results in less muscle mass, and with less muscle mass, it's much harder to burn fat (thus leading to weight gain). The cure: resistance exercises. The sign that your testosterone levels are dropping: if you have to shave (your face or legs) less often than you used to.
- Growth hormone levels can decrease as you age, leading to weight gain. The best ways to get it naturally: getting proper sleep (see more in chapter 6) and exercise (see our band workout on page 351).

But some medications can help control these problems, as well as the accompanying fat. So if you can't figure out what you're doing that's contributing to weight gain, it's worth talking to your doc about.

(found in some simple sugars, especially the sweetener high-fructose corn syrup). These two hormones interact through a complex series of events that occur in your brain, but if you can make leptin knock ghrelin on its rear, then it's your body shape that will have the look that the other gender will perceive as healthy enough to be a parent of her or his children. (For a more detailed explanation of ghrelin, leptin, and related chemicals, see *YOU: On a Diet*.)

Your Muscles

Muscle cars, muscle shirts, and muscle heads—they all connote the same image. Big, strong, powerful. And for good reason: Muscle is what provides your body's power (see Figure 5.3). It gives you the ability to lift, to run, and to make eyes pop. But the immediate connection many people make between "muscle" and "meathead" is the wrong one. Muscle actually gives you the ability to change your

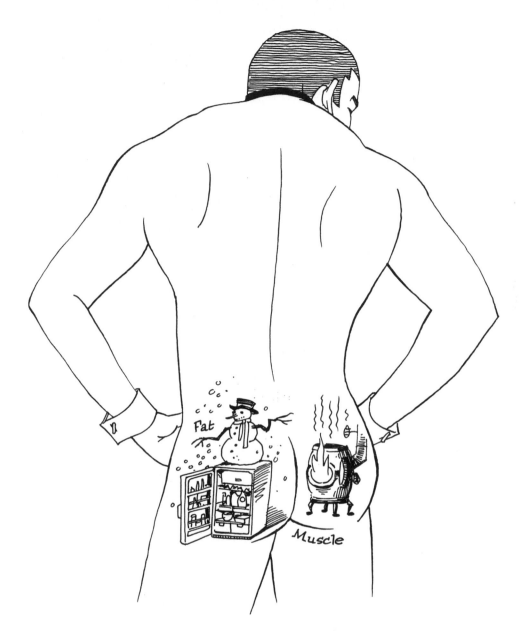

Figure 5.3 Muscle Up Muscles may help you shot-put pianos, but they also serve a more important role: Besides giving you strength, they help burn fat. Adding some lean muscle mass to your body will help your body burn more calories, especially compared to fat, which contributes to your storing more fat because it takes very little energy to maintain.

Drugs That Make You Fat

You already know that alfredo sauce and buttered biscuits can plump you up. So can the drugs you take. In a small percentage of people, medications can work against you by increasing your appetite or making you drowsy so you burn fewer calories during the day. Some of the most common offenders include certain antidepressants, antipsychotics, antihistamines, migraine meds, steroids, some blood pressure meds, and insulin. You should check your weight constantly when you start a new drug and let a five-pound gain be an alarm that something's going wrong, so you can talk to your doc about other options.

body in a couple of different ways. Of course, on the outside, a lean and toned look can imply a message of health and strength more than a lumpy, fluffy, or fatty body. Even more important, we all need muscle for the metabolic machine that it is. Simply, muscle helps your body burn calories. That's because your body burns 50 to 100 calories per pound of muscle every day, compared to less than a handful of calories per pound of fat. So the result is that you burn fat by adding muscle.

We know what many of you are saying: That sounds all well and good, but the fact is that I really have no desire to look like an Eastern European shot-putter, thank you very much. Understandable concern (though we have nothing against Eastern European track and field athletes), but somewhat of a mistaken one. Adding muscle—by doing strength training—doesn't mean that you're going to develop arms the size of Hummers or legs the size of redwoods. Why? Muscle requires something else to feed it to really bulk up. That substance? Androgens, relatives of testosterone, which cause muscle fibers to grow. That's why men get bulky when they build muscle, while women can lift weights, build muscle, and remain Jaguar-like sleek. So if what you're trying to do is just tone, shape, and tighten, you can still lift weights and do resistance training (see the ideas below and our complete workout on page 351).

FACTOID

We don't have an issue with cellulite, but if you do, it seems that some massage therapies can help change the appearance *temporarily* (and we mean temporarily, hurry up and snap that picture), but no creams, gels, or other easy solutions have been shown even to assist. More invasive procedures (such as body lifts) can help, but you have to ask yourself whether the treatment is really worth the cure.

YOU Tips!

You've got quite a few options when it comes to getting the body you've always wanted. To make real changes, you need to change the food you eat and the way you exercise. (Of course, there are also surgical options, some of which we'll discuss in detail in the appendix.) But even if you know what to do, you also have to know how to do it. That's where these tips and tricks come in: They'll give you the firepower necessary to change from belt-popping to jaw-dropping.

BUST YOUR BODY. You can't spot-reduce body parts when it comes to frying fat (your body decides where it comes off first). Forget those ads for "electrostimulation" that promise to reduce two inches of fat in an hour. But that doesn't mean you can't target the muscles in your hot spots. How? You do it by incorporating some resistance training into your workout. Men can change their chests from a feminine to a masculine appearance by just pumping their pecs for five minutes a day. (And ripped abs look good on everyone.) Building muscle will help you burn fat because it takes more energy to maintain muscle than it does fat, and it will also help give you that toned (not bulky) appearance. You can see a complete workout on page 351.

The best way to tone your muscle: Do each exercise with a higher number of repetitions (say, 15 to 20) and using a lighter amount of weight than you'd be able to lift for 8 or 10 repetitions. In addition, you can help create that long look by lengthening your muscles through stretching and yoga, which is one of the reasons we've included a complete yoga workout as well, which begins on page 361. Make sure that you train to exhaustion so that you really struggle with the last few repetitions. Achieve this goal either by using higher weights or by lifting them more slowly so that your muscles are really taxed by the exercises and get the message to build themselves up in preparation for the next battle.

If you already have a routine you like, here are some fun exercises that can target your particular problem areas.

BUTT/THIGHS

Clock Lunge: Stand with your feet shoulder width apart with your hands on your hips (or holding light weights). Looking straight ahead, lunge straight out in front of you (the 12 o'clock position) with your right foot so your thigh comes parallel to the ground but your knee does not extend past your

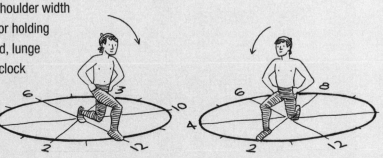

toes. Your left knee should nearly touch the ground. Next, lunge to 2 o'clock, then backward to 4 o'clock and 6 o'clock. Continue the lunge pattern, starting with your left leg to 6 o'clock, then around to 8, 10, and finish with 12 o'clock.

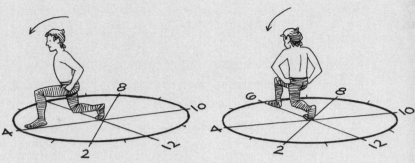

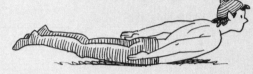

Locust (from yoga): Lie on your stomach on the floor. Raise your straight legs behind you as high as you can without putting excessive strain on your back. You can do both legs or one leg at a time. Lift your arms and leave them behind you. Hold the position and repeat.

Squeeze Squats: Hold a medicine ball (or beach ball or basketball) between your lower thighs. With your hands on your hips or out in front of you, squat down, keeping the ball in place and not allowing your thighs to go farther down than parallel to the floor. Come back up. This works your legs and butt and is great for developing balance.

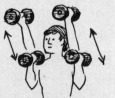

ARMS/SHOULDERS

The Shoulder Matrix: Hold a dumbbell in each hand (or other household objects such as jugs of water), at your shoulders. Press them straight up over your head. Bring them back down to your shoulders. On your next repetition, press them up and slightly to the left. Next time press to the right, then forward, then slightly backward. Repeat through all the moves.

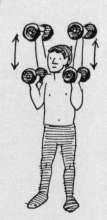

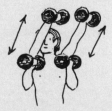

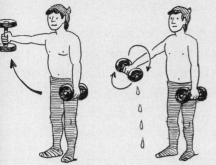

Empty Can: Hold dumbbells down and by your sides. Keeping your arm straight, raise one arm forward (thumb stays up toward the ceiling) until your arm is parallel to the ground. As you lower your arm, rotate your wrist as if you're emptying a can. Repeat with the other arm and alternate repetitions. This emphasizes different parts of the shoulders.

ABS/CORE

Dead Bug (from Pilates): Lie on your back with all fours straight up. Lower your left leg and right arm at the same time, and then bring them back up. Then repeat with the opposite arm and leg.

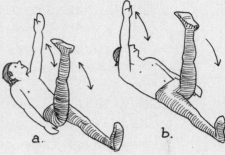

Punching Bag Crunches: Do a traditional crunch, with your knees bent and feet on the floor. When you crunch up, have someone lightly punch your abs (while wearing a boxing glove, preferably). That forces your abdominals to stay tight and contracted throughout the movement. The abs-alicious Janet Jackson has been reported to do these.

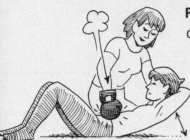

Turkish Getup (advanced): Lie flat on your back with one arm straight up, perpendicular to the floor (you can be holding a weight). Keeping your arm above your head the whole time, stand up, using your legs and free hand. Then get back into the down position (all while keeping the arm up). Repeat with the other arm up. It works the entire core—and is a true fat burner.

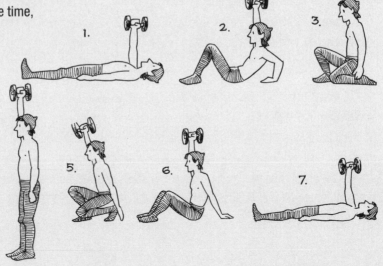

ADD INTENSITY. When it comes to cardiovascular exercise and stamina training, you may know our stance: Walk 30 minutes a day, and then (if you have risk factors for heart disease, ask your doctor) find a way to break a sweat (cycling, swimming, running up stairs, etc.) a few days a week to improve your cardiovascular health. But if you really want to kick up the fat burners to DEFCON 1, you'll want to add some more intense cardiovascular training. How? Through interval training. That is, pick a cardiovascular exercise and, after warming up, alternate periods of high-intensity work with lower-intensity work. Here's how: In the next to last minute of a ten-minute phase of exercise, push yourself as hard as possible for a minute, then slow back down to the usual rigorous rate. That kind of workout has been shown to burn more calories after exercise than workouts in which you train at the same level of intensity during the entire period.

FIGHT FAT WITH FOOD. In movies, it may not always be easy to tell the good guys from the bad, but in refrigerators, it can be—as long as you know what you're looking for. These nutritional cops and robbers will help you achieve your ideal body shape, as long as you know who's on your side and who's out to hijack your thighs.

The good guys. Eat foods with fiber, healthy fats (monounsaturated omega-3 with DHA and some polyunsaturated fats, such as olive oil), 100 percent whole-grain carbohydrates, fish and nut protein, fruits, and vegetables. It's also smart to eat a little healthy fat (such as a handful of nuts) 30 minutes before meals to allow the satiety signal to go from your stomach to your brain so you avoid overeating. Drink buckets of water to do the same (we're kidding about the buckets here and really don't want you to get what we call water intoxication, but you get the point). No matter what diet you choose, water helps you lose weight.

The criminals. Avoid five aging foods: trans fats, saturated fats (aim for 0 and never more than 4 grams per serving), simple sugars (they end in -ose and include syrups, such as high-fructose corn syrup, rice syrup, molasses, or cane sugar), and any starch or grain with less than 100 percent whole grains.

GET CALCIFIED. You already know that calcium is good for your bones, but more and more research is showing that there's a link between calcium and weight loss. It seems that 1,000 milligrams a day of calcium help both reduce fat intake and increase fat metabolism—a double whammy in the world of weight loss. You can get the calcium (which is absorbed better through the liquid form of milk, called the whey, than the solid part, the curd) through the usual suspects such as low-fat dairy products or supplements. But don't rule out the stealth sources either, such as spinach, sardines, beans, sesame seeds, and oranges.

FILL ON UP. Here's a medical fact: The hungrier you are, the more likely it is that you're going to go on a feeding frenzy and gnaw on any candy, chips, and hunks of fat-laden pork products in sight.* And the more you gorge, the more likely it is that your body shape is going to change—for the bigger. That's why one of your jobs as a healthy eater is to eat the foods that fill you nutritionally without causing those roller-coaster spikes of blood sugar and other chemicals that lead you to feed uncontrollably. In an index that ranks the satisfaction levels of various foods, vegetables score pretty darn high. You'll want to include plenty of fiber (35 grams a day for men and 25 grams for women), as well as lots of protein. Protein-rich foods are the most filling foods because protein induces the hypothalamus to let you know that you're satisfied. Besides fish, another good source of protein is nuts. Nuts reduce appetite, and only 85 percent of their fat is absorbed, so enjoy a few ounces daily. Another alternative: soup (broth-based, not cream-based). Soup has been shown to take longer to traverse your GI tract (and thus makes you feel fuller) than when food and water are consumed separately.

TRICK YOURSELF. Truth is, we don't listen to our stomachs when it comes to eating. We listen to our eyes. Ideally, if you eat right, you'll be able to stop eating if you eat slowly, have that little bit of healthy fat before a meal, and listen for the stomach signal that says you've had enough. The way most of us eat: Down it until it's done. It's why we have to pay attention to portion size when we're eating. We can do it by using smaller dishes or by doling out servings onto a plate rather than eating right from a bag. (Researchers found that people ate more soup when they were served a bottomless bowl—that is, a self-filling bowl that filled slowly as people ate from it—as opposed to when they finished the bowl they were served.) Another good way to let your eyes help your body: Leave a candy wrapper on the kitchen counter. It's a visual cue that you've indulged in a little postdinner chocolate— and reminds you that you don't need to do it again when *Grey's Anatomy* begins.

GET FITTED. While the two main prongs of the body-shape fork are exercise and eating, you also can't ignore a third prong: your clothes. As you well know, clothes can't change your body shape per se (*pants that burn fat!*), but they can certainly change the way your shape appears to the rest of the world and how you feel about your body. Women, this advice is for you. More on other guidelines for clothes in our toolbox on page 149.

    Bras. It's estimated that 80 percent of women don't pick the right bras. How so? Some pick a cup size too small (perhaps to give more lift). Some pick a band that's too tight or too loose.† The

---

*It's not worded quite that way in the scientific journals.
†Some smaller studies suggest that tight-fitting clothing (including bras) affects the nervous system and hormones such as melatonin. It's probably nothing to be too alarmed about, but it should be a bit of encouragement to find the best fit.

effect: Besides being a source of pain, a poorly fitted bra can change the shape of your breasts over time. And unsupported breasts actually sag faster. Since much of the droop comes at night while you sleep braless, you might even consider wearing a bra to bed. For the best-fitted bra: Get a professional fitter to take your measurements (measure from under the breasts for the number and around nipples for the cup size). You can get a good idea for yourself with these guidelines: If the straps fall down, the band size is too large, and if the breast does not fit within the cup, it's too small.

Jeans. We've got the same problem on the lower half as we do on the upper—with about 90 percent of us wearing the wrong jeans for our body type. Wrong jeans and bad fit equal an unattractive look. You should expect to try on at least a dozen pair of jeans (and even alter the ones you choose). What you're trying to avoid: jeans that appear cellophane-tight or jeans that have too much room, which makes it appear that you have more body squeezed in there than you actually do (look for bumps or creases in the crotch area at the rise to the waist). Get boot-cut if you're tall and straight-leg if you're short; a dark wash can make you look thinner, whereas a stone wash can put a spotlight onto your thighs.

YOU Tool: Fashion Statements

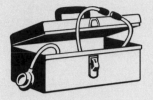

A lot of times, we assume that the mind's eye works like a copy machine or a camera: We see something in the world, process it, and form an exact representation of what that object is. The reality is that your mind is hardly as mechanical as a copy machine or as exact as a camera. Your mind extrapolates, interprets, and perceives. So one very concrete thing can look two different ways to two different people when it's processed—it's the ol' optical illusion at work. Just take a look at the illustration of tables. They're the exact same drawings, but your mind perceives them in totally different ways. And sometimes we can't see subtle changes between two similar things, as in the image of Margaret Thatcher on the next page. Notice how similar it is (though it's different—just turn it upside down). That can be attributed to something called a saccade—a fast movement of the eye that lasts between 20 and 200 milliseconds. These movements refresh an image—meaning that we take chunks of that image and process it, rather than reprocessing the whole thing. The phenomenon helps explain why our vision is synthetic—and unlike a camera's.

Tables

all the same.

Why all the hubbub about perceptions and interpretation? Because that's a fundamental principle of fashion—something that can play a role in how our body shape is perceived: Every component of what we see in the world—namely, shape, depth, color—is an interpretation of what is actually there. When it comes to our skin-covering methods of beauty, it helps to know a few guiding principles (ladies, please pass this along to your men, because they're the ones who *really* need it).

Beauty BOOSTERS	Beauty BUSTERS
Clothes with vertical lines to make you look taller and slimmer	Stiff, bulky fabrics, which will give you a boxy look
Dressing in one color, which gives the impression of one long, vertical line (why the little black dress is so effective)	Shiny fabrics, which will make you look bigger when light reflects off you
Dark neutrals, which have the ability to absorb light and recede into the background	Wearing dark on top and light on bottom; switch them
These fabrics: crepe, silk, cashmere, knits, jersey, rayon, gabardine, Lycra, synthetics	Pleated pants, which emphasize your belly
Clothes with SPF protection	Tan-through shirts, which have a loose weave that exposes your skin to more UV light

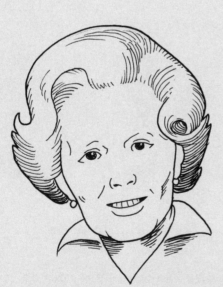 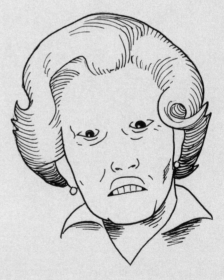

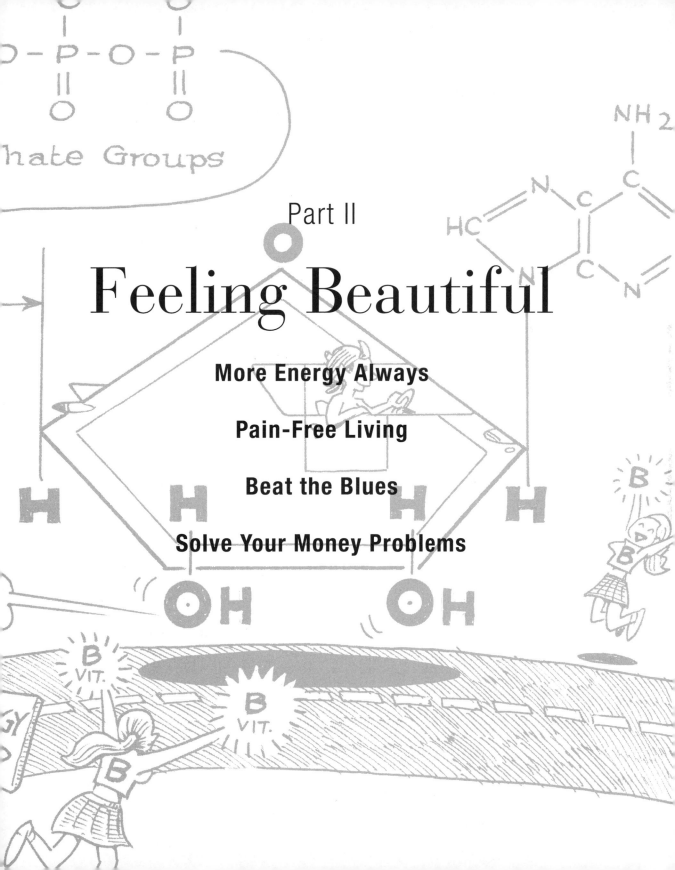

Part II

Feeling Beautiful

More Energy Always

Pain-Free Living

Beat the Blues

Solve Your Money Problems

If we decide to stop by your house at random (we've been known to do that, you know) and ask you how you're feeling, it's likely that you'd answer in one of three ways: fine, great, like dog dirt. The funny thing is that while most of us limit ourselves to these three nondescript categories, the possible answers to the question how you're really feeling are about as nuanced as it gets. The way you feel when you're in pain is a lot different from the way you feel when you're stressed, which is a lot different from the way you feel when you've had three hours of sleep, which is a lot different from the way you feel when you've just lost a loved one, a bundle of cash, or the use of your back.

So as you enter this section about feeling beautiful, you'll see that we'll cover quite the gamut of topics. Specifically, we'll dive into the big things that really affect how you feel at your core—things like your aches, your emotions, your stressors, and your energy levels.

The goal of feeling beautiful really centers around how well you harness energy and manage pain. In some cases, we're talking about physical pain—the pain that keeps you in bed or sends you to the sidelines in the game of life. In other cases, we're talking about managing intangible pains, such as depression, grief, frustration, financial despair, or hopelessness.

How we feel—and how we cope with the pains that affect how we feel—really just comes down to biology (see Figure B.1). Any information our brain receives stops at the emotional part of our brain (the amygdala) before it reaches the logical, decision-making side (the neocortex). As well it should—we ought to run from the tiger *first* and think about why we're doing so *second*. Because the amygdala receives a limited amount of information, it has to do a quick-and-dirty scan for danger—therefore triggering an emotional-cognitive response.

Take this example: Let's say you walk out in your garden and out of the corner of your eye, you see a long, coiled black thingy. *A snake!* You jump, move away, and make sure it doesn't strike. Upon closer inspection, you realize that the anaconda slithering through your mulch was actually your ratty ol' garden hose. While it may seem that the end result is that you look and feel like a dolt, the reality is

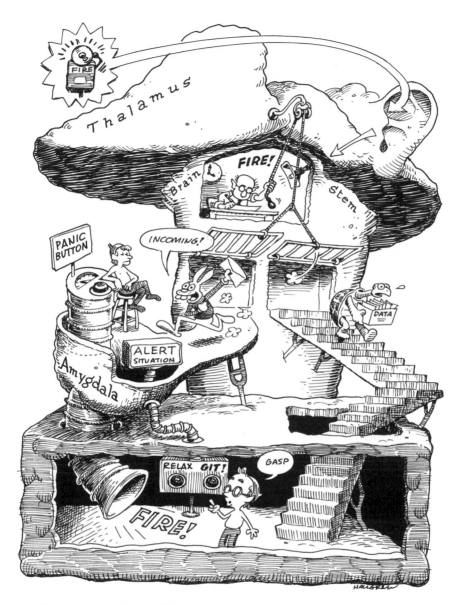

Figure B.1 **Sound the Alarm** The reason we react emotionally to beauty is because of a process in the brain that starts with the thalamus relay station: When we get news of something happening (such as a real smoke alarm), the messages first get sent to our emotional center (the amygdala), rather than our logical side (cortex). Those emotional responses are good in some situations (the smoke alarm) but may not be so much so in others (such as when you make hasty financial decisions).

that your jumpiness makes a vital point about beauty: We are hardwired to respond emotionally to situations. Rather than go over, touch it, and see if that sucker had fangs instead of a nozzle, you reacted with emotions, not logic. There's an evolutionary reason for this: It doesn't hurt you if you overrespond by jumping from a hose ten times; it does hurt you big time if you don't jump from the poisonous snake even once.

That's the biological reason why your emotions influence how you make decisions. The net result of all this is to unleash a neurological cocktail of chemicals that make the emotions of fear, aggression, and desire so passionate, so robust, and so thoughtless that they often create addictive behaviors, such as dependence on cigarettes or drugs or alcohol (all three are actually drugs and dysfunctional coping mechanisms). Or they manifest themselves in trends like gambling or depression and anxiety. And all of these problems and accompanying emotions have a huge impact on how we feel and live.

Just as we have an automatic reaction to appearance, we have the same kind of response to pain: You're hardwired to feel pain instinctively so you can quickly move your hands from a burning coffee cup without having to think through the process. It's the ultimate biological smoke alarm—the signal to get us away from trouble that can move quickly from an acute problem to a problem that pulls the plug on life. This pain response comes in many forms, both physical and emotional.

Both responses have a very direct relationship with beauty. When you're feeling sluggish (from no energy) or run-down (from overwork) or in pain (from sore muscles or back) or just plain ol' blue (from feeling depressed), it's harder for you to look, feel, or be beautiful. That's because how you feel influences every other aspect of your life.

Our goal in this section is to address (and sometimes attack) those things that may be the source of your physical and emotional pains. Because it's hard to feel beautiful when your body, brain, pocketbook, or heart is aching, we'll give you the biology behind some of life's biggest physical and emotional stressors and then strategies for defusing them. Once you identify and erase the nagging downers in your life, you'll be better able to enjoy the natural highs.

6

Energized and Revitalized

Power Up Your Body by Resetting Your System

YOU Test: Zapped

When's the first time you feel tired during the day?

a. When I awaken, even after sleeping a full eight hours every day for a week.

b. Morning, or at the latest midafternoon.

c. Whenever I move.

d. Whenever I have to deal with my boss.

e. Not until after a day of working 12 hours or more.

Results: If you answered anything other than E, it could be a sign that the energy systems in your body are either slightly or completely out of whack—causing you to tire even at times when you should feel vital and energized.

Ask anyone who's ever succeeded on a diet or similar change-your-life health plan about the benefits, and they typically say the same thing. Some may say that their clothes fit better. Some may say that their sex life got hotter. And some may even say that with every footstep the world's seismographs got quieter. But you know what almost all of them say when you ask them the biggest change they felt? More energy.

Yep. Stronger, zippier, peppier. Happier. With a "can do" attitude and enough confidence to conquer the world. Oftentimes, people in that scenario have a hard time explaining what *more energy* really means—except for the fact that they feel better getting up and going rather than lying down and snoring. But that key phrase—*more energy*—lies at the heart of what feeling beautiful is all about. You can be in the best relationship in the world and have celestial-quality facial features, but if you'd rather lie on the couch watching 12 hours of trashy reality shows than moving, living, loving, and passionately doing, then, well, your life may feel about as satisfying as a one-bean dinner. And isn't that what feeling beautiful is about—having passion for life and the energy to act out that passion?

So that's what we're going to talk about now—how to increase your energy so that you can not only manage life but bathe in it. We all have varying degrees of energy levels. Some people are perpetually peppy, some people are about as animated as an anchor, and many of us live life in the large gray area in between—as we battle bouts of fatigue, sluggishness, and the occasional aches and pains that slow us down. Our goal here is to make sense of all those gray areas and understand how we can manipulate, tweak, and nudge our biology to make ourselves feel better.

Let this chapter serve as your literary caffeine—drink up! And then see if any of the tips might benefit your situation.

Your Energy: In Crisis

We all know what happens when there's an energy crisis: There's chaos. Think back to the long lines at the gas stations in the 1970s. Or a citywide blackout. Or when just one Christmas light goes and the whole strand blows right along with it. One small problem, issue, or incident triggers a domino effect that has lasting effects. That's really what's happening when you can't maintain your energy levels, which may eventually lead to a major short-circuiting of your energy system. These kinds of massive energy drops are ultimately an energy crisis in your body, much like having a blown fuse in your body that needs to be reset. The most common causes of lack of energy are detected the old-fashioned way—and you can make the diagnosis with a little insight. Culprits include not enough sleep, too much food, too much saturated fat and sugary foods, too much stress, not enough fun and passion in life, or an infection or other chronic disease. Even seemingly mundane things such as sinusitis, gingivitis, and vaginitis can stimulate this.

Once your resilience is gone, you're more prone to being attacked by bacteria, viruses, or fungi. Even the ensuing insomnia and stress that come as a result of those attacks can wear down your adrenal glands, creating a vicious cycle where smaller and smaller problems cause progressively larger challenges until you experience a complete health shutdown. This chapter is meant to help you understand where your energy really comes from or doesn't.

To see how your energy levels dip, let's look at how energy works. The energy in your body is stored in packets called ATP as well as phosphocreatine, which are made up of a number of chemicals including a sugar called ribose, adenine (which used to be called vitamin B4), and derivatives of B vitamins. Ribose—which you'll learn more about in our tips—serves as the lumber of your energy-producing house, while other substances help support it (like hammer and nails). What is inside your cells (nutrients and genes) and other substances (hormones and chemicals from nerves and from your brain, etc.) act like fuses and switches to control the power factory you have. Your mitochondria and their component ribosomes take that ribose, sugar, and helper B vitamins and use electron trans-

Stocking Stuff

Sometimes, after a hard day, your legs may feel as though they have about as much zip as if you were a napping cat. They feel heavy, you feel tired, and the only thing you want your legs to do is hang out on the ottoman. One solution: socks or stockings that compress your feet, calves, and thighs. Besides giving you the benefit of decreasing the chance of developing varicose veins, these stockings—after a day of wear—will make your legs feel stronger and more well rested. How? They decrease the pooling of blood in your legs, letting your heart function better. Though the best stockings are custom-made, off-the-shelf ones work well, too; choose ones with pressures starting at 10 mmHg and work up to 40 mmHg. The higher the pressure, the better they work, but the more expensive they will be and the harder they are to put on. If you have no symptoms, choose 10 mm; if you have mild swelling in your feet and legs, choose at least 20 mm. You can wear compression stockings every day for about four months (that's when they usually wear out), washing them in cold water at night.

UNH

port to crank out ATP—your energy packets. Once you have enough ATP, your body can crank out activities. Now, if you blow the fuse that allows you to produce ATP—through infection, hormonal dysfunction, not getting enough sleep, having a diet that diverts energy rather than stimulates it, or many other causes—your body produces energy inefficiently, using all its energy to, well, produce and store energy.

But ATP is only part of the body's energy portfolio. Even if you have plenty of ATP, you also need abundant blood flow to provide your body nutrients and take away waste products—and that comes down to doing the things that help keep your arteries dilated and your blood pumping. What's good for your heart and arteries, in essence, is good for your energy levels, too. For example, nitric oxide—that short-lived gas lining your arteries and breathing tubes and in your brain that rapidly changes according to your diet and activity level—helps open up your arteries and lung passages to improve blood flow and increase the transfer of oxygen.

Problems with these systems really contribute to all energy deficiencies, yet the onset, cause, and treatments of lack of get-up-and-go are hard to nail down. You know when you feel slow and low, but it's hard to pinpoint what exactly is tripping you up—or if it's just a normal part of running through the rigors of life. While fatigue, lack of energy, and inability to sleep can explain other problems, the truth is that when put together, this constellation of symptoms makes it hard to navigate through our daily lives.

So what starts the process that steals your energy? What sets up the dominos, and what causes your first domino to fall? We don't know all the answers for sure, but we do know a few things that make your cellular energy plants—those mitochondria—inefficient. Three big ones:

FACTOID

In the next chapter, we'll discuss the pain of TMJ disorder, which can make your jaw feel like concrete. Research has shown that this condition can also be a cause of or caused by chronic fatigue, by causing chronic subconscious stress. Here's a self-test: Put a small finger in your ear and lightly push in while performing a chewing motion. If you hear or feel cracking, your jawbone is displaced and the resulting stress can contribute to such things as poor posture, dizziness, hunched shoulders, and chronic fatigue. Another trick to help disrupt the pain cycle: Put a cotton ball or soft-rolled paper between your upper and lower first molars (the teeth in the back) and walk with an upright posture—this helps correct the contracted, hunched shoulders that afflict some with pain issues and relieve some of the associated pain and long-term effects of TMD.

INSULIN RESISTANCE: We become inefficient in getting the sugar to our production plants and distribute it into fat storage rather than into cells that need to use it to produce energy, such as muscle cells.

VIRUSES AND OTHER INFECTIONS: Acute infections as well as chronic, low-grade infections can eventually cause the fuse to blow. We often see the buggers

YOU Test

What's Causing Your Sugar Cravings?

There are three main kinds of sugar cravings, and here's how to tell what's causing yours.

A: Feed me now or I'll kill you. If this is what your cravings are like, this usually reflects low blood sugar from an exhausted adrenal "stress handler" gland. Eating sugar helps in the first few minutes but makes things worse in the long term. Even sucking on a Tic Tac or two can be enough sugar to break the attack; then eat more protein and fewer sweets to keep your blood sugar stable—and treat the adrenal as we discuss (see page 167). If you want a sweet, eat a small amount of dark chocolate, as the flavonoids in dark chocolate improve energy and immunity. Multiple small meals through the day instead of three big ones also decrease cravings.

B: The happy Ho Ho hunter. You feel OK but often find yourself going through your cabinets looking for a Twinkie. Holistic docs say (without great evidence save some successful treatments) that this often reflects yeast overgrowth in the gut—a controversial area. Treating the presumed yeast overgrowth with probiotics can help improve your fatigue and pain, and may also eliminate your chronic sinusitis and spastic colon. We like to repopulate your gut with bacteriodes coagulans from spores. Try Digestive Advantage or Sustenex. By the way, new data also indicate these could increase serotonin levels (see next point).

C: I'm having my period and I'm depressed. Low levels of serotonin (the "happiness molecule") around your period can cause you to carb-crave. Eating dark chocolate will supply a natural antidepressant (called PEA) as well as the carbs you crave.

Good Vi-vi-vi-vi-brrrrrr-ations

A new technique called biomechanical stimulation is getting more and more attention for its effect of giving muscles more energy. How does it work? You stand on the machine or plate, as it's called (more advanced ones like Swiss Wing allow you to train your muscles more actively and you don't need to stand on them), and the machine vibrates to stimulate muscle energy and strength. Early research shows that the technique provides the benefits of flexibility, energy, and better coordination and balance. These machines are used in gyms, by professional sports teams, and by patients suffering from chronic fatigue or fibromyalgia.

invade and fray the wires from your fuse box, reducing the amount of energy that can be supplied. Or the lines get frayed from lack of nutrients to keep them repaired (for example, lack of the healthy fat DHA). That starts the "out of energy" cascade after a pregnancy or after an injury, when your immune system is vulnerable. Viral particles have been identified in the nuclei and mitochrondria of many cells of folks with serious energy deficits like fibromyalgia. Once one area feels less energetic, you put more demand on another area, furthering that cascade, so a little wire fraying by viruses can make you feel exhausted much of the time.

SLEEP PROBLEMS: Many people always have trouble falling asleep. Additionally, many of us (yes, we are guilty here at times) develop less than optimal habits that worsen our ability to sleep or obtain full sleep time and then we have to fight a vicious cycle. And when your immune system needs all the energy it can get—such as when it's fighting an infection for you—not resting your energy supply adequately acts to overheat those wires and worsen your energy problem. That weakens the energy your immune system can borrow from other parts of your energy stores. So you feel more tired. When your body gets too little sleep or poor-quality sleep (not deep enough or not enough dreaming), you tend to have more pain (the lack of sleep doesn't allow you to refresh fully the neurotransmitters you have that normally suppress pain). And that extra pain drains the line of energy, too—so you feel wiped out very near the start of the day. Sleep is important to feeling beautiful.

HORMONAL IMBALANCES: Your hormones are like the dimmers on your headlights—when you need bright lights, you turn on certain hormones to in-

The End Point of Low Energy

Chronic fatigue and fibromyalgia (which is chronic fatigue coupled with insomnia and total-body aches and pains) are somewhat misunderstood even by well-meaning docs. Because we cannot measure "energy levels," it's difficult to study these ailments well.

In fact, it used to be that docs would hear either of those two phrases and lots of things would come to mind: It's all in his head, she's a hypochondriac, it's just a politically correct way to be lazy. For years, the medical and lay communities didn't believe that these conditions really existed. But now there's not much debate about the fact that these are very real and very devastating illnesses that are marked by such symptoms as fatigue, insomnia, aches and pain, loss of libido, weight gain, and occasional brain fog.*

The tricky part in diagnosing the two is that the conditions are triggered by many causes, ranging from hormonal to infectious, but they all have the same effect: That one little problem starts a process that causes your entire system to short-circuit. Why? Because people with these conditions spend more energy on producing energy (as we explained on page 157), so they have no extra energy for life.

This lack of energy to do anything but process energy especially plays out in the hypothalamus gland in your brain—which balances the energy budget in your body. That little neurological doodad, which links your nervous system with your hormonal system, uses more energy for its size than any other place in your body. So when the systems that produce energy falter, you can feel exhausted, yet suffer from insomnia. In some cases, it also plays out in your muscles, which seem to get stuck (hence the aches and pains associated with the extreme form, fibromyalgia). How? As you can see in Figure 6.1, when muscles don't have energy, they get locked in a contracted position and you're unable to relax them, unable to supply them with fresh oxygen and blood or remove waste materials, and that's what causes the pain (think writer's cramp or rigor mortis). Once the muscles unlock, the pain flees faster than a graffiti artist in a cop's headlights. To top it off, that decrease in usable energy also means that you lose energy in your heart; like other muscles, it struggles, too. When you waste energy all over the place, your body falls behind and you can never really get going.

Not only do people without their usual energy feel sluggish and less beautiful, they fulfill that feeling by gaining weight. The average weight gain of patients diagnosed with fibromyalgia or chronic fatigue syndrome is 32.5 pounds. It is as though you need more energy and try to provide that with more calories, but the calories do not do any good.

Want to figure out if you have CSF or fibromyalgia and tailor a treatment protocol to your case? Do the free short online program at www.vitality101.com or at www.RealAge.com. These computerized tests will analyze your symptoms to help you assess the most likely causes of your fatigue and give you a detailed program tailored to your case.

*I.e. . . . you blanked out for a moment and thought you were reading *Harry Potter*.

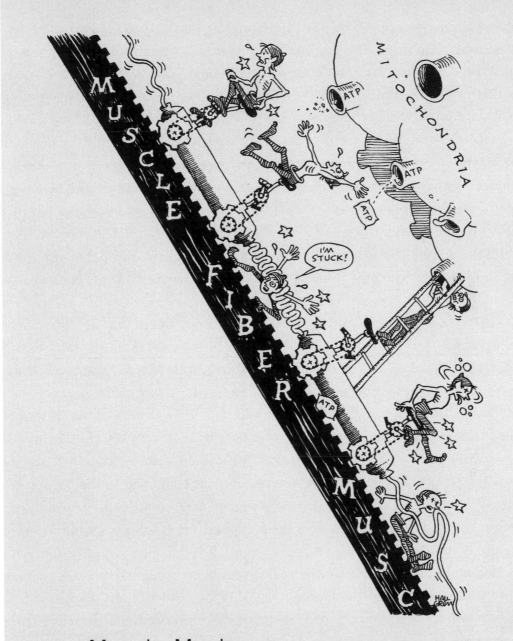

Figure 6.1 Muscle Mania Without enough energy, muscles lock up in a tense, contracted position that causes the pain felt by fibromyalgia patients. One of the ways to work through the pain is by strengthening, releasing, and feeding (with ATP energy) the very muscles that hurt—a tough irony but an effective solution.

crease the energy sent to that area (for example, your immune system) and to de-crease usage elsewhere. This fine-tuning starts in your hypothalamus and pituitary. Thus, there's a strong association between hormonal issues and energy issues. We see these changes primarily with slow-functioning adrenal and thyroid glands, but small, important changes happen minute to minute. Stress causes increases in cortisol, which increases sugar in the bloodstream and insulin resistance—and that wastes energy in distributing sugar into fat instead of where it is needed to produce ATP. The tough part here is that it's not always clear what the best ways are to deal with hormonal issues. Case in point: We physicians aren't sure whether to treat the numbers or to treat the symptoms patients have. We often try to "nor-malize the numbers from blood tests" even if we're not eradicating the symptoms. The so-called normal range of blood levels for many hormonal levels is defined as the middle 95 (95!) percent of people with those levels; the top 2.5 percent are considered high and the bottom 2.5 percent are considered low. Unfortunately, that's just not good math for the individual. It's like saying that if the number that is normal is size 6 to 11 in shoes, then a 6 shoe will be okay for you, even if you have a size 4 foot. Not a good fit, but you'd be wearing a "normal"-size shoe.

Instead, we docs can choose to treat the symptoms as long as the treatment doesn't cause levels that are very abnormal on blood tests. Here's one example of why treating the symptoms (it's what docs learn to do—most important, listen to the patient) and not just getting a number on your blood test in the 95 percent range is important. If a T3 (free thyroid hormone) level up to 1.4 is normal but we have to get up to 1.5 to eradicate your symptoms, we think we should listen to you and do that, periodically backing off to see if you can be symptom free with less thyroid hormone. Because when hormones aren't regulated to levels that are right for you, you've got a dimmer that keeps flipping from producing power full-time to producing power half-time. So that lack of thyroid hormone means your energy factories can't use the food you've eaten to produce those ATPs efficiently. That makes you feel tired.

Since your hormones do more than keep your muscles pumped and your sex-ual engine revved (they're prime regulators of how you feel from day to day and hour to hour), if you feel a lack of optimal energy, talk with your doc about these:

Thyroid. Your hypothalamus is responsible for making the hormone that causes your pituitary to produce thyroid-stimulating hormone—a marker for thyroid disease. The problem is that most docs treating the symptoms of thyroid problems (such as weight gain and fatigue) treat based on a number that really doesn't make perfect sense (like that 6 to 11 shoe size). We docs should be looking at both forms of thyroid hormone (free T4 and T3 levels) as well as TSH levels. Your TSH levels are from your pituitary; they're your internal dimmer trying to make the lights bright enough to read by. So your TSH levels go up when your thyroid isn't pumping out enough T4 and T3, in an effort to increase your thyroid gland's production of T3 and T4. But sometimes your pituitary fails to succeed or the wires in your thyroid are frayed, so you cannot produce all the T3 and T4 you need. We docs try to help by giving you more—but many times we are guided by that 95 percent target rather than that target and your symptoms. To boot, we often treat it with a drug that doesn't always work in everyone's body:

FACTOID

"Energy" drinks seem to have taken over the world—you can get them everywhere from convenience stores to nightclubs. But the question is, do they work? We wish we could give a definitive answer, but there are just not enough data to be sure. If you are going to indulge, go for the ones with the lowest sugar content. Many are loaded with caffeine or its equivalent, which, of course, can explain why drinkers feel a boost, no matter what the other "energy" ingredients are (things like taurine and guarana). While it doesn't appear that they're unsafe (though there have been some links to heart problems in rare cases), we do know of one definite warning: Don't mix them with alcohol. By getting you "up," they allow you to drink more booze before you feel its negative effects— a dangerous combo indeed.

YOU Test

Thyroid Tester

The thyroid gland is your body's gas pedal, so it controls how much get-up-and-go you have. Since blood tests for thyroid function are not always reliable, how do you know to ask your doc if you need a trial of natural prescription thyroid? Just take this test:

1. Are you tired even after a low-key weekend?
2. Have you gained more than ten pounds since your fatigue began?
3. Do you often have a body temperature under 98 degrees?
4. Are you achy more than one hour a day?
5. Do you have high LDL cholesterol or low HDL cholesterol?
6. Do you like the house warmer than your spouse does?
7. Do you have dry skin?
8. Do you have thin hair?
9. Do you have heavy periods?

If you have chronic fatigue or pain and have at least three of the above symptoms, you should ask your doc to consider testing your blood for thyroid dysfunction. If it's positive, she might give you a trial of Armour Thyroid by prescription. This form has the active thyroid hormone (called T3) in it, and many experts in this field find that it works better than the more commonly used Synthroid. No data prove this difference, but some patients swear it made the difference to them.

There's a complex and delayed reaction to many drugs that can vary among people. (It takes four to eight weeks to arrive at stable levels of these drugs after you make a change in doses.) Many times, you need to help your doc know how you feel and maybe push to get treated (if other treatments fail) with a bioidentical thyroid hormone that doesn't just adjust the numbers in your blood test but helps the way you actually feel.

Adrenal. This symptom sound familiar? When you're hungry, do you quickly switch to feeling so ravenous and irritable that if you don't get something to eat immediately, you'll commit a felony? That's a sign that your adrenal glands—your fight-or-flight glands—may not be working properly. A blood test picks up only very dangerous levels (not just abnormal ones), so you need to address the signs that malfunctioning adrenals are making you feel bad. (See page 385 for a list of tests we do when our patients are feeling as if their energy factories are off-line.) If all else fails (and we mean *all else*), talk to your doc about taking 5–20 mg every other day of a cortisol type of medication called Cortef or its cousin DHEA (not DHA) (your doc will need to measure levels before and frequently). See our YOU Tips for more on treatment options.

Sex Hormones: Perimenopausal women who experience worsening of their pain and fatigue around their periods are probably also experiencing a drop in estrogen. Cause and effect? Maybe. Remember, pain diverts your energy, too. A bioidentical estrogen such as estradiol combined with a micronized bioidentical progesterone and preceded by two baby aspirin has benefits we think exceed risks for most women* and can help your fatigue, pain, and brain fog. Women and men who have decreased shaving frequency (legs and face, respectively) should also consider testosterone if they need it for the associated elevation of LDL cholesterol, triglycerides, decreased HDL cholesterol, or loss of libido.

Of course, with declining energy, the issue isn't just having one symptom; it's having one overriding problem (an energy crisis) that plays out in many different

---

* See *YOU: Staying Young*, for our lengthy discussion on hormone therapy.

Warning for Those with Chronic Fatigue or Fibromyalgia

If you ask a brain surgeon to repair an ACL, she probably won't be able to do it. Or if you ask an ear, nose, and throat specialist about the bunions on your big toe, he probably won't be too much help. But somehow, we expect our general docs to know how to treat the general-sounding symptoms associated with fibromyalgia and chronic fatigue syndrome. Truth is, most docs don't know much about these conditions and can leave you feeling more frustrated than a laryngitic opera singer. So what do you do? Find a specialist. Find the docs who can piece together your medical puzzle and help you come up with a plan that combines the lifestyle changes we've suggested with any needed medication and hormonal treatments. You can find a specialist at www.vitality101.com (initial appointments may be in various centers around the country, but you can often do follow-ups by phone).

ways—specifically either having low energy and/or having high pain, two things that will certainly make you feel about as beautiful as a wart-dotted, hairless cat. Many muscles feel tired and then pained as you start to use them. This description doesn't do justice to the problem. Remember how low you felt when you had the worst flu you ever had? That's how people with chronic fatigue syndrome and fibromyalgia feel at their best. The good news is, we have some solutions that seem to work in a large percentage of people with these syndromes and may work for little energy boosts that many of us feel we need even if we aren't as devastated as these patients. Remember, as we discussed in the introduction to this section, pain and a lack of energy aren't the enemies. They're the smoke alarms— the warning signals that your body has some kind of fire raging—and that you, my friend, better find the way to put it out if you want to function with the passion of a beautiful being.

YOU Tips!

If you blow a fuse in your house, you can't expect to get power back by lighting a few candles and searching for food with flashlights. You've got to find the bad one, replace it with a good one, reset the system, and power up. Same goes here. To restore your energy—both at the "feeling great" level and at the chemical level—it just takes some awareness and action to get your body headed in the right direction.

SCOOP UP, POWER UP. Some ill-advised folks might say that the greatest nutritional discovery of the last decade has been the Baconator (at a whopping 830 calories, we don't think so). The real nutritional heroes: DHA and ribose.

> **DHA:** The active form of omega-3 helps constitute nerve membranes and keeps the nerves to your muscles firing, as well as helps encase muscles. You can get this in fish oils or from the algae that fish eat. Try 600 mg of DHA a day (equivalent to 2 grams of fish oil if you like that taste better).
>
> **Ribose:** This special sugar is made in your body and doesn't come from food; it helps build the energy blocks of your body. Of all the things you can do to combat the effects of knee-dragging fatigue, taking a daily ribose supplement is the one that seems to really turbo-charge some people who have diseases associated with low energy. (The only side effect is that some people feel too much energy, if that's possible.) The data aren't good enough to recommend ribose for all of us. But if you want to give it a try, start with 500 mg three times a day for a week or so until you get used to the taste (or find a smoothie, coffee, or tea to put it in). Then go to 5 grams three times a day for three weeks to get a sense of the effect. Then you can scale back to 5 grams twice a day. By the way, since we know you're wondering: Each 5-gram scoop contains only 20 calories, since ribose isn't metabolized as a sugar. Taking it won't increase your chances of becoming mistaken for a Sea World attraction. In fact, since it is a bit sweet, you might think of it as a sugar substitute. As an aside, ribose has been shown to relieve fatigue, soreness, and stiffness after exercise, and some professional athletes have reported muscular benefits after taking ribose (again, the data are too weak to say it does or doesn't work well, since the studies just haven't been done).

MOVE MORE TO MOVE MORE. One of the best ways to increase your energy is to jump-start it with some physical activity such as walking; that brings in more nutrients since nitric oxide is released from the linings of arteries to allow blood vessels to move blood more freely. One of the greatest things about your body is that it responds to what you're doing through mechanisms called feedback loops. You tell your body that you want to watch *Scrubs* reruns all night, and it responds by

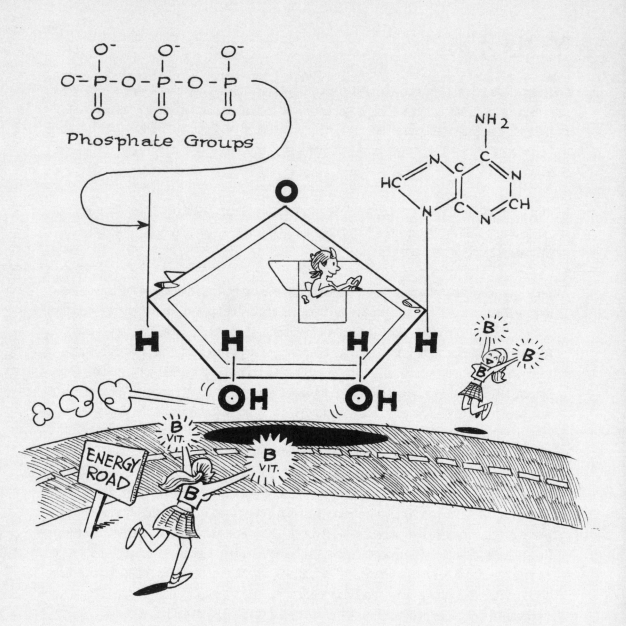

Figure 6.2 Sugar Smack The sugar ribose helps give us energy by feeding the power plants of our body (ATP). Don't worry; it's not a high-cal sugar. If you take it as a supplement, you may feel an increase in your energy level.

downshifting energy production (don't need much muscle power to change channels). But tell your body that you need to walk around the neighborhood or swim a few laps or do an early-morning stretch-to-the-ceiling routine, and it responds by giving you the energy you need. And we know it's sometimes tough if you have pain or sore muscles, but it's the best way to get rid of the pain or sore muscles—to strengthen those muscles and bring nutrients to them (and take away waste products). So take advantage of these feedback loops by integrating more exercise into your routine. And start early in the day, when you have the energy to exercise. Ideally, aim for 45 minutes a day of physical activity with at least 20 minutes a day involving the sore muscles. Start by doing gentle exercise such as walking or warm-water stretching. The trick is to do only the amount or intensity that makes you feel "good tired," not "bad tired" or in pain afterward. Tell your body which way to go, and it's going to follow. By the way, the average person who walks a dog for 60 minutes gets only 8 minutes of physical activity when actually measured by a pedometer.* You should get 100 steps on the pedometer for every minute of walking.

SLEEP EIGHT. Blame it on the invention of electricity, more demanding jobs, or great late-night TV on F/X, but we sleep a whole lot less nowadays than we used to. On average, Americans awake at 5:47 a.m. and do not hit the bed (not when we actually sleep) until after 10:15 p.m.; that's not enough. While you may think that sleep is just a good way to let McDreamy enter your subconscious fantasies, sleep has the ultimate restorative powers and you need it for your hormonal balance and for increasing the rejuvenating human growth hormone, which is needed to choreograph the looking and feeling beautiful dance in your body. Growth hormone is secreted primarily when we sleep and is dependent on your sleep. We're just not doing enough of it. Eight high-quality hours a day will help you restore energy, decrease pain, and lose weight. If you have trouble falling asleep, you may need to include some sleep tactics in your bag of bedroom tricks.

- Do nothing in your bedroom but sleep and have sex. If you work, watch TV, or work out to fitness DVDs in the room, you're basically training your body to be alert in the bedroom space. Your bedroom should be a sanctuary from the normal hustle and bustle of life.
- Practice good sleep hygiene. That means you should make a sleep schedule (plan your eight hours); before that eight-hour period starts, give yourself ten minutes to do the quick chores absolutely needed for the next day (such as making lunch), another ten minutes for hygiene, and ten minutes for meditation (all before starting the eight hours). Some people even dim the lights in their bedroom an hour before sleep to transition from artificial light to darkness.

*A great pedometer is one of the four things we think you should overpay for—the other three being a heart rate monitor, a pair of cross-training shoes, and an eight-inch chef's knife.

Another helper: Make sure your room is cool; the ideal sleep temp seems to be around 67 degrees.

- Add in a power nap. Just make sure to keep it under 30 minutes. Any longer than that, and you'll slip into a stage of deeper sleep so close to the dreamy REM phase that when awakened from it, you'll feel hung over and drowsy (that feeling, by the way, is called sleep inertia and is associated with making bad financial judgments and getting into auto accidents). At less than 30 minutes, a nap can be invigorating. Naps enable your body and brain to reboot and are commonly practiced in societies that boast great energy and longevity.

- In terms of sleep supplements, the data aren't good enough to love these, but some patients like valerian root (though it has an energizing effect in 10 percent of people), passion flower, theanine, hops (ask any college student), and melatonin, 0.5 to 3 mg (especially if you're jet-lagged or working weird shift hours). Calcium (1,200 mg divided between two doses) and magnesium (400 mg) are also helpful. These can help you get to sleep and wake up refreshed with no hangover (which some sleep drugs cause).*

CHECK YOUR PLATE. You know us when it comes to food. We think it's nature's best medicine. These are the dietary tactics that seem to work best for increasing energy:

- Drink as much water as it takes to keep your mouth and lips moist throughout the day, so that your urine is clear enough to read through. If you have chronic fatigue or fibromyalgia and have low blood pressure, you can increase your salt intake (try sea salt, when convenient, for the added minerals) when your body craves it. One hidden cause of fatigue is a little bit of dehydration. It's something that many people can't quite identify, so if you're feeling a little low, a glass of water (and not a bag of M&M's) may be the jolt you really need.

- Avoid simple sugars—they end in -ose, like glucose, sucrose, maltose, dextrose, etc. (except ribose!)—syrups (another word for sugar), any grain but 100 percent whole grains (since grains turn into simple sugars), and saturated and trans fats.

- Aim to consume high-quality protein such as nuts and fish and a low-carb diet, and include lots of fruits, vegetables, and 100 percent whole grains.

FIND YOUR CHIA. Say the word *chia,* and most of us immediately think of little green pets. But we want you to think of chia for another reason: A whole grain used by the Aztecs as their main energy source, chia can help restore energy levels and decrease inflammation because of its omega-3 fatty acids. Similar to cornstarch, chia can be used as a thickening agent and as a substitute for whole

---

* See *YOU: Staying Young* for more details on which sleep supplement may be right for you.

grains in your diet. Whole grains, of course, are especially important because they help stabilize blood sugar levels, as opposed to causing the spikes and falls that can occur when you eat sugars and refined carbohydrates. Here's one way to use chia.

CHIA MUFFINS

1 tablespoon chia seeds, ground (use a coffee or spice grinder)

$1^1/_2$ cups whole wheat or whole grain flour

2 teaspoons cinnamon

$^1/_2$ teaspoon nutmeg

2 teaspoons baking soda

$^1/_2$ teaspoon salt or salt and pepper to taste

16-ounce can organic pumpkin (make sure there is only pumpkin listed in the ingredients list)

2 egg whites

$^1/_4$ cup high-quality canola oil

$^1/_2$ cup agave nectar

1 tablespoon vanilla

$^1/_2$ cup of chopped walnuts

Preheat oven to 350°F. Mix dry ingredients together in a bowl. In a separate bowl, mix all wet ingredients. Fold the wet ingredients and nuts into the dry ingredients, stirring only until dry ingredients are moistened (don't overmix). Spoon into paper-lined or greased (with canola oil) muffin tins. Bake for 25 to 30 minutes, or until a toothpick inserted into the middle of a muffin comes out clean. Store completely cooled muffins in resealable plastic bags in the freezer. Makes about a dozen.

GO PERUVIAN IN THE MORNING. In the heights of the mountains, Peruvian tribesmen get energy by sucking on maca (*Lepidium meyenii*) plants. This turnip- or radish-shaped vegetable from the mustard family has been used as food and medicine, to promote endurance and improve energy, vitality, sexual virility, and even fertility. The data on its increased energy effects seem strong, but the reported side effect is insomnia. It can be obtained in a powder at many stores (Whole Foods, etc.) or from reputable dealers on the Internet, and 1 teaspoon (that's the dose in the studies) can be added to blender drinks, pancakes, and other food products. The teaspoon keeps you going all day long. For you pill lovers, take $^1/_2$ gram of the extract twice a day.

GO RUSSIAN IN THE EVENING. Hunted in Siberia and extracted from chips, *Rhodiola rosea* anecdotally promotes energy, stamina, and sexual function and libido. Stuff chips into a pint container, and fill with vodka. Then try a tablespoon a night (if beet red, it will have 200 to 600 mg of the extract). How good are the data? Not solid enough to recommend to everyone, but we know a little alcohol every night keeps your cardiovascular system younger, even if it's not red wine.

GET RID OF INFECTIONS. While most of us want to treat infections because of their acute symptoms, we can't ignore that they can have chronic implications as well. Since inflammation and infection can be two of the dominos in the cascade of low-energy symptoms, one of your goals could be to monitor your body so that infections don't linger. That means regular flossing to decrease the risk of gum inflammation, regular use of a neti pot to reduce sinusitis, and probiotics for treating such infections as prostatitis, bowel infections, and vaginitis. Many infections are viral, in which case good sleep, frequent hand washing, and food choices that avoid all simple sugars and saturated fats can help.

GO B. You need B vitamins for your mitochondria to produce energy from glucose. Most of us absorb the B vitamins well (in either liquid or pill form), but 99 percent of us don't get enough from our diets. Take a multivitamin in the morning and evening (twice a day to keep stable levels, since we pee the water-soluble ones out) to keep you energized. If you're having symptoms, check your vitamin B12 and D levels. Get your vitamin B and D levels checked yearly. You may be the rare person who doesn't absorb them well from your stomach and intestine and needs a B12 vitamin injection yearly. Much of the world is short of vitamin D—and you need it to help fight cancer, to keep arteries young, and to aid brain function. So make sure you get it measured and take what is needed to keep its level normal.

GO GREEN. Green tea has been shown to have the highest content of polyphenols, which are chemicals with potent antioxidant properties (believed to be greater than even vitamin C's). They give tea its bitter flavor. Because green tea leaves are young and have not been oxidized, green tea has up to 40 percent polyphenols, while black tea contains only about 10 percent. Another interesting note: Green tea has one-third the caffeine of black tea. Even better, it's been shown to yield the same level of energy and attentiveness, but in more even levels than the ups and downs associated with other caffeinated drinks. Just don't drink milk with it; the casein in milk has been shown to inhibit the beneficial effects of tea.

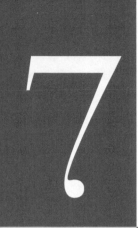

7

That's Gotta Hurt
How to Manage Your Major Aches and Pains

YOU Test: Pain Threshold

Stick your hand in a bucket of ice water and see how long you can keep it under before you feel that you have to take it out (you should get your doc's permission before doing this, because it can increase your blood pressure and change your heart rate). See where you fit on the scale on the next page. If you have lesser amounts of substance P in your pain-sensing nerves or greater amounts of serotonin in your brain, you're likely to be able to tolerate pain longer, even 30 percent longer than normal, on this test.

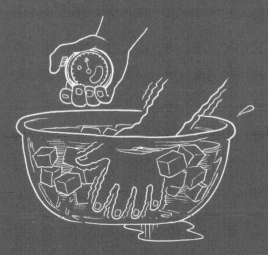

Race, Gender	Age	Shortest Time for Normal
White male	under 27 27–39 40–52	75 seconds 60 seconds 45 seconds
Nonwhite male	under 27 27–39 40–52	60 seconds 50 seconds 35 seconds
White female	under 27 27–39 40–52	40 seconds 35 seconds 30 seconds
Nonwhite female*	under 27 27–39 40–52	30 seconds 30 seconds 30 seconds

*Not atypically, the sample was small so it was difficult for the study to establish norms.

So your skin radiates, your hair is soft, and your body is the object of desire (or envy) of every man, woman, and model scout in the world. Excellent. Be proud that you look like a million bucks. You know what? All of that doesn't mean a lick if it takes you 36 minutes to pick yourself up off the couch. Suddenly, your million bucks feels more like 80 grand in credit card debt. After all, that's what pain—no matter what kind it is—does to us: It debilitates us, it slows us down, it's the leading reason we go to the doctor, and it makes life feel more miserable than a dreary December rain. And if you don't *feel* beautiful, frankly, who gives two hoots about how plump your lips are?

Pain saps your energy—you get dressed and are ready to face the world for, oh, about 15 seconds. Chronic pain makes you look old and haggard, which makes you feel old no matter what your age. You can't bounce back the way you used to, and that's why you need a pain management plan.

In this chapter we're going to cover the three big chronic and nagging pains that affect the typical person—back pain, joint pain, and headaches (and throughout we'll throw in a dash of a few other common pain-producing ailments). And if you allow us a slight deviation from our typical chapter structure, we're going to do this: Instead of piling up our change-your-life YOU Tips at the end of the chapter, we're going to divvy up this chapter into separate parts, so that those of you who are concerned about one form of pain and not another can get what you need in each succinct section. Our goal here—no matter whether your pain occurs above the neck or below the belt—is to get you feeling the way you want to feel every day.

What Is Pain?

You already know that pain differs from other sensations like touch or sound—pain hurts instantly. Why? It's nature's way of catching your attention and alerting you that something is wrong. But pain is even more complex than hearing, seeing, or touching, because it takes on a life of its own. When it is prolonged and when tissue is damaged, pain worsens over time. It even modifies how you sense it in the brain and changes the way your DNA is expressed.

So let's explore how pain really works. Just as a mosquito bite triggers us to scratch (itch is like less severe pain, which serves as a hint of a problem without sounding a big alarm and which gets more intense if you do not get rid of it), pain is a similarly useful behavioral and biological response. That's especially true when it comes to physical pain: If someone drops a hammer on your foot, the impact causes various nerve endings in the foot to fire, and these signals immediately cause your muscles to contract and you to move your foot away fast and then maybe writhe in pain so you can remember to get the heck away from the next stray hammer. Yet, even after you treat the physical pain, that physical pain eventually evolves into an emotional pain—a pain that's actually not a pain at all but rather what we think of as fear.

It may help to think of fear as pain remembered, and that memory works quickly and subconsciously to help us avoid the same situation in the future. Our nervous system operates using this kind of smoke detector principle: False alarms,

Alternate Routes

In this chapter we outline many different therapies to help relieve the fire, the knives, the cramps, and the strobe lights that are making you feel about as good as the bottom of a shoe. As in many areas of medicine, there are also some alternative therapies that can prove to be helpful. Though they're not all well studied, some of them show enough promise that they may be worth trying; just make sure they're the real thing. A few of our favorites:

- Devil's claw (200 mg). The name *devil's claw* comes from the herb's unusual fruits, which are covered with numerous small clawlike appendages. The roots, or tubers, of the plant are used in herbal preparations. Devil's claw has been used as a tonic to relieve arthritis, tendonitis, and rheumatism and ease sore muscles.
- Boswellia (900+ mg/day). Boswellia, or olibanum, is a close relative of frankincense, the biblical incense, and has been used historically in the ayurvedic medical system of India for various conditions, including arthritis and other inflammatory conditions.
- Arnica (1–10 grains or more in gel for direct application). Popular in Europe, this homeopathic remedy seems to have some benefit for those suffering from osteoarthritis and muscle aches.
- Capsaicin (twice a day in higher than 0.075 percent preparation) rubbed on your skin: The active principle of hot chili pepper, capsaicin depletes the pain-causing neurotransmitter substance P over time—so you'll have some burning for a while until the substance P is almost undetectable in your nerves.
- There's some promising evidence that other therapies might be helpful also. Specifically: green algae and SAMe for fibromyalgia, willow bark and ginger for arthritis, and thunder god vine for various pain conditions.

though annoying, are still less costly than failing to react to a real crisis. The cues to a threatening situation may not always be obvious. If your reaction is delayed until danger is a certainty, it may already be too late. When dealing with life-threatening situations, a single lapse can be fatal. So a selective advantage goes to those who gear up the fear response and become more responsive and vigilant at the slightest evidence of danger. Better to hide in the bathtub during a tornado warning and not have it come than to ignore the warning and wind up flying down the street in the middle of the twister.

Your body senses pain through two sets of nerve endings in the skin that transmit pain. Slow ones without a myelin sheath around them give us burning or deep pain, while fast ones have that fatty sheath around them (the sheath speeds the pain sensation's transmission to your spinal cord and your brain so you can react faster) to tell you that you put your hand on a hot burner or your god-blessed elbow hit a doorknob. These sensations are mainly in the skin, but almost every tissue has them (such as those in the esophagus).

Your body really reacts to pain in one of two ways. You know how when you put ice on a sprained ankle, it's cold at first, but then you get used to it. Some pains are just like that—you get used to them and tolerate them. But some are the exact opposite. Those cause your cells to produce more neurotransmitters and/or more receptor sites so the next pain or the pain gets less bearable with time.

That's why it's so important to learn to break the pain cycle by using the tips we present in this chapter. You need to have a completely pain-free day every two weeks to break the pain cycle. If you don't, your body will build up too many pain receptors, and that causes your pain to increase.

FACTOID An older theory of pain sensation (but one that many still believe useful to understanding) is the gate-control theory. The gate consists of specialized nerve cells in the spinal cord that act as gatekeepers to filter the pain messages on their way to your brain. For severe pain that's linked to bodily harms, such as when you touch a hot stove, the "gate" is wide open and the messages take an express route to your brain. Nerve fibers that transmit touch also affect gatekeeper cells by decreasing the transmission of pain signals (it's why rubbing a sore part of your body makes it feel better). It's one reason why acupuncture may work: by closing the gate and not letting pain sensations through.

While acute pain can contort you or make you writhe in a less than beautiful way, at least most acute pain is preventable. Chronic pain also prevents you from acting in other ways that can help you feel beautiful. After all, pain is very commonly associated with depression—both of them serving as cause and effect; they're wake-up calls and force a change in the status quo. What we want to teach you is how to prevent things such as back pain, joint pain, neck pain, and headaches from occurring and recurring. The great news: You can do plenty of things to control or prevent pain so you can get back to feeling like seven figures again.

Part 1

Back Pain: Get Back In Shape

We're creatures of adaptation. If we lose some vision, we get glasses. If we survive a heart attack, we drop the bacon burgers from our diet. If our skin starts flaking off like an upstate New York snowstorm, we goop on moisturizer by the fistful. Faced with a problem, we find a solution as quickly as we can so we can get back to our daily routine. But one of the problems most likely to interrupt and interfere with that daily routine is the health problem that sends more people to the doctor's office than just about any other. Millions of Americans suffer from all kinds of back pain—some of it chronic and throbbing, and some of it so debilitating and sharp that it'll send them to the floor yelping for their mamas.

FACTOID

While mattress preference is about as subjective as music preference, some research shows that people with medium-firm mattresses are the most likely to have their back pain improve.

In many ways, back pain is a metaphorical gunshot wound to your body because, depending on its intensity, it can paralyze you and prevent you from doing anything—even walking, tying your shoes, or using the toilet. (In fact, 72 percent of people who sought treatment for back pain gave up on sports and exercise and 46 percent of people with back pain say it was enough to have them give up sex. And not just for a day.) Back pain is so prevalent that it's spawned multimillion-dollar industries that are trying to deal with it. Any time you have a lot of treatment options, it means none of them is perfect or else the others would die off (we hate to use that word in a medical book). Luckily, there are things you can do, too. In general, less is more.

Your Lower Back: Nature's Girdle

The price we pay for having the ability to stand up straight and walk upright is that much of that pressure and shock absorption that used to be distributed among our limbs when we walked on all fours is now transferred to our lower backs. But since we're sort of content with our two-legged mode of transportation

YOU Test

Lie on the floor in standard push-up position with your toes on the ground but your elbows on the ground instead of your hands (the classic "plank" position). Maintain a straight line through your body with no arch in your back. Keep your head down and in line with your back. Hold that position for as long as you can.

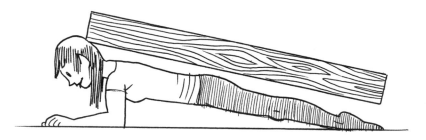

If you lasted less than 15 seconds: The core muscles in your abdominals and lower back are on the weak side, meaning you're more vulnerable to suffering from acute or chronic lower-back pain.

If you lasted 15–45 seconds: You've got a nice foundation of strength, which will help protect your back, but there's still room for improvement.

If you lasted more than 45 seconds: Wow, can we see your abs?

(and willing to trade off wear and tear on our knuckles for an erect spine), we have to train our lower backs to deal with it.

Of the numerous risk factors for back pain (including smoking, your job, age, and certain diseases such as arthritis), omental obesity (obesity around your abdominal tissues and organs) and core muscle weakness are the biggest. With obesity, it just makes anatomical sense: The bigger your belly, the more likely it is that your center of gravity is pulled forward, putting excess strain on your back. The solution's simple (at least in principle): Drop the weight, and you'll ease the tension.

Even if you're skinnier than a chopstick, you can still have back problems—especially if you have a weak set of muscles in your core, the area that includes your hips, abdominals, and lower back. That core tissue—made of muscles, ligaments, and tendons—acts as your own natural back brace. If you have a tight anatomical back brace, you'll absorb shock and provide a strong foundation for all the different kinds of movement you do throughout the day. But if you have a brace that's loose, weak, and as unsupportive as a size XXL jacket on a size S body, even reaching around to hand your kid a bottle in the back of the car (don't try it now) could result in your writhing in kill-me-now pain.

Your back is made up of an intricate system of bones, nerves, and tissues. These are the main ones we want you to learn about.

VERTEBRAE AND DISCS. Your spine is made up of small stacked bones (the vertebrae) that form a column separated by discs (see Figure 7.1). Think of your spine as a column of doughnuts separated by nice wedges of Havarti cheese: The vertebrae are the doughnut portion, and inside the holes travels the spinal cord;

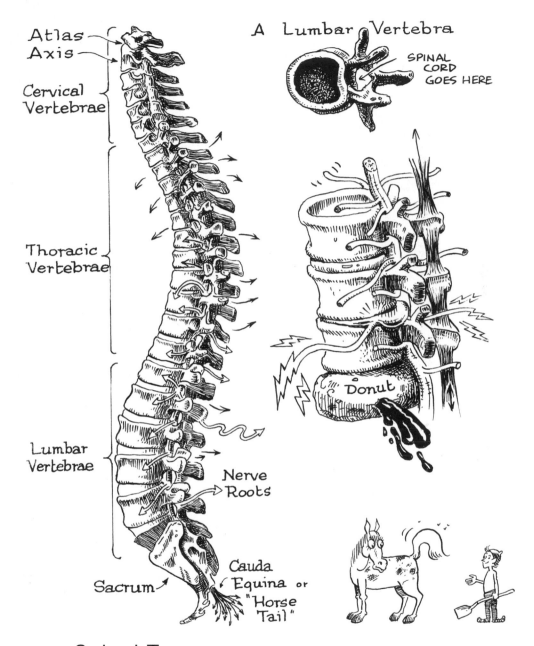

Atlas
Axis
Cervical
Vertebrae

A Lumbar Vertebra

SPINAL CORD GOES HERE

Thoracic
Vertebrae

Lumbar
Vertebrae

Nerve
Roots

Donut

Sacrum

Cauda
Equina or
"Horse
Tail"

Figure 7.1 Spinal Trap Your vertebrae are a lot like a squishy jelly doughnuts; in between the vertebrae are discs, which, if they come out of alignment, can lead to intense back pain. It seems that some medications can help relieve pain by providing fluid to the area around the spine to relieve some of the pressure.

the Havarti wedges are the discs. A bulging disc happens when you put too much weight and twist on the spine and the disc of Havarti squishes out, pushing against and then compressing either the spinal cord itself or the nerve root on either side. Even without compressing, the oozing discs can leak irritating chemicals that cause inflammation and zowie-wowie pain. Diluting or washing away those chemicals (with steroids or other liquid injections) seems to relieve pain rather successfully. The curvature of our spines is for shock absorption. If the spine were straight, all the impact would be passed directly from our feet to our head. We walk with our legs rather than our spine, and this provides us the advantage of a narrow, fast gait.

MUSCLES. Surrounding your spine, there's a large and complex set of muscles that have the job of an anatomical administrative assistant; they're all about providing support (see Figure 7.2). These muscles are broken into three broad categories: extensors, which are attached to the back of the spine and give you the strength to stand; flexors, which are in the front of the spine and help you bend forward; and obliques, which are attached to the sides and help you win twist contests. Also important in this complex are the abdominal muscles—actually the most important front muscles of the lower back.

When you injure your back, it's not just the injury itself that causes problems but the collateral damage that can come in the form of straining other muscles as you try to compensate for your bad back. In addition, you can also develop inflammation around the nerves (which is why such things as rehab, fish oil or the DHA equivalent, and anti-inflammatory meds such as naproxyn or ibuprofen or sometimes even steroids can be helpful). Also, having a bad back means you subject yourself to a dangerous domino effect: You can't exercise and can't have sex, and then you become depressed because you can't exercise or have sex. And it hurts

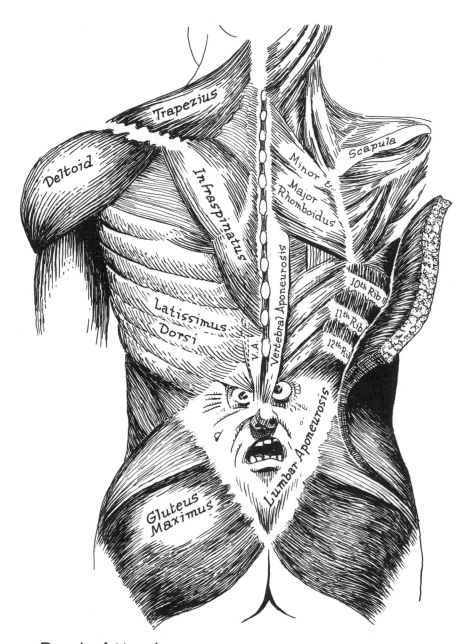

Figure 7.2 Back Attack In many cases, back pain is really a muscular problem more than a problem that needs to be corrected with surgery. Strengthening your abdominals and lower-back muscles can help prevent a lot of chronic back pain.

Back Under the Knife

It used to be that you heard the words *back surgery* and you'd think body casts and five months of recovery. But these days, newer techniques are making back surgery a quick procedure— even outpatient in some cases. For example, vertebroplasty and kyphoplasty are minimally invasive procedures where a collapsed vertebra that's been weakened by osteoporosis or cancer can be strengthened with a cementlike mixture that's inserted through a tiny skin cut with special tools under X-ray guidance. There's also a similar procedure done to burn the painful nerves inside the discs and to reinforce the collagen fibers of the discs. Nevertheless, back pain sufferers without neurologic complications should usually avoid surgery until they have worked with pain therapy and rehabilitation specialists for at least a few months. And the truth is that surgery is rarely needed for general lower-back pain, which can be treated through therapy.

even to cough or go to the bathroom. If you don't take care of the problem, your health may begin a downward spiral.

Now, you'd think that the people most prone to back pain would be professional contortionists and those playing contact sports. While you can certainly suffer from acute injuries to your lower back from moving the wrong way, it's much more common to suffer from back pain from doing something that seems harmless—sitting. People who sit for long periods of time are prone to back pain because of the strain of being in a fixed, slumped position (which is why you need to maintain good posture). Sitting increases pressure in the discs, even more than standing. Sitting also leaves back muscles weaker than watered-down coffee, since sitters don't actively use and engage those muscles much throughout the day—it's what's called disuse atrophy (in other words, you lose it if you don't use it). Standing with poor posture also puts your back at risk, since belly muscles are lax and your spine bears the brunt of any unexpected or awkward movement.

NERVES AND MYELIN. Nerves exit the spine through a small space called a foramen. Sometimes nerves are trapped in this small space as they exit the spine, are inflamed by recent trauma, or are surrounded by fat, and the delicate myelin sheath that coats our nerves to prevent short circuiting is compressed, with resulting inflammation (see Figure 7.3). Since the nerve that comes out from that area of the back innervates the muscles of the lower leg and foot, you usually feel

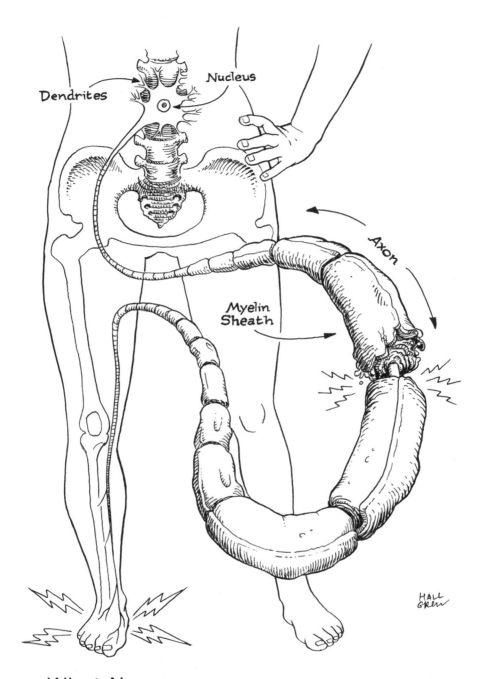

Figure 7.3 **What Nerve** Some back pain originates from your nerves. When the myelin sheath that surrounds the nerve is compromised (like the coating of a wire that may break), the nerve is exposed and the resulting pain can shoot down your legs.

low-back nerve compression and inflammation in the leg, accompanied by shooting pains down the leg or a dull aching pain in the buttocks or back. Our nerves, like many other parts of our bodies, simply get inflamed and have less room to move about as fat fills the space as we age so they lose insulation (like a copper wire without insulation). Muscle spasm, by contrast, is the sustained contraction of a muscle supplied by an inflamed nerve, which may fire repeatedly. Without new oxygen, the contraction results in pain and weakening of the muscle. The sequence of contraction without more oxygen then repeats itself and gets worse if you can't break the cycle.

The solution to both of these problems is to rebuild the insulation and/or restore normalcy with nutritional support (and a little time) so the inflammation can resolve. If your core muscles are strong (and we show you how to make them so in the Band Workout on page 351), you stand less chance of a muscle spasm (sustained muscle contraction) and nerve trauma from disc injury.

Back to the Solutions

Back pain is one of medicine's true anatomical enigmas. As common as back pain is, it's often difficult—if not impossible—to diagnose what caused it. In fact, some of the diagnostic testing we use, such as MRIs, only makes the medical mystery more confusing. Some people with lots of symptoms have normal or near-normal MRIs, and some people with MRIs that would seem to suggest terrible back pain have absolutely no pain at all. About 20 percent of people younger than 40, and at least 50 percent of people older than 50, have MRI or CT scan (diagnostic tests used by docs) evidence of degenerated spines and disc abnormalities. But not all of them have pain, making an already complex and hard-to-diagnose issue even tougher.

For many sufferers, nutritional deficiencies promote inflammation and pre-

Let's Get Some Structure

If you are so stiff that you feel as if you're stuck in your own body with a block of cement, then you should consider trying Rolfing—a yoga and massagelike technique that's used for such things as chronic tissue pain, tightness, and poor posture. The technique aims to work on a muscle called the deep psoas muscle, the only muscle that attaches the upper five lumbar vertebrae to the lower body, via your pelvis and the upper and inner aspects of your upper leg bone—the femur (the thighbone). This allows your body to be realigned and stack up efficiently. That way, your weight will be supported by skeletal structures rather than overworking your muscles. Although Rolfing is concerned mainly with structural changes in the body, many patients report positive changes in their outlook on life and in their ability to handle emotionally challenging situations.

vent them from making normal myelin nerve coatings, so even a little pressure from a disc or twist results in shooting nerve pain. For these folks, instead of focusing on the mechanical problems (i.e., the disc), we're better off resuscitating your anti-inflammatory powers and your ability to coat your nerves with appropriate B vitamins and DHA-omega-3 fatty acids.

Fortunately, pinpointing the exact cause of a back breakdown isn't what's important, since most back pain can be alleviated with the right therapy. Many times, there's no need to push your doc for a definitive answer about the cause. He'd be guessing with the expertise of a Las Vegas oddsmaker—an educated guess, but there's still a lot left up to chance. Focus instead on what you can do to alleviate the pain and prevent it from crippling you again. The real key is having some level of postural intelligence—that is, being aware of your posture and the muscles in your trunk, so that you can not only support your back but also prevent other structural damage, for example to your joints.

FACTOID Chiropractic treatments can be as effective as conventional medical management for back pain. Chiropractic theory aims to realign vertebrae and establish normal spinal mobility, which in turn alleviates the irritation to the nerves and surrounding muscles. Multiple sessions are usually required to alleviate pain.

YOU Tips!

No matter what kind of tattoo might be adorning your lower back, it's not going to be all that appealing if you can't clip your own toenails. That's why now's the time to make sure your back has the strength to handle the load you ask it to carry—at work, on hikes, through the mall, while dancing on poles, all the time. With these tactics, you'll develop a muscular back brace so that you can prevent pain—and bounce back from it faster in case you can't.

DEVELOP THIS TO THE CORE. Sure, working out your biceps and calves may be nice for showing off at the pool, but if you want to stave off the crippling effects of a lower-back meltdown, the most important thing you can do is work the foundation muscles in your body's core. These muscles—especially the ones in your abdominals, which oppose your back muscles—help provide the support, muscular strength, and stamina to prevent back injuries. Do core exercises three days a week to work your abdominals and lower-back muscles (we cover them in our workout on page 351). And don't forget exercises such as lunges and squats, which strengthen your core by placing them on a firmer foundation.

The exercise philosophy preferred by more than 9 out of 10 rehab specialists is Pilates, which emphasizes movement through the use of the core muscles, those closest to the spine. Instead of performing more reps, Pilates focuses on performing fewer, more precise movements that require concentration, control, and proper form. The most successful programs for back rehabilitation are those that creatively integrate traditional Pilates with props such as big balls, resistance bands, or balance disks.

STAY LOOSE. You want to team up strength with flexibility, so include yoga, which also helps build up the collateral muscles that can protect you from injury. Even cardiovascular exercise has been shown to help with lower-back pain because it keeps you moving, so you can strengthen your back muscles to help protect you from injury.

STOP INFLAMMATION. If you experience one of those oh-my-lord moments when your back gives out on you like a plastic bag filled with too many cans, you know the first line of action:* Grab the ice. Applying ice for 20 minutes at a time will lower the inflammation that's occurring from the strain. After you remove the ice, the blood flow increases in a way that takes away toxic chemicals from injured tissues. Use for the first 24 to 48 hours, then switch to heat (be it through pads, sauna, wraps,

---

*After weeping like a crate-locked puppy.

heating pads, or fire-breathing dragons), which will help promote blood flow to speed healing. By the way, when you use ice, your back will feel better afterward as it works to warm itself up. When you use heat, it feels better during the treatment and then tends to stiffen up when you stop using it as the area cools down. Use heat for only 20 minutes at a time, or else you can overheat the muscles.

Of course, you can also use anti-inflammatory drugs such as ibuprofen to reduce pain and inflammation, and docs may prescribe a muscle relaxant or shoot local anesthetic into the muscle (trigger-point injections) to keep the darn things from spasming and feeling tighter than a cyclist's shorts. For a natural alternative, willow bark, from which aspirin was derived, is often as effective as ibuprofen, without the risk of irritating your stomach if you rub it on. Another way to help heal: Lie on your back flat on the floor with a small towel in the small of your back and stretch out your back muscles. It takes 15 minutes to realign and stretch your back muscles with this position. Use the time to meditate, and you'll be doing your body two goods instead of one. If your back keeps tightening, it may be worth also trying massage therapy.

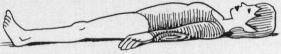

GET UP AND GO. Constantly lying in your bed or on the floor with back pain is going to do one thing and one thing only—make it worse. The way to bounce back is to make sure that you're up and around, moving your muscles, working them back into shape. We're not suggesting that you sign up for the local rugby team if you just pulled your back. But walking around the house is more productive—and more healing—than sitting around in it. That's why married folks recover more slowly than those living alone; if you're being waited on hand and foot, why give up a good thing? But you might be penalizing yourself by lounging in bed and taking advantage of your loved one's concern.

BE A MARINE. And stand up straight, would ya? Good posture promotes strong core muscles. Bad posture? Well, let's just say it teaches your muscles to crumble like a cookie. This goes not only for standing but for sitting, as well. It's also worth noting that you should be aware of your posture whenever you use any exercise equipment, such as stationary bikes or stair climbers. Correct posture should be practiced with your back against a wall. Tucking your chin under slightly will allow a larger area of the back of your head to touch the wall, as well as the top of your back, buttocks, and legs. The small of the back should not be against the wall (the spine is naturally curved). Pretend a string attached to the top of your skull is pulling you skyward and feel yourself becoming taller. When you're standing for a long time, elevate one foot on a step or curb to help alleviate some pressure. And if you're sitting for a long time, put your feet up on a stool, so your knees are higher than your hips; that will decrease the pressure on the discs in your lower back. You can also get a small kid's ball, rolled-up towel, or bag of frozen peas (wrapped in plastic and used for only 20 minutes) to place in the small of your back when sitting for additional lumbar support.

GET SHOT. A cortisone shot in your lower back can help reduce pain. When the steroid is injected around the spinal column, it helps reduce the inflammation. It's thought to do so either through the medication itself or simply from the fact that fluid is injected. Talk to your doc about this treatment.

SIGN UP FOR REHAB. The key to recovery from back injury or chronic back pain is working with a specialist who can develop a good rehab program—so you can build your back better than it was before. These specialists focus on muscles upstream from the injury, since it's the weakness in those muscles that eventually leads to imbalances that culminate in the holy-Crayola moment. (Much leg pain can actually originate from problems in the back, since the nerves to the leg and foot traverse the small spaces from the spine in your lower back.) Predicting the best exercises for your recovery requires a physical medicine specialist who understands the asymmetries of your body. These folks have tons of knowledge about how our muscles (and habits) pull a body out of balance—making us human slingshots ready to blow out our backs.

By the way, research shows that active exercise (you working your own muscles) tends to be more beneficial than passive therapy (such as massage and spine manipulation), which is particularly effective for reducing symptoms that may be preventing you from getting moving. More important, this movement may prevent additional or recurring injuries. Certainly, spine manipulation is better than just rest but way inferior to active therapy. And be patient, since it takes time to build up surrounding muscles. It may hurt in the beginning, since these muscles aren't used to being exercised. The data suggest that actively exercising the very core muscles that have pain 20 minutes three times a week for 10 weeks is the fastest way to be pain free for a long time, and much better than hanging out on the couch.

PICK IT UP. Bending over might work if you're playing offensive line for the Browns. But in most cases we all make the same mistake every time we accidentally drop a crumb, paper, or binky on the living room carpet. We bend at the waist and pick up whatever it is we need. But basic physics would dictate that 90-degree flex is the source of a lot of trouble. The 90-degree flex puts the most strain on that cheese wedge in your back—which means the flex is more likely to cause the cheese to crack and ooze out or a piece to break off and rub against your nerve. Instead, bend at the knees into a squat position and then pick the object up. This is another reason lunges and squats are good exercises: They keep the leg muscles strong so you can use good technique when picking things up. Or just walk around with a pooper scooper (a clean one, preferably) or one of those handy-dandy reach-assist things, so you rarely have to bend over.

ROLL AROUND. Use your spare tennis balls for something other than Bluto's game of fetch. Put one or two balls in a sock. Put the sack under the painful spot in your back and lie on the balls. It works like an ultrafocused deep-tissue massage on the area, sans the hands of Sven.

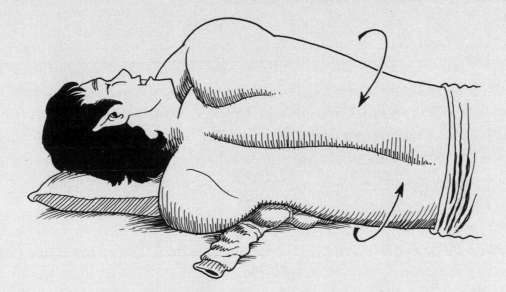

Part 2

Joint Pain: Revel In The Joy of Flex

Most of us treat our joints like our uncles—we take them for granted. So forgive us for a second while we think of what life would be like without them. No turning, no twisting, no bending, no typing, no yoga classes, no craning our necks to gawk at beautiful passersby, no sex positions involving the backseat, no running, no playing leapfrog, no nothing—except a life of stiltlike or snakelike movements. As soon as our joints start to deteriorate, however, we're well aware of their importance. Maybe you can't lift the bag of dog food anymore, or maybe your knee pops every time you bend down to say your prayers, or maybe your ankles feel as crackly and crumbly as stale piecrust.

There's a good reason for that. We didn't start out as a species standing upright (or being able to perform tango steps or dunk from the free-throw line), and because hardly any of our ancestors lasted longer than 40 years, there was never any need for our joints to function beautifully for longer than that. Now, of course, that's not the case, and you need those joints to do everything from tie shoes to thumb-type on your BlackBerry phone. To be able to use your joints—and enjoy all that life plans on offering for the next few decades—you need to know how they work and how to keep them bending as smoothly as possible. Joint injuries are only predictable with 20/20 hindsight, and sometimes we wish we protected them better in our youth. So read on to learn how to minimize the pain.

Your Joints: Motion Is Lotion

The light changes to red. You mash down the brake pedal, but it feels soft. Later you get the news: Your brake pads are completely worn down, and it'll cost you hundreds of dollars to replace them. Not so bad, you think; they lasted 30,000 miles. Now substitute a 55-year-old, stiff, painful knee joint for the brake pad. Like its car counterpart, the knee has simply worn down due to prolonged use. Simple, right? Though it's tempting to compare the wearing out of a machine to

YOU Test

Add Flex

Flexibility is like real estate—it all depends on location. Some people can twist their necks around like a horror-movie monster, while others probably have hamstrings that are tighter than football pants. If you want to test your flexibility, try these exercises. But do not force them or elicit pain—the YOU tests are not designed to cause you disability, just to test your current state, so if you have doubt, do them only with the guidance of a professional. You can also perform these tests routinely to improve your flexibility.

FOREARMS. Place your hands against each other upside down with the backs of your hands against each other (see figure) for 30 to 60 seconds. If any numbness or tingling develops on the surface of the thumb, index, or middle finger, it may mean you have carpel tunnel syndrome.

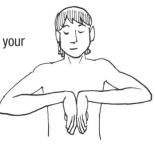

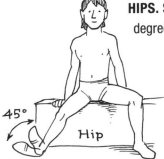

HIPS. Sit and rotate your legs approximately 45 degrees in both directions. Normal rotation is 45 degrees.

45°

Hip

SHOULDERS. Test both internal and external rotation of the shoulder. Reach behind you with one arm and touch the opposite shoulder blade. Reach up over your shoulder, touching your reaching hand to the inside of the same shoulder. If you can't reach those points, you likely have tight muscles or weak rotator cuffs.

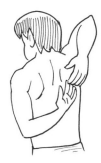

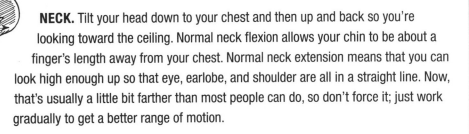

NECK. Tilt your head down to your chest and then up and back so you're looking toward the ceiling. Normal neck flexion allows your chin to be about a finger's length away from your chest. Normal neck extension means that you can look high enough up so that eye, earlobe, and shoulder are all in a straight line. Now, that's usually a little bit farther than most people can do, so don't force it; just work gradually to get a better range of motion.

the wearing out of a body, the similarities are at best superficial. Both are more vulnerable to breakdown the older they get, but in very different ways.

You could think of gasoline as "food" for the car, but the gas doesn't become part of the car. In humans, about 60 minutes after you've downed a cheeseburger, it's well on its way to becoming a new lipid plaque in one of your blood vessels, or part of a muscle—part of you. We're constantly renewing ourselves; the car is not. The car isn't growing new brake pads (at least not yet), ready just in time to replace the old ones. To stay beautiful, humans have to renew their joints.

Human joints are subject to wear and tear from the minute we start to use them, but for the first few decades of life, our body's repair mechanisms can keep up with the damage. When we begin to feel the effects, it's more likely due to less-effective repair and regeneration of what has been worn down than to just accelerated wear and tear. To understand, let's take a look inside our joints.

Joints—particularly hinge joints such as the elbow and knee—are made up of bone, muscles, synovial fluid, cartilage, and ligaments (see Figure 7.4). They're designed to bear weight and move the body. Here's how the different parts function.

Collagen. A type of tissue that serves as the scaffolding upon which everything else is built.

Tendons. They're collagen fibers that attach muscles to bones.

Ligaments. These soft tissues connect bone to bone. Joints with few or weak ligaments, such as the shoulder, allow more motion (and provide more work

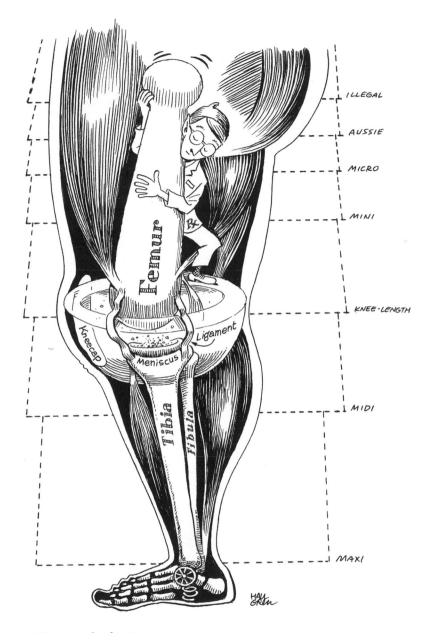

ILLEGAL

AUSSIE

MICRO

MINI

KNEE-LENGTH

MIDI

MAXI

Figure 7.4 Nice Joint As you age, the soft tissues in between your bones can deteriorate, leaving you at risk for crushing your meniscus and painful bone-on-bone grinding that can severely limit the way you move. The vulnerability of your joints can be decreased by having strong surrounding muscles that can absorb some of the shock and wear that come from everyday living.

for orthopedic surgeons), while joints with more supporting structures, such as the sacroiliac joint, are more stable but have a smaller range of motion.

Cartilage. It gives us form before our bones are mineralized after birth—and continues to give structure to our ears and nose. In the rest of the body, it serves as the glistening plate of soft tissue at the end of bones that prevents bone-on-bone clanking. Articular cartilage (the cartilage between bones that acts as the body's shock absorber) does not have a blood supply of its own, so it needs to get nutrients from the surrounding synovial fluid. The meniscus—cartilage that's especially vulnerable to injury—works as a key shock absorber in the knee.

Synovial fluid. The surfaces of the bones that touch each other are covered in articular cartilage and are bathed in synovial fluid—joint oil, if you will. In a normal, healthy joint, the articular cartilage is smooth, and the synovial fluid is as pure as spring water. Cells called chondrocytes in the articular cartilage help to repair and regenerate the cartilage as it wears away. Glucosamine, synthesized in the body from glucose, provides the building blocks necessary for chondrocytes to repair the damage and affects the rate of breakdown of the cartilage. Like most things, your body balances putting new fluid in with getting rid of the old fluid. But if a joint becomes injured or inflamed from wear and tear, you can produce too much synovial fluid, which leads to painful swelling. Over time and as we age we produce less synovial fluid and our cartilage breaks down. The

FACTOID

Uric acid is the most abundant liquid antioxidant you have. It accounts for as much as two-thirds of all free-radical-scavenging capacity in the blood and may be able to help prevent damage from a stroke, but it can do a real number on your joints. Uric acid can form crystals that wind up in the fluid in your joints. These crystals mar the smooth cartilage surface as a diamond would scrape a piece of glass. The result—the joint condition called gout (which can also come from your parents, medications, renal disease, and eating a rich diet full of meat and red wine)—is the price we pay to keep the free radicals away. Glucosamine and chondroitin sulfate seem magical in reducing the uric acid and treating the pain.*

*We state "seem" here because there are not enough data to determine if these really work well or magically or do not work magic for the typical patient.

breakdown of cartilage and loss of synovial fluid can lead to painful bone-on-bone grinding because of the loss of your shock absorbers. The knee is especially illustrative in this case. Your knees each have two shock absorbers that form the shape of a C—called the medial and lateral menisci. They should be plump like grapes, not dried out like raisins.

Over time, your joints can take a beating from a variety of things—from running too much, from weighing too much, or from playing too many contact sports. And as you age, the shock-absorbing cartilage and synovial fluid thin and you gradually lose their protective cushioning—just as old running shoes lose their ability to absorb shock and minimize pounding.*

Nevertheless, don't give up on exercise. Muscles suspend the bones in joints, so the bones don't touch each other and there's less pressure on the joint. When muscles get weak, joints deteriorate and bones lose their ability to slide smoothly, so they end up rubbing against each other like stick on stick. When you have pain, you start hobbling and your muscles immediately get weaker, so when you start moving around again, guess what? The ability of your muscles to suspend your bones is lost and you feel bone hit bone with only the thin Teflon cartilage in between. That process triggers painful inflammation, which can make even walking tough. Joint deterioration (osteoarthritis) is so prevalent that it already affects 40 million Americans. Osteoarthritis can occur in any joint, including your hips, hands, and spine. But there's a prevalence of joint deterioration in the knees—mainly because we rely on them so much to carry our body weight up stairs, around the house, and everywhere we go.

---

*We should quickly note that there's no proven link between running and the joint condition osteoarthritis.

YOU Tips!

Oh, you might think that to protect your joints, you have to treat them like superstars—pamper them, guard them, let them soak for hours in warm, rose-petal baths. While there's some truth to that, you do have to let joints do their job. And with that, you will experience some wear and tear over the years. The key, however, is to find the middle ground between exercise and rehabilitation. There are also specific things you can do to help protect your joints from injury and expedite repair when wear and tear take their toll.

CHECK YOUR BOTTOM. One of the largest and most preventable causes of joint destruction and ligament tears is misalignment (it happens more in women, who generally have wider hips). If your bones and joints are slightly misaligned, which is common in people who walk bow-legged or knock-kneed, or if you had a leg bone fracture that was displaced, or if you don't have what you think is typical range of motion in a joint, get yourself to a physical therapist who specializes in this area. In the meantime, you can get some insight into your biomechanics by looking at the wear pattern of your running/walking shoes. You should see two wear patterns on the bottom of the shoe—where the heel strikes and where the forefoot (front of the foot) falls. At the forefoot, if the wear is to the extreme inside, that means you're a pronator (rolling your foot in). If it's to the extreme outside, that means you're a supinator (you don't roll in enough). Running shoes are constructed to compensate for and correct some of these biomechanical issues.

COVER YOUR FEET. Invest in the right kinds of shoes. Your feet don't have natural shock absorbers, so some of that shock you experience when you're walking will go right up the leg to the knee. That's why it's crucial to have well-cushioned walking or running shoes when you'll be on your feet for extended periods of time (even if you're just standing). Running shoes are usually a good option because they're well cushioned in the back—where your heel strikes the ground first and absorbs most of your body's weight. We suggest that you go to a specialty running shoe store, have your shoes fitted by an expert, and buy a shoe that's made for your particular gait. Try on at least five pairs and walk around. Pick the one that feels the most comfortable. And comfortable, supportive shoes aren't just for exercise anymore; look into the myriad of cushion-soled shoes that you can wear to work.

HIT THE WEIGHTS (AND THE MAT). Resistance training not only strengthens your muscles and bones and helps you burn fat but also helps your joints. In addition to reducing the weight your ankles, knees, and hips carry (every pound less you weigh, your knee and ankle joints carry four pounds less going uphill and seven pounds less going downstairs), resistance training increases the protection and shock absorption you get from strong muscles surrounding your joints.

FLEX MORE. You also need to increase the flexibility of your joint-muscle units, so that you're better able to adapt to the awkward positions that life may put you in. Strength training itself does not increase flexibility, but yoga does and also builds strength, balance, and elasticity—so that muscles can better absorb shock in a shorter range of motion. Our program starts on page 361.

SPIN FASTER. Biking at rapid revolutions appears to strengthen cartilage without the dangers of injuries that you can get from some weight-bearing and running exercises. Plus, look at any biker and you can appreciate the thickness of his or her quadriceps. Remember, the muscles surrounding (above and below and alongside) your knee are the shock-absorbing differences between you and a squished knee.

SAVE YOUR KNEES. The best gift you can give to your knees (not to mention your heart and your pants) is dropping weight. Being overweight or obese—or, as we call it, waisted—exponentially increases the risk factors associated with a host of diseases and conditions, including joint pain. Having extra weight on board leads your cartilage to break down faster, even in the fingers, which don't bear the burden of carrying the pounds. Why? Because fat is hormonally active and stimulates inflammation, which affects all of your joints.

The second-best gift: being careful about playing high-impact sports. People who have knee injuries have a five times greater chance of developing knee arthritis sometime in their lives than those who don't. High-intensity or high-impact sports—such as high-intensity aerobics, aggressive skiing, and basketball—increase the risk and damage associated with osteoarthritis.

HAVE SOME RICE. If you do experience joint pain or related strains and sprains in the surrounding soft tissue, it's best to follow the RICE protocol:

Rest. Stay off the injured area.
Ice. Ice the area of injury (a bag of frozen peas on the injured area for 20 minutes four times a day is ideal for keeping inflammation and swelling down. Put it inside a plastic baggie to avoid messiness when the pea bag breaks, as it eventually will. Protect your skin with a thin washcloth or towel).
Compression. Wrap the joint in an elastic bandage to help support weakened tissues. Fit it snugly, but not so tightly that it causes pain or cuts off blood supply.

Elevation. When you're at home, keep the injured part up off the ground (higher than the heart) to decrease blood flow and prevent swelling.

Now, rest means taking a break from the tennis or basketball court right away, but it doesn't mean lying on the couch all day. The optimal healing of ligaments and cartilage actually requires some movement. That may cause some pain, but the flip side is that staying totally immobile can lead to joint stiffness, weakness, and undernourished cartilage—meaning that the ligaments, tendons, and other supporting structures can lose their strength and form. So you need small movements to increase blood flow and promote healing. We call this biomechanical stimulation. The trade-off for this activity or stimulation is that the little bit of pain you may feel in the short run will give you optimal flexibility and strength in the long run. That's why many walking boots and braces these days allow you to have some range of motion (casts not so much). This, of course, is an example of a biological trade-off, like breaking an addiction or dieting: The short-term pain is small compared to the long-term gain, which can be huge.

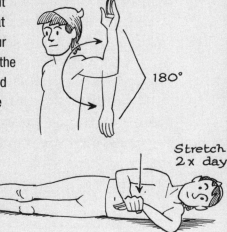

180°

Stretch
2 x day

GET CUFFED. To prevent a shoulder injury, one of the most important things you can do isn't wearing shoulder pads (they don't look all that swell with silk blouses after all). It's strengthening and stretching your rotator cuff muscles to help give you a good range of motion around the joint. To test your own range, stand with your arm out to your side and your upper arm parallel to the floor (as if you're taking an oath on the witness stand). Without moving your upper arm, rotate your shoulder forward and backward—you should be able to get at least 180 degrees of rotation. If you can't, try this move to help give you some flexibility: Lie on your side with your upper arm on the floor and your elbow bent at 90 degrees. With the opposite arm, push down on your hand and hold the stretch for 30 seconds.

GET WET. If it hurts too much to walk, exercise in a (preferably) warm swimming pool. The buoyancy of the water takes the weight off your joints and allows you to recondition. Pool exercises have been shown to be as effective as land exercises for healing arthritis, as well as being less painful (and more fun) to do.

OIL UP. Turns out that fish oil is good for joint oil. The good fats found in fish such as salmon and mahimahi, and in walnuts, canola oil, flaxseed, avocados, and DHA supplements as well as the omega-9s and/or polyphenols in olive oil, are good for just about every part of your body. Omega-3s are believed to help provide lubrication that the joints need to function at an effective level while decreasing inflammation. By keeping the joints lubed, you experience less friction, less grinding, and less pain as you age. Another bonus: Fish oil (DHA—docosahexaenoic acid, for you chemistry fans—is the key component) and fish protein have been shown to regenerate the membrane of the meniscus, which can help if you suffer a painful tear or have chronic meniscus discomfort. If you don't like fish, try fish oil capsules—about 2 grams a day is the equivalent of 13 ounces of fish a week (and usually comes without the contaminants some fish have). Even better, if you just want the active oil with even less chance of impurities, you can take smaller capsules of DHA; all you need is 400 mg for women and 600 mg for men. You can get these purified, from algae (also called a vegetarian or plant source). That's where the fish get these oils from. If you're taking fat-soluble vitamins such as vitamin D3 and want to absorb them, you need some fat in your stomach and intestines first—so taking DHA before the rest of your vitamins helps absorb the fat-soluble ones.

POP THE JOINT SAVERS. Glucosamine, which is naturally synthesized in the body, is critical to formation of collagen and preservation of cartilage, which can then better flex and absorb shock. Since glucosamine levels decrease with age, injury, and stress, it's smart to supplement with glucosamine sulfate at 1,500 mg a day. Chondroitin is also a building block for cartilage and is often given at 800 to 1,200 mg a day. Adding methylsulfonylmethane (MSM) at 2,500 mg a day helps absorption of glucosamine while also decreasing inflammation. Cartilage regenerates slowly, so you need to take the supplements for six months before declaring the experiment a success or failure. Avocado-soybean unsaponifiables (ASU) also have demonstrated some evidence for decreasing inflammation and stimulating cartilage growth. (There are conflicting studies; some indicate great benefit, and other studies show none.) A few of our patients swear that either or both of these (glucosamine-chondroitin and ASU) preparations saved their joints.

SAY HY. Hyaluronic acid (HA), a skin filler, also has another use: It seems to improve the quality of synovial fluid as both a lubricant and a shock absorber. Because oral hyaluronic acid is broken down into simpler substances and can't get into your joints, it has to be sent there by your doc through a needle. HA in the form of Synvisc or Hyalgan coats the surface of cartilage to help it maintain its strength, and it may help to prevent inflammatory cells from entering into the joint space when there is damage.

ADD VITAMINS AND MINERALS. Vitamins D3 (1,000 IU a day), C (500 mg twice a day, less if you're taking a statin), and E (400 IU a day, 100 IU if you're taking a statin) have the potential to protect against damage to connective tissue, especially when buttressed by calcium (600 mg twice a day) and magnesium (400 mg a day). Research shows that people consuming high amounts of vitamin C have up to a 70 percent reduction in risk of osteoarthritis. High vitamin C intake levels have also been found to be associated with a reduced risk of knee pain. Vitamin D3 is essential for calcium absorption and is a very common vitamin deficiency.

PUT A CHERRY ON TOP. Bing cherries have been shown to reduce inflammation and may help with arthritis pain. They contain substances with anti-inflammatory properties. Have a couple of Bing cherries—fresh or dried—a day. We're told cherry juice works, as well. Add boswellia (aka frankincense) at 1,000 mg a day and willow bark so you get 120 to 240 mg of the active component called salicin, which is also, by the way, the active component of aspirin—we like the aspirin itself. That's a powerful herbal mix for settling down inflammation.

GET A SECOND OPINION FIRST. When it comes to joint injuries, healing with steel is not the first choice, unless your athletic career depends on it. The major benefit of surgery is to remove the pain quickly so you can rehab the joint immediately. An alternative approach for a lot of people is to skip the surgery and still rehab the joint immediately. Option two requires a gentle approach for the first two months, but it's nice to avoid losing a piece of you (even if it's only your meniscus). But always get a second opinion from someone not associated with the first doc—as sometimes leaving the damaged meniscus or cartilage part can cause more damage.

YOU Tool: Orthopedic Injuries

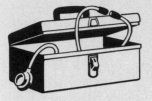

We all know the downsides of being couch potatoes—not enough exercise and way too much TV. But there can also be some downsides to being more active than a Labrador puppy. This tool will help you decode very common muscular aches and injuries, so you can figure out how to help heal your body—to make you feel beautiful.

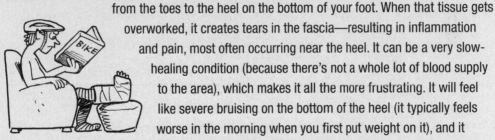

PLANTAR FASCIITIS. One of the most common injuries among runners, this condition doesn't just affect those who gallop for a living or for recreation. The result: intense pain in the foot and heel (and a lovely-looking limp to boot). The plantar fascia is a thick bundle of tissues that runs from the toes to the heel on the bottom of your foot. When that tissue gets overworked, it creates tears in the fascia—resulting in inflammation and pain, most often occurring near the heel. It can be a very slow-healing condition (because there's not a whole lot of blood supply to the area), which makes it all the more frustrating. It will feel like severe bruising on the bottom of the heel (it typically feels worse in the morning when you first put weight on it), and it typically happens because of overpronation of the forefoot (rolling the front of the foot too far to the inside). To stretch and strengthen the area, sit in a chair with your affected foot crossed over the other leg, so your ankle is resting on your knee. Grab your toes and bend them up toward your shin. This will stretch the fascia to help relieve or prevent some of the pain. Make sure you get good running shoes that can help control your overpronation; cushioned heel inserts and rubber-soled shoes can help. You may also want to add anti-inflammatories.

ANKLE SPRAINS. These constitute 20 percent of all sports injuries. No wonder, since the ligaments in the outer ankle aren't very stable. The treatment is RICE (see page 201), and to recover, you must include strengthening exercises. The aim is to regain full range of motion by bending your ankle in all four directions and then doing so while pushing against it as it goes in those directions. You'll need to strengthen the surrounding ligaments and muscles as well, such as those in the back of the ankle, since they are dynamic stabilizers of the joint. Proprioception—knowing where you and your limbs are as you move around—is also important to help you regain motion, so practice walking with your eyes closed.

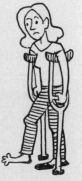

ACL STRAINS AND TEARS. These days, it's not just football players and skiers who are tearing the anterior cruciate ligament of the knee. A lot of people are doing it—and menstruating women are doing it eight times more often than other people. Why? Two reasons: Because women have wider hips, the angle of the femur into the knee is sharper, making them prone to putting more torque on the ACL when they abruptly start and stop. Then, during menstruation, hormones (progesterone and relaxin) cause the soft tissue to become like a wet rubber band—and thus more likely to rupture. In order to keep pressure off the ligaments, it's important to build muscle around the knee (for example, in the quadriceps and hamstrings), so your muscles—and not the joint—can take on some of the force that you'll experience, be it through sports activity or tripping on a curb.

ACHILLES TENDONITIS. This happens when you torque the Achilles tendon, which connects the two large muscles of the calf to the heel—usually by rotating the knee and foot in opposite directions. This tendon, which is the largest and strongest tendon in the body and can withstand a force of 1,000 pounds, is especially vulnerable when you increase your training dramatically (or fall into a hole). After a tear, you'll need surgery and/or immobilization. You can reduce the chance of tears and inflammation with stretching and by warming up the area, along with wearing good, stable shoes.

HAMSTRING PULL. The hamstring—a group of muscles that support the hip joint and attach to the lower leg—is injured by overuse, especially if you're overstriding during a run. Reinjury rates are 80 percent because scarring of injured areas creates more tension, so stretching after a warm-up is especially important. Stretch by putting your foot on a chair and leaning forward while bending at the hip until you feel tension in the hamstring. Hold for a minute and switch legs.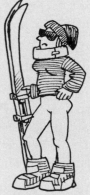

GROIN PULL. This partial tear of the adductor muscle group (your inner thigh) between the pubis bone and femur is especially common when the muscle is cold and you've overexerted yourself. Stretch and strengthen the area by lying on your back and spreading your legs (i.e., the butterfly position). Allow your knees to fall apart so you feel the stretch. Put a ball between your legs and squeeze to strengthen.

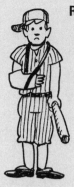

ROTATOR CUFF STRAIN. The rotator cuff consists of four muscles and their tendons that originate from the scapula and form a cuff over the upper end of the arm (head of the humerus)—your shoulder joint. The cuff helps lift and rotate the arm and stabilize the humerus within the shoulder joint, and it's vulnerable to tears after a fall or after repetitive overhead arm activities. You can prevent the injury by strengthening the area. And never lift weights without being able to see your hands.

Part 3

Headaches: Noggin Problem

Some headaches are debilitating enough to send you right to bed. Other headaches? They prevent any funny business from happening once you're there. Though headaches can range on the pain scale from annoying to debilitating, they do share one important trait: They make you feel like mushroom fertilizer—and, except to pigs, that's not a beautiful sight. No one looks healthy or feels beautiful when their hands have a vise grip on their temples.

So what can you do? Pop a few pain pills and hope the pounding stops? Not quite. To lessen the throbbing, let's first take a look at the primary kinds and causes of headaches.

As you can see in Figure 7.5, much of the biology of headaches stems from the function of a nerve that sounds like the name of a Jedi knight. The trigeminal is a large nerve that comes directly from the brain and divides into three branches to cover the face. A variety of triggers can stimulate inflammation and irritation of this nerve and surrounding tissues. And that erupts into the pain we sense as a headache. Another major cause is a dilation of blood vessels. Too-large blood vessels can be painful themselves or can cause pain by allowing various chemicals to ooze slowly out of the blood vessels and seep into the tissues around and in the brain and cause inflammation.

About 15 percent of us are born with a small hole in our heart called a PFO (patent foramen ovales). If that hole doesn't close, blood shunts right past the lungs to the brain. (If it doesn't close naturally, it can be subsequently

FACTOID

Some of the vitamins, minerals, and supplements that may help prevent headaches include the herb butterbur (50–75 mg twice a day for prevention or 100 mg every three hours for the first three doses during an active migraine), vitamin B2 (riboflavin at 400 mg in the morning), coenzyme Q10 (200 mg three times a day), and magnesium sulfate (200–400 mg twice a day—less if you have loose stools). There's a hung jury on the effectiveness of these, but if you have chronic problems, they may be worth a try. They take six weeks to work.

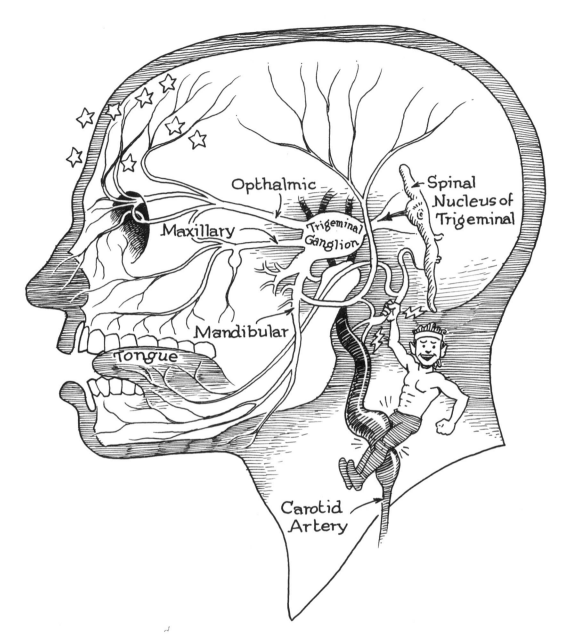

Figure 7.5 A Real Pounding The exterior cause of your headache may be the kids or the job, but the interior cause is the trigeminal nerve, which branches out to three other ones. Various triggers can cause irritation of the nerve, as well as dilation of the arteries, which contributes to the pain and the pounding.

Pressure Points

Yes, let your fingers do the talking. Developed in Asia more than 2,000 years ago, acupressure works when your fingers press points on the body that release muscular stress. Get a shiatsu massage, or do it yourself next time your head is pounding. However, lots of the experts warn against using these points if you are pregnant.

- **Belly of your temporalis muscle:** Located in the center of your temple region. Palpate this region with your first and middle fingers pressed closely together until you find a tender, muscular zone. If you have trouble locating this point, place your fingers against your temples and then clench down on your molars a few times. You should feel the main belly of your temporalis muscles bulge in and out.
- **Behind the ears:** Locate the points at the base of the skull in the back of the head, just behind the bones in back of the ears, and apply rotational pressure for two minutes with your thumbs.
- **Between the eyes:** Pinch the tissue just above the nose with your middle finger near one eye and the thumb near the other and slowly push upward so you feel the pressure near your eyebrows.
- **The hand web:** Using the thumb and index finger of the other hand, apply a pinching pressure to the soft fleshy web between the thumb and index finger, on the back of the hand.

closed with a procedure using a catheter threaded from the groin, in which an umbrella-shaped device is fed up through the body and covers the hole.) Maybe you didn't know it, but the lungs serve to detoxify and clear a lot of irritating chemicals from the blood. Without going through a detoxification process in your lungs, those chemicals can go right to the brain to trigger headache pain by dilating brain arteries.

During a headache, levels of the feel-good chemical serotonin drop. This may cause the trigeminal nerve to release substances called neuropeptides, which cause blood vessels to become dilated and inflamed. In migraines, serotonin first elevates, then drops—making you even more sensitive to pain (remember the pain threshold test on page 175). Migraine medications mimic serotonin or block serotonin reuptake so cells can use it more effectively, and they also stop the release of those neuropeptides to prevent the dilation of blood vessels.

When thinking about a headache, treat it like a perp in a police lineup: Make a positive ID. Head-

FACTOID
It may seem that the only value of a migraine is to keep an overactive husband on the other side of the bed, but they actually do have another survival value as well. People who get migraines tend to be meticulous people who are acutely aware of their environments, so they're extrasensitive to pain and everything around them. That sense doesn't serve a huge purpose now, but way back when, it came in handy when these people could use this sixth sense to intuit whether predators or other dangers were threatening the tribe.

aches can come in lots of forms, and knowing which kind you have will help you stop it and prevent it from happening again. The first thing to do is make sure you don't have a secondary headache—that is, a headache that's not the problem itself but rather a sign of another potential health problem, such as severely high blood pressure, infection, stroke, sinus problems, temporomandibular joint problems, a hole in your heart, a brain tumor, or an aneurysm. It can be helpful to have a doc figure out the cause, but you can assist big-time by identifying the triggers of your headache. Keep a log that has the date, time, and what you did and ate for the immediately preceding 48 hours (and, if you're a woman, what time in your menstrual cycle it occurred). If you can find out what committed the crime, you can execute it before it attacks again. The three most common primary headaches are:

Migraine. If you've experienced one of these, then you don't need us to tell you that it feels as if your gray matter is going to ooze out of every orifice in your head. These disabling mothers of all headaches—which occur in 17 percent of women and 6 percent of men—also may come with the add-ons of nausea, tingling in your arms or legs, an aura (flashes of light), the smell of ammonia, or tingling beforehand. Stress, bright lights, a change in sleeping patterns, coffee, chocolate, medication, even changes in the weather have all been linked to migraines. The two biggest triggers: food and hormones (not on the same plate, mind you). Some dietary culprits include aspartame, MSG (monosodium glutamate), chocolate, aged cheeses, nitrates, and alcohol (especially beer and red wine). And, although the link isn't perfectly clear, it does seem that many women seem to experience migraines when there's a fluctuation of estrogen (before or after their periods, during the first trimester of pregnancy, postpartum, and at perimenopause). And great sex is reported to make migraines better, though you might have a problem readying for sex if you can't stop vomiting.

Tension. You know how your belly feels after Thanksgiving dinner when your belt is too tight? A tension headache is the same feeling, but in your head. With 9 out of 10 women and 7 out of 10 men experiencing a tension headache sometime during their lives, it's clearly one of the most common pains around. The good news is that it's usually not there all the time and is usually mild or moderate, not drop-to-the-ground severe, like migraine pain. It used to be thought that tension headaches came from muscle tension, but it's now believed these headaches occur when fluctuations in serotonin and endorphins activate

The Story of Jaws

Nearly 10 percent of the population suffers from pain in the temporomandibular joint (TMJ, so the disease is called TMD). The TMJ is the joint between the upper jaw (called the maxilla) and the lower one (mandible) that purposely dislocates itself with every bite to increase your chewing force. The TMJ is like a hurried business exec—it's constantly on the move. It moves when you're eating, moves when you're talking, moves when you're kissing the neck of your beloved. The edges of these jawbones are coated with slippery connective tissue that allows the bones to move, almost like a silicone pad on a chair leg.

If you have some pain in your jaw, you can actually diagnose the problem yourself (untreated, it can lead to headaches, tooth and gum disease, and other problems). Open your jaw. If you feel pain, hear a pop, or can't open your mouth fully, that means you've got some kind of joint problem (causes can be muscular, joint dysfunction, teeth clenching, poor alignment of the teeth, and stress). You should see a TMJ specialist. Besides medication, mouth guards and massage have been shown to be effective treatments. And more recently, even Botox has been injected into the muscle that clenches the jaw to help relieve the pain.

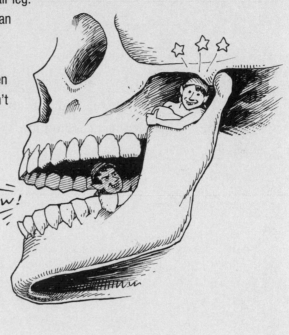

pain pathways in the brain. Tension headaches have more triggers than a rifle range: stress, lack of sleep, skipping meals, bad posture, clenching your teeth, medications, and being about as active as a comatose slug. Your role if you're susceptible to a lot of headaches? Isolate the triggers to see if you can ID the cause and avoid it.

Cluster. The least common of the major headaches, the cluster headache is the surprise party of the bunch—it comes with little warning (but no party hats!) and bunches or clusters (thus the name). It strikes quickly, and the pain is sharp, burning, and excruciating within minutes; people who have them describe the feeling as being like a hot poker being stuck in the eye. Pleasant,

Do You Have a Tic?

Another painful condition that can affect the head and face is called trigeminal neuralgia (TN; also called tic douloureux). This involves a disturbance of our old friend and nemesis the trigeminal nerve and usually affects women over calendar age 50. At the onset many people complain of a toothache, but the tooth is fine. Symptoms can also include stabbing or lightning bolt–type electrical jolts in the head and face. A telltale sign of TN: The pain is only on one side and one side of the face will often droop, resembling a symptom of a stroke. Some meds, such as anticonvulsants, can help, as can lifestyle and dietary changes. Good news is that many people recover.

we know. The pain may also come with excessive tearing, redness in the eye, stuffy or running nose, and sweating because the autopilot nervous system of the body is often turned on in the neurologic cacophony of the cluster headache.

YOU Tips!

PULL THE TRIGGER. Some of the foods that are known to trigger migraines include coffee or caffeine, wines, cheese, smoked meats, sugar, chocolate, and anything with the chemical MSG. Most of them aren't all that good for the rest of your body, so it should be no surprise that they can wreak havoc on your head, too. If you're prone to headaches and regularly indulge in ache-inducing foods, eliminate them one by one from your diet to see if you can find the link between what you put in your mouth and what you feel in your head. Same goes for some of the other triggers we mentioned. For example, if your migraines might be caused by fluctuations in estrogen, talk to your doc about stabilizing medications that have a lot of estrogen, such as birth control pills—several are available that cycle only four times a year; Seasonique and Seasonale are two common ones. For once-yearly periods, consider Lybrel. While you can treat your headaches with pain meds (see next tip), the better course of action is to find the cause and stop them from occurring in the first place.

STOP THE PAIN. For many people, the natural reaction when they experience pain (after yelping) is to reach for the pill bottle. And that's okay. Here are your OTC choices: ibuprofen, aspirin, and medications that are marketed for migraines (they include acetaminophen, aspirin, and caffeine,* which are actually as effective as Imitrex can be). But if OTCs don't work, your doc may opt for a prescription-strength version of the same drug or may recommend a popular class of drugs called triptans, like sumatriptan or rizatriptan (an older version of drugs called ergots are cheaper, but they're not considered as effective and have more major side effects).

STOP IT EARLY. Suffering may have been something that got you a merit badge in the Middle Ages, but prolonging head pain today leads you to, well, more head pain. The neurons that respond to pain are like patrons at a free food buffet; they come in waves. If the pain can be stopped early, you close the door on the mad rush of neurons being activated in an ugly way and you gain more control over your pain.

WEAN OFF. Rebounds might be great if your name is Shaq or Yao Ming, but not if you're having a lot of headaches. Many people who experience cranial rock 'n' roll concerts fall into a dangerous trap: You have a headache, so you take pain medication. Fine, but if you stay on it too long, you set yourself up for rebound headaches when you try to withdraw from the medication. You need to limit your pain meds (including OTCs) to less than three days in a row or ten pills total. Any more than that, and you

*Yes, caffeine can be both a trigger and a treatment.

increase your risk of experiencing a rebound headache. Try a three-day detox with no pain meds to reset your system; exercise also helps, since the natural endorphins you get from exercise can counteract the pain.

BE SPECIAL. There are some topics in medical school that students (and subsequently when they become doctors) never revisit again once they learn about them. That's true for headaches: Once the ins and outs and the basic treatment for headaches are presented, those treatments are typically never discussed again. So what? Well, that points to the fact that many docs can get caught in a diagnostic rut when dealing with people whose heads hurt. If you're experiencing headache pain that changes your life, then you need to see a headache specialist—someone who has the most current treatments and insight available. Having fewer than five headaches a year is about average. If you're continually sidelined because of them, you really ought to have your head examined. If you have an excruciating headache—the worst of your life—you may need a CT scan to be sure your noggin is okay.

STRENGTHEN YOUR NECK. Headache pain can come from weakness or spasms of the neck muscles—you feel the pain in your upper back and it goes to your lower neck, then upper neck, as progressively weak muscles compensate for too much computer or bridge time. If the muscles of your upper back are sore, it may be weakness of the trapezius muscle. Getting symptomatic relief and taking analgesics so you can exercise is the first order of business. See our workout on page 351 for moves that will help strengthen the area. Strengthening that area takes five minutes three times a week for ten weeks to reduce such pain by more than 80 percent. Rare types of headaches arise as referred pain from arthritis of small joints between the vertebrae of the neck called facet joints. Exercise, analgesics, and sometimes nerve blocks are required to eliminate this type of headache.

SWEAT IT OUT. Walking, swimming, and biking aren't just good for your heart health, your waistline, and your sexual magnetism. Regular aerobic exercise also means that you'll have less regular headaches. How? It helps relieve stress and increases the levels of painkilling endorphins. Similarly, yoga, stretching, and meditation also help reduce tension and thus relax the chemical wackiness that can cause headaches.

Female Pains: Cramping Your Style

Periods are great when they come at the end of sentences, not necessarily when they come every 28 days. As you and the people you live with are fully aware, the menstrual cycle can come with a fair share of side effects—the most common of which is known as "primary dysmenorrhea." * Essentially, that's marked by the recurrent, crampy pain that occurs in the lower abdomen during menses. Cramps are thought to be caused by decreased blood flow that accompanies prolonged uterine contractions to get rid of the excess uterine lining when an egg doesn't implant. The decreased blood flow means the tissues don't get enough oxygen, and that causes pain.

Of course, these cramping symptoms and other side effects such as mood swings are part of your three least favorite letters in the alphabet—PMS. Several different theories exist about how PMS symptoms occur. Some say that PMS symptoms are brought on by changes in estrogen and progesterone levels that occur during the menstrual cycle. Others say that PMS is caused by an inability to properly metabolize fatty acids, by a calcium deficiency, and even by the use of chemicals, fertilizers, and pesticides. So which is right? Probably a little bit of all of them. And that can often make PMS a PIA to treat. Now we do know more about causes and effects. For example, women who have more pain and cramping are ones who smoke, have longer cycles, irregular or heavy menstrual flow, and a BMI under 20. Luckily, the flip side is also true, and you can do plenty to keep the cramps and other side effects at bay.

> **FACTOID**
>
> Breast cysts lead to a lot of pain, fear, and biopsies, and they're thought to be present in 60 percent of women and believed to be associated with ovarian hormones. To help, you might try reducing dietary fat and limiting caffeine.

REDEFINE PMS. Instead of calling it premenstrual *syndrome,* think of it as premenstrual *supplements.* Why? Because you can reduce your pain and symptoms with some of these choices by taking them for the entire month. For menstrual pain: vitamin B6 (4 to 6 mg a day), magnesium (200 mg twice a day), and omega-3 fatty acids (2 grams a day, or 600 mg of the DHA version). And avoid all foods with saturated and trans fats.

For PMS prevention: magnesium 200 mg twice a day, vitamin B6 (200 mg a day), plus borage oil or evening primrose oil (3,000 mg a day for 4 months), and then for the week before your period. Give this recipe three months to start working.

---

* Sounds awfully close to "primarily, the men are diarrhea," oddly enough.

Problems Down Under

Vaginal pain can come from a number of different problems, including immune issues or even excessive use of antifungal medications. Vulvadynia—a collection of various ailments, which manifests itself as pain or discomfort around the vaginal opening—can be tough to diagnose. (It's actually like back pain in that way.) Different from pain that's associated with deep penetration (which is usually caused by fibroids), vulvadynia keeps women from enjoying (or even having) a sex life. Besides medicine and surgical options, another treatment focuses on increasing blood flow to the area, since reduced blood supply causes some of the pain. Kegel exercises (targeting the muscles you flex when you stop your pee midstream) can be helpful. Avoid excess hygiene like douching, scrubbing, and soapy baths. The reality is that it can be a difficult condition to treat, and women suffering from it see an average of three docs before getting a diagnosis. Since there are no skin changes, it's tough for gynecologists to pinpoint it. See a pelvic pain specialist if you have these symptoms. Some women find that applying a bag of frozen peas to the area around the vagina helps reduce inflammation and ease some pain.

GET THE NEEDLES. Acupuncture, which has been shown to be effective for many pains including back pain, is also a good option for menstrual pain. Traditional Chinese medicine suggests that PMS is caused by a basic energy imbalance in the body, and acupuncture can help restore that balance (and provide instant relief from cramping).

GO 12 TO 1. On average, women today have 400 menstrual cycles in their lifetimes. Historically, they had 100 cycles during adulthood (you do the math, assuming 12 pregnancies and breast-feeding for a year for each child). So it's really not that far-fetched to imagine cutting down the number of cycles per year. How can you do that? By using birth control pills—several are available that cycle only four times or even once a year.

More Pain Relief

Quick Tips on Two More Big Pains in Your Life

Irritable Bowel Syndrome

Funny name, irritable bowel syndrome. Think about all the other diseases and conditions there are, and none of them is named like this one, with an adjective describing the organ. We don't call heartburn "angry esophagus syndrome." We don't call depression "melancholy hypothalamus disease." And we surely don't call erectile dysfunction "stubborn penis condition." But get yourself some innards that growl, grumble, explode, and erupt, and you've got yourself one irritable bowel.

Most of the people who have irritable bowel syndrome (and there are plenty of them, with 10 to 15 percent of the population suffering from it) know they do through the very persistent— and very frustrating—symptoms that go with it: the bloating, the cramping, the pain. Some people experience constipation with IBS, while others experience the opposite effect and get diarrhea. And some people flip-flop between the two extremes, living in a world where one moment they couldn't poop if they tried and the next moment they couldn't stop it if they wanted to. Irritable indeed. That's because the gut is where one of the body's most intense civil wars takes place. It's where your body has to interact with, process, and react to all kinds of outside chemicals and nutrients—not to mention with the gazillions of foreign bacteria also living there.

People with IBS experience some dysfunction of the immune and nervous systems that regulate the lining of the bowel; this lining (called the epithelium) is what regulates the flow of fluids into and out of the intestines. When stuff moves too quickly from start to finish, the intestines can't absorb fluids from it (hence it ends up in the toilet). And when the last meal moves too slowly, the bowel absorbs too much fluid (hence it stays in your system). The second aspect of IBS involves the neurotransmitter serotonin (which is found primarily in your gut, with only a small amount in your brain). People with IBS have abnormally low levels of serotonin, which causes all kinds of digestive problems and makes these people more susceptible to feeling pain when those problems arise. To be specific, even if you have exactly the same amount of gas as the next gal, you will sense more pain if your serotonin levels are low. Similarly, the same stress that everyone else feels will cause you depression if your brain serotonin levels are low (see Chapter 8). (Irritable bowel, by the way, is not the same as acid reflux; to treat that, elevate your head at night and be careful not to eat acidic food late at night.)

Potential culprits for spastic colon and irritable bowel syndrome are hidden infections that we historically have not checked for. Colleagues of ours who specialize in this area look for two main ailments:

- **SIBO (small intestinal bacterial overgrowth).** The small intestine gets the first shot at digesting food and should not have as many bacteria in it as the colon. If your bowels are sluggish, the bacteria can move upstream to the small intestine, causing the bowel symptoms. These doctors use a hydrogen breath test (HBT) to look for SIBO. If it is positive, taking an antibiotic such as rifaximin (400 mg a day for 7–10 days) will often eliminate the spastic bowel. If the sluggish bowel is not treated, it may come back. A low thyroid (despite normal labs) is a common cause of SIBO, with half of those with a low thyroid having a positive HBT.
- **Yeast overgrowth.** Although still a controversial area, many holistic physicians (see www .holisticmedicine.org) find that treating for yeast overgrowth in the gut will eliminate both spastic colon and sinusitis (the yeast causes swelling in the nose). This means avoiding sugar (which feeds yeast) and taking probiotics plus 6 weeks of the antifungal Diflucan at 200 mg a day.

Some tips for easing the pain:

- If your gut twists and turns like an amusement park ride, you need to throttle down. And one of the best ways to do that is to eat foods that help calm the entire digestive process. If you're suffering from IBS, eliminate foods that are high in fat or fried foods, alcohol, caffeine, carbonated drinks, and gum (swallowing air makes matters worse). Instead, substitute foods that are high in fiber, and don't forget to add loads of water.
- Many people with the diagnosis of spastic colon actually have difficulty digesting milk (lactose intolerance) or sugar. There are some ways to test for the problem, but it is easier to simply avoid all milk and sugar (especially sodas) for a week and see if the symptoms go away.
- The worst thing you can do to an angry bowel is to make it angrier. So your job is to make the little fella as happy as can be. One way: Eat slowly and regularly—to avoid the roller-coaster highs and lows that come from overeating and starving. You can also identify eating issues (as well as trigger foods) by keeping an eating diary that allows you to pinpoint the patterns that make you feel better or worse.
- Peppermint doesn't just come in handy to neutralize a garlicky meal. It also helps calm the digestive system by relaxing the smooth muscles in the intestines.
- Probiotics are probably your best allies. The best (in spore form so the stomach doesn't destroy them) come in small capsules at less than $10 a month. We like Digestive Aide,

Digestive Advantage, and Sustenex, which decrease IBS symptoms (some believe that one of the causes of the condition is a lack of good bacteria in the intestines). Also, decrease inflammation and strengthen your team of fighters. We may sound like a broken record, but much research supports the use of omega-3s (2 gm a day of fish oils or 400 mg of algal DHA for women, 600 mg for men) and vitamin D3 (1,200 to 2,000 IU a day) in IBS.

Neuropathies

In a lot of cases, tingling can be a very good thing. But in this case, a little tingling can cause a whole lot of problems. Pain and numbness in the body's nerves—primarily in the hands, feet, and face—are called neuropathies. They're typically classified by a tingling sensation that feels a lot like when a part of your body falls asleep or when you hit your funny bone (numbness or pins and needles). What's happening in this case is a malfunction of the nerves—either peripheral nerves like ones in the hands and feet, or central ones like in the spinal cord. If you think of your nerves as electrical cables covered in protective sheaths, you can see how this numbing happens: When something causes the sheath to constrict, it puts a lot of pressure on the inside cables and wires. And that disruption of messaging (as in conducting electricity) causes the nerves to short-circuit, leading to your tingles. So what causes that constriction? Lots of things, unfortunately, such as diabetes, nutritional deficiencies, and cancer chemotherapy.

The big problem with neuropathies isn't necessarily the tingling or numbing itself but rather the domino effects if you don't break the cycle. For one thing, the pain can worsen and eventually become debilitating. For another, the numbness can mean that you're more susceptible to developing infections (if you cut your foot on a stray shell and don't feel it, you don't know the cut is there, so it gets dirty and infected). And that's not even mentioning that neuropathies can lead to bowel and bladder pain, itching, and numbness—and that, well, is about as fun as it sounds. Luckily, you can help improve the symptoms with such things as exercise, avoiding secondhand smoke, and following other guidelines for healthy living. Some tactics:

- If you're feeling numbness in various parts of your body, don't assume it's your only symptom—even if it's the only thing you're feeling at the moment. Neuropathies are a sign that something else is happening inside your body, so you'll need tests (such as for diabetes) to determine the root cause. Docs can also prescribe certain medications that can help relieve the pain (some classes of antidepressants and antiseizure medications have been shown to be effective).

- If you have neuropathy, you can strengthen the surrounding sheath to improve the ability of messages to travel from the brain to your limbs. How to do it? By taking omega-3s and some vitamins. The best vitamins for strengthening the sheath are B6, B12, and folic acid. But remember, it often takes months to regenerate this protective covering, so be patient. In addition, lipoic acid (300 mg) plus acetyl-L-carnitine (1,000 mg twice a day) is also often helpful for nerve pain.

- A more extreme approach: The nerves have sheaths on them (like sausage casing). There's been some success with surgery that cuts the sheath to free the compression of nerves. To see if you're a candidate, a doc will tap your nerves to see if it re-creates the symptoms.

- While you're still diagnosing the problem, it's vital that you protect your hands and feet so that you decrease your risk of developing—and then not being able to detect—an infection. That means wearing gloves in the yard and sandals or water shoes around the beach, and never sticking your hands or feet in places you wouldn't want your kids to go either. Most important, work to control your blood sugar because diabetes is a major cause of neuropathies.

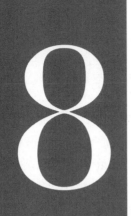

8 Get in the Mood

What You Can Do to Straighten Out Your Mind

With more than 6 billion people on the planet, it'd be a pretty boring place if we all loped around like robotic machines—each with the same appearance, the same fashion sense, and the same preference in coffee flavors. There'd be little spice in life if every single person was a five-foot-four, purple-skinned, helmet-wearing latte lover. The beauty of life centers around the fact that we're not just different from one another, but that we're quirkily different. We have nuances, subtleties, and personality traits that make us three-dimensional. Some of us are laid-back, some are stuffy; some of us think jokes about bowels are funny, some don't; some of us like sports, some like soap operas; some of us like chicken parmesan, and some like chicken parmesan only if it's grilled with no cheese and served with extra sauce.

In fact, minor versions of personality quirks are part of what makes us beautiful. You can be very sensitive on the way to becoming depressed, you can be very thoughtful on the way to becoming compulsive, and you can hold yourself back from acting out inappropriately and escalating interpersonal conflict on the way to becoming passive-aggressive. But extreme versions of mental illness destroy our sense of self-worth and make us feel ugly and useless.

If you look into your own personality stew pot, we're sure that you (and your family and friends) can pick out the main ingredients—the stock that forms your core moral and value system, the chunks that form your personal characteristics, and all the subtle aromas that give you the heat and flavor to make you the only one of your kind.

In this chapter, we want to take a deeper look into the emotional roller coasters you may be riding to find out if there are any ingredients that don't belong or if you've added too much spice in some key areas. That is, we want to explore the areas in which personality quirks and traits can develop into things that actually can be harmful to you and to others. Namely, we want to talk about things such as depression, addiction, and other behavioral disorders that stem from the mind—the things that can make you feel "off" in life.

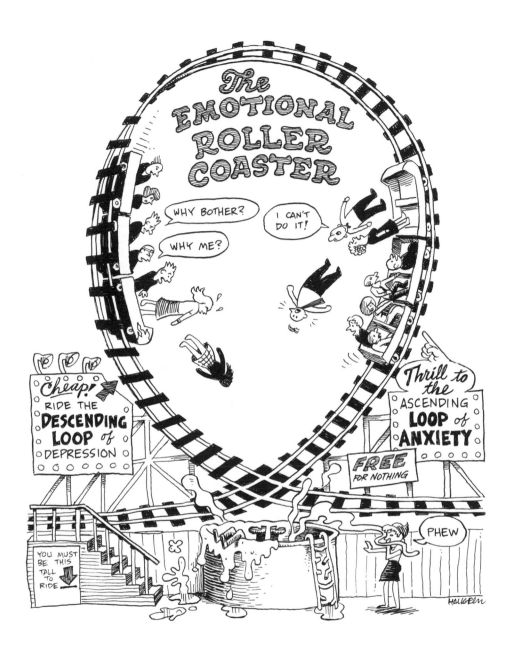

Figure 8.1 On a Roll Personality disorders and depression are often characterized by severe ups and downs—and extreme ends of the emotional spectrum, especially when it comes to fear and anxiety. In smoothing out the highs and lows, talking about problems with others and developing a greater sense of community seem to have a major benefit.

YOU Test

Are You Depressed?

While diagnosing depression isn't always easy, you can get some insight into whether your foul mood is due simply to hormonal or situational issues as opposed to a more clinical state of depression. Ask yourself the following questions. If you answer yes to more than two of them for more than two weeks in the last month, it may be a sign that you should talk to your doc further about your symptoms that may be associated with depression.

Are you unsatisfied with your life?
Do you often get bored?
Do you often feel helpless?
Do you prefer to stay at home rather than try new things?
Do feel worthless the way you are now?

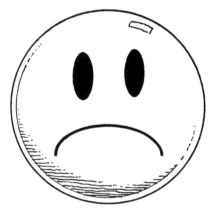

The biology of such mental problems involves your neurological gatekeeper—the part of the brain called the amygdala. Almond-shaped, the amygdala takes all of the information from the part of your brain called the thalamus relay station and pushes it to the cortex—the part of the brain that helps you make decisions, such as running out of a burning home. It's the amygdala that assigns meaning to that smoke alarm—so that you actually jump when you hear it (see Figure 8.2). How? The amygdala assigns emo-

FACTOID

Scientific studies have shown that as many as 40 percent of divorces are caused by genetic factors that affect personality and behavior. The relationship between personality and divorce is clear: Extroversion is related to risk of divorce, particularly in men. Neuroticism elevates risk of divorce for both men and women.

tion, so that the alarm isn't just some buzzer from some appliance affixed to the ceiling. That buzzing and beeping means your little derriere might be best off humping it right out the front door. And here is where the beautiful biology shines through. The amygdala recognizes that there might be an emergency; the cortex decides what to do about it. So, in essence, your amygdala establishes what science-heads like to call "salience"—that is, it chooses which stimuli or pieces of info to prioritize.

The cortex is the rational part of the brain; the amygdala is the emotional part. The amygdala controls fear and anxiety, which are at the root of most emotional disorders. While the amygdala can send lots of messages to the cortex, the cortex can't do much in return; in fact, in adults, the amygdala has ten times more neurons headed toward the cortex than it receives. So we can't *will* ourselves to be calm just because we want to. Right? We can't *will* ourselves out of depression, we can't *will* ourselves not to wash our hands 300 times a day, and we can't *will* ourselves away from a powerful addiction. But what you can do is understand a little more about how these emotional disorders work and learn ways to flip the switch so that we reduce our fear and anxiety.

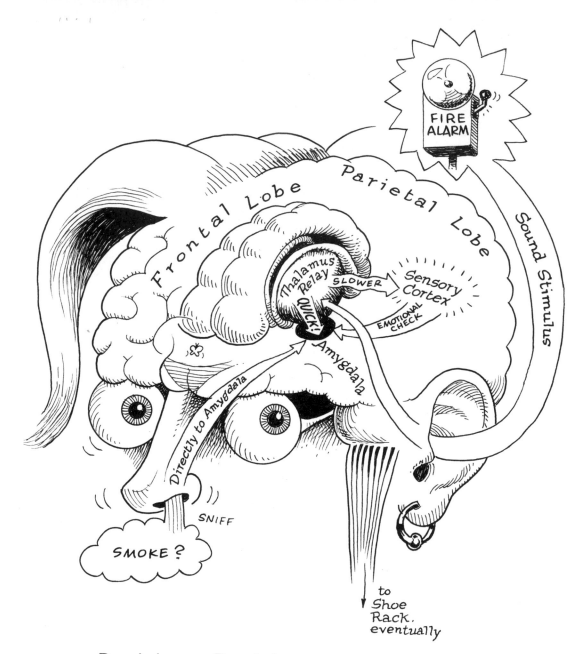

Figure 8.2 Decisions, Decisions The thalamus relay station dumps information more quickly into the amygdala than the cortex. Therefore, the emotional part of the brain (the amygdala) makes our initial decision before the rational side (the cortex) even gets a chance. So, we're hardwired to react emotionally to people and situations. That response is heightened in people with emotional issues.

Mood Swing: Depression

We all throw around the word *depression* with the same nonchalance with which we get a cup of coffee. You're depressed because the Buckeyes lost. You're depressed because *Sex and the City* ended. You're depressed because your doughnut-addicted friend wears size 4 jeans.*

But when you say these things, you're actually referring to daily ups and downs—not more global or long-term alterations in mood. Clinical depression is not a momentary sadness but a persistent feeling of despair triggered by an imbalance of chemicals in your brain. Yes, it's a physical disease—and one with potentially lethal outcomes. Suicide is one of the top four killers of Americans between the ages of 15 and 44. While the elderly overall are less depressed (and happier) than their younger counterparts, white men over 65 have a suicide rate five times higher than that of the general population. Women try more often, but men succeed more often (if you know someone with suicidal tendencies, get them help now).

We have to start thinking of depression the way we would any so-called tangible health problem, such as heart disease or cancer. Catch it early, and you've got a good shot at curing it. Let the problem linger, and you'll increase the chances that your brother-in-law is going to be drafting your eulogy pretty darn soon. The myth about depression and other mental conditions is that they're "soft" diseases, that you can will yourself out of them, that all you have to do is suck it up and be happy, dagummit. But depression isn't a "mental" disease—you can't control it, as you can your moods; it's a "chemical" disease, no less a threat to your health than HIV/AIDS or diabetes.

Depression is associated with all kinds of

FACTOID People tend to think that bipolar disorder is one disorder, but it's actually more a kaleidoscope of different personality disorders. People who suffer from it typically have extremely elevated moods (and along with them, high energy) and also suffer from extremely depressive moods. Genetics play a huge role, and medications can help sufferers find more of a middle ground, rather than the extreme opposites of emotion.

* The high-metabolic witch.

Boys and girls cry an equal amount until age 13, and then guys cut down to once a month while gals stay at once a week. The women must realize that tears lubricate the soul. According to the research, crying may serve as a request for help or to communicate the presence of a problem such as hunger, pain, or loneliness, and it may serve as a signal of empathy. Tears flow in response to watching a fellow human being in trouble, as well as through some sort of destressing mechanism after arousal. Technically, the parasympathetic nervous system is what shoots out tears via nerve messages. The program is especially active when people experience moods and emotions characterized by helplessness—which explains why we cry when we're sad or hurt. The actual content of tears, in case you're wondering, is a chemical cocktail of various hormones such as estrogen and prolactin (the same stuff that helps women breast-feed offspring) and proteins. What's even more amazing is that the substance of tears actually differs depending on whether the tears are generated by emotions or simply for the purpose of lubricating dry eyes.

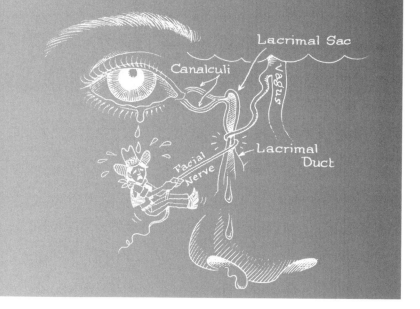

life-altering symptoms, such as lowered mood, lack of self-esteem, lack of interest in sex, weight changes, sleep problems, and fatigue over a period of two or more weeks. Depression suppresses your immune responses so that you're more vulnerable to infections. It increases inflammation in your body (your CRP levels—a marker of inflammation—more than double, in fact). It increases your chances of cardiac disease (maybe through disrupting your automatic nervous system), which means that you have a higher chance of developing lethal arrhythmias. And if that's not enough to make you feel less than marvelous, we don't know what is.

Here's the stunning stat of the day: About

15 percent of us have clinically significant depression at some time in our lives. Depression, particularly as we get older, can be especially confusing to diagnose. For one thing, it shares many symptoms and is often diagnosed in tandem with anxiety. For another, depression is often associated with dementia* and other physical illnesses. Depression is associated with increased physician office and emergency room visits, increased drug use, and high costs of health care. Plus, depressed mood may be the first symptom of a number of medical conditions including stroke, diabetes, cancer, hypothyroidism, heart failure, and other heart diseases. Depressing, isn't it?

Depression is reported to be more prevalent among women, but that may be because women are more often classified as depressed, while men are classified as alcoholics (that's because men are more likely to self-medicate their blues with the bottle). So, although the prevalence of diagnosed depression is higher in women across all age groups, this may be an artifact of how depression is defined and symptoms are elicited (men are more likely to present with anger, irritability, withdrawal or apathy, and alcohol abuse, and less likely to acknowledge sadness or psychological symptoms).

The truth is that depression is a lot like hot sauce—there are all different kinds and nuances, but they can be dangerous just the same. There's postpartum depression, which 10 to 15 percent of recent mothers experience. There's seasonal affective disorder, which is brought on by lack of exposure to sunlight—most notably in northern climates during the winter (although some people have the reverse pattern—a summer depression with improvement in the winter). There's depression brought on by medications, ranging from steroids to narcotics to alcohol to sleeping pills, which suppress dopamine and serotonin, mimicking the chemical reactions that cause depression. Generally, depression is classified in three categories:

Major depression: This is a major depressive episode longer than two weeks with at least five of the seven following symptoms:

* Dementia's nickname is actually pseudodepression.

- sleep alteration
- decreased interest in activities
- feelings of guilt
- decreased energy
- difficulty concentrating
- alteration in appetite
- thoughts of suicide

Situational depression: Greater than two months with the above symptoms after suffering a significant life change, such as bereavement or retirement. Significantly, your symptoms improve with time after the major event, so most therapists feel that your long-term functioning is better if you can manage to get through this without drugs.

Vascular depression: Depression that commonly occurs after a brain or blood-vessel disorder, such as a stroke, or after a heart attack or heart surgery. Patients with lesions in the left hemisphere of the brain, especially of the left prefrontal cortex, tend to have increased frequency and severity of depression. The greatest risk period of depression following a stroke appears to be the first two years afterward, peaking within the first three to six months.

Some believe that depression may be related to an abnormality in the functioning of hormones in the brain. That's because people with severe depression tend to have higher levels of the stress hormone cortisol, and the size of their hippocampus actually decreases (see Figure 8.3).

Though different kinds of depression may be brought on by different triggers or may have different symptoms, depressed minds have similar qualities. Most of us tend to think that depressed people must have brains that are murkier than a muddy pond—that they can't think straight, that they're not able to put life's ups and downs in perspective. Yet the opposite is true. Depressed people see the world extremely clearly (and accurately for them); they have a very crisp perception of reality, which is why they often feel down—because they see life's toughest moments so vividly. Because of their hypersensitivity, depressed people are often quite

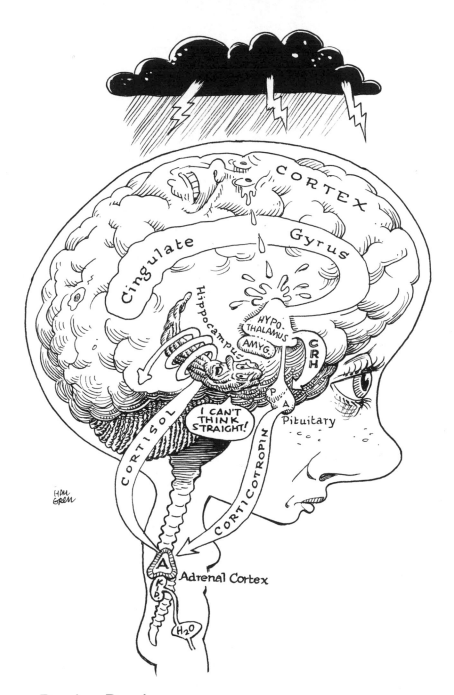

Figure 8.3 Brain Drain Stress hormones affect the hypothalamus and shrink the size of the hippocampus, showing us that depression can be both a hormonal and a structural issue.

creative. Lots of beautiful people, artists (Hemingway, for example), and some very productive statesmen (Abe Lincoln) thrived between episodes of depression. Another silver lining in all this? There's actually a survival benefit to depression, in that it gives individuals the self-awareness to know their limitations and not take certain risks—the old idea of knowing when to hold 'em and when to fold 'em.

While some signs of depression are self-evident, many of us hesitate to call ourselves depressed. We'll write it off as being too tired or too stressed or justifiably sad because Boozer, our 18-year-old cat, couldn't hang on anymore. But here's the thing: Depression is actually one of the ways that your body sends a signal to you that something isn't working quite right—and that you should be thinking of coping strategies to get your mind and body on the right track. One under-the-radar symptom of depression is that early-morning awakening (we're talking 3:30 a.m., not 5:15 with a normal 5:35 alarm clock). While most of us would say that's simply a sign of stress, it's actually one of the more subtle signs of depression. If you experience it chronically, and not because you have to pee, it's something worth mentioning to your doc.

Depression is trickier than a David Blaine stunt because some of the symptoms are on the subtle side. Your doctor—trained to be a medical detective—can put together a good treatment plan, but only if she knows the whole picture. In an exam, she'll ask you about medical problems that could be related to depression. But you also want to be up front about your recent history—the changes in your life that might not be medical but can certainly influence your mood. While it may sound as though you're going to confession, you should talk to your doc about major life events (such as deaths in the family or financial stresses, and, yes, changes in sexual pleasure or frequency), as well as changes in job and family situations (retirement, for example).

Sometimes you might need medication. Listen, if you have an infection, you take an antibiotic. If you have a headache, you take a pain reliever. If you tear your ACL, you rehab it and/or get it repaired. So if you have a chemical imbalance in your brain that's altering your mood and leaving you bluer than pen ink, you should get it treated. Your doc will prescribe drugs that best match your symptoms. Your doc may prescribe medication based on symptoms alone, or she may do further testing, such as blood tests to ensure you are not short on normal quantities of thyroid hormone and B12, which are linked to depression, as well as brain imaging in some cases.

Antidepressant drugs should rarely be given without psychotherapy because they dull us to the realities of life. In some cases, they're essential to turn back the tide. Typically, they take three to six weeks to have substantial effects. This delay occurs because the brain accommodates (or appears to accommodate) to the accumulation of drug in the brain. Thus the drugs are usually used for six to nine months for the first episode of depression. (The recurrence rate after that is the same whether you continue the medication past nine months or not). Recurrent episodes require longer-term treatment. Selective serotonin reuptake inhibitors (SSRIs), such as Prozac and Zoloft, are especially effective if you're experiencing anxiety. SSRIs work by boosting serotonin in the brain, with one nasty side effect—decreased libido.* That can be addressed with a few options, including decreasing the dose, switching to another SSRI, switching to a different class of antidepressant drug, or using a second drug to offset the sexual side effects. Viagara seems to work for both women and men. Other side effects of SSRIs include nausea and weight changes.

Good non-SSRI choices are Wellbutrin or Remeron, which appear not to have much of an effect on sexual function or desire. Different drugs affect different parts of your brain, which is why you should discuss changing drugs or drug classes with your doc if you're feeling that you're sacrificing quality of life at the same time you're trying to restore it. Remember you have to tell the doc; she can't

---

* Which can be depressing in itself.

guess which side effects you're having, if any, and which are bothersome or not to you or to those with whom you associate.

Let's Get Personal: Other Emotional Issues

Look around your home, office, or neighborhood. We bet you can quickly rattle off five people you've thought were just a little bit off. Auntie Hilda has 4,000 apple decorations around her house. Bob from the next-door cubicle folds his papers into fours before he puts them into the trash. Old man Johnson washes his car four days a week and twice on Saturdays. The question really becomes: Are these people suffering from a disorder, or are their actions simply part of who they are? Good question, and sometimes hard to answer.

We do know that emotionally based disorders are estimated to occur in about 18 percent of the population and that these people fail to see themselves as others see them. And that means that their behavior—whether it's lining up paper clips just so, being afraid to be in rooms with more than three people, or keeping the Weather Channel on approximately 17 hours a day—is labeled as sick, not to mention making them very unattractive to possible partners.

The end of this spectrum—obsessive-compulsive disorder—means that those affected suffer from a fear that the worst is always going to happen (which is why they take such precautions as washing their hands so often). And for these people, their fears interfere with their everyday lives (these people are different from those labeled as compulsive, who may be perfectionists and highly organized). Often accompanied by depression, obsessive-compulsive disorder can be quelled with medication, support groups, and even a form of therapy called exposure therapy, in which sufferers must confront their worst fears. Ironically, a fear of life prevents them from living life.

The consensus is that all of these kinds of mental issues are caused by a mixture of genetics, general temperament, and childhood experience. This is the important point: You need the genetic predisposition, but you also need the environment. That is, someone with naturally low self-esteem can develop personality problems when exposed to the wrong environment. But again—though not always—you can control your environment.

Without question, we're all unique creatures, but researchers have found that there are some common patterns associated with personality types, broken down into five categories and each, of course, consisting of various degrees of that characteristic. When these types reach the high end of the scale, it may be a sign that it's more than just a trait; it is a type of disorder.

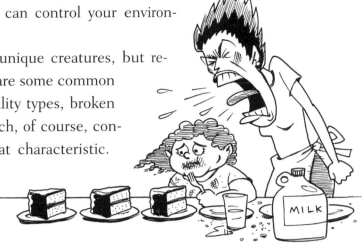

Extroversion. You know them well. They're loud, they drive fast, they approach strange ladies at the bar, and they're unafraid to be the ubiquitous lampshade wearer at the company party. They like talking and actually tend to be happy.

Agreeableness. This "Kumbaya" group is the "never say no" type. They'd rather negotiate than fight. They'd rather retreat than engage in conflict.

Conscientiousness. Look over there at the next cubicle: Julie is busting her tail, working on next month's report. Conscientious people work hard, are on time, and are reliable. No surprise that this group of do-gooders also reports greater job satisfaction and more positive relationships.

Emotional stability. What's the marker for this? How people handle stress. Are they the rock that can think through a situation in an emergency, or do they shrivel up into a pool of protoplasm the minute a crisis comes? The stable person stays the course with a steady mood, while emotionally unstable people get more tired throughout the day because they're constantly battling life's ups and downs.

Openness. People who are open to new ideas and new things process information a little bit differently. They're stimulated by everything, meaning that they don't mind experimenting with new foods, new vacation spots, even new extramarital affairs. Those who are less open have more tunnel vision—because it's easier for them to ignore all the stimuli that are competing for their attention.

So, back to the big question: How do you know whether old man Johnson is a wacko or just really likes his car? How and when does a quirk become a form of craziness? The standard is whether that personality trait causes adversity in your relationships: Does it hinder your ability to do a job or form intimate bonds like all the other beautiful people?

One other thing worth mentioning about personality disorders: In the right dose, these disorders can be incredibly important. Think back especially to our ancestors. Someone who was bold and assertive would be able to fight off predators. Someone who was obsessive-compulsive could build a weatherproof hut. Someone who was paranoid likely saved her family from threats that would be undetected by others. You just have to figure out whether these traits cross the line. Washing your hands after you go to the bathroom is a good thing. Doing it ten times in a row so that the skin sloughs off and you look like a horror-flick monster? Not so good. In the tips below, we'll help give you some guidelines to help you figure out if you or someone you love is more than just a little bit kooky.

The Crave Rave: Addictions

We all know people who have their boutique "addictions"—they may say they're addicted to eBay, *CSI*, or all things Cheddar. You can love something, adore something, and want to surround yourself with that thing, person, or experience at all times, and automatically you say you have an addiction to it. And you just may. While there's nothing terribly wrong with being addicted to some things (like the smell of your lover), there can be something terribly wrong and destructive if you're addicted to booze, drugs, plastic surgery, shopping, porn, gambling, or any sauce including the word *alfredo*.

Much in the same way that the diagnosis of personality disorders can be unclear, so can the diagnosis of addictions. Is it an addiction or just a whole lot of love? Generally, you can tell if you or a family member has an addiction if their behavior falls into three categories:

- They have a compelling need to engage in that behavior or activity.
- They lose a little control as a result of the use or activity.
- They continue to do it even if there are adverse consequences (such as causing conflicts in a marriage or job).

We get addicted to such things as nicotine, caffeine, and whiskey through the reward-seeking chemical of dopamine. As you can see in Figure 8.4, addictive substances stimulate the release of dopamine in a key area of your brain that makes you feel higher than a mountaintop. The way you can tell whether you're prone to addiction is by assessing first-time use of alcohol/nicotine/nudie magazines. If that first-time use took you to a rapturous place (rapturous, as in it feels better than your best orgasm ever), then it's likely you have the genetics to get hooked on something. But you can get hooked even without the genetics.

Once you get addicted to anything, the dependence is either physiological, psychological, or both. Psychologically, you need the rapture your addiction creates. Physiologically, you'll experience painful withdrawal symptoms if you stop the behavior. In people with nicotine addictions, everyone experiences the physiological dependence, but only a third of people have a true genetic addiction in which the psychological addiction is present. (For our quit-smoking plan, which also serves as a prototype for stopping other addictions, see our YOU Tool.)

Smoking, of course, is the classic example of addiction because not only is it legal, but it's detrimental to your health as soon as you puff (unlike other addictions, which in a nonaddictive form may be OK in moderation, such as alcohol). It's a maladaptive response to stress or something else that is bothering you. Why maladaptive? Because when you finish the cigarette or the chaw of tobacco, the stress or boss is still there. And while the hydrocarbons do damage to the rest of your body, the vehicle of nicotine is the addictive part. Regardless of how nicotine

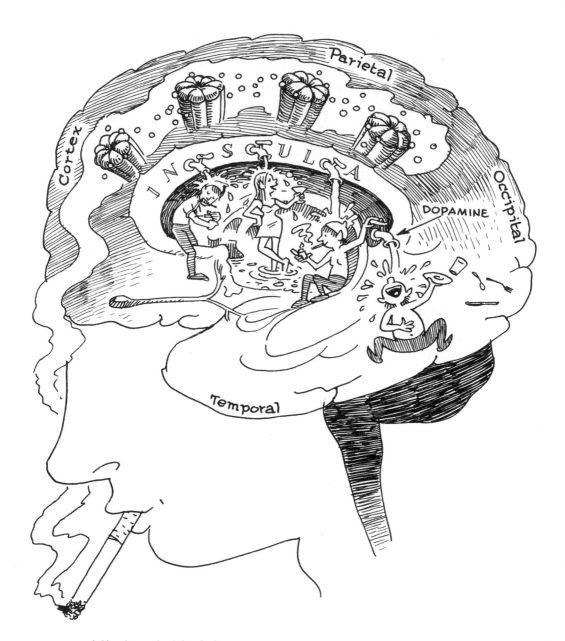

Figure 8.4 Kicked Habit For some people, the insula may be the part of the brain that's nicknamed party central, but it's really the part of the brain that influences your cravings and, along with dopamine levels, helps determine whether habits become addictions. Our addiction-busting plan on page 246 addresses not only the chemical influences on addiction but also the emotional ones.

reaches the bloodstream, it's distributed through the brain and body, where it activates cholinergic receptors. Nicotine changes these receptors so that a regular user needs to continue to get nicotine to have a normal functioning brain—and stopping can trigger withdrawal symptoms. Plus, nicotine stimulates the release of the reward-seeking chemical dopamine—which supports the pleasure that many smokers feel and makes it so dang hard to stop. That underscores the point that addictive behaviors can change our brain chemistry in ways that make the addiction nearly impossible to break (especially with willpower alone).

As you know from TV shows, movies, and perhaps your own personal experiences with addiction, addictions that are harmful to the abuser and the abuser's family are harder to break than Joe DiMaggio's hitting-streak record.* And, unfortunately, addiction isn't one of those areas where you can just pop a pill to make it go away, because all addictions have physical, emotional, and social influences (as you'll see in our Breathe-Free Program). So you often require a pro who can get you off the wrong track and on the right one and a buddy who can help you stay there.

FACTOID Some of the supplements that are purported to help anxiety and depression are omega-3 fatty acids (which are so safe that this supplement should be a no-brainer, and it helps make you brainier—600 mg a day for adults makes a big difference). By the way, the reason that 99.7 percent of infant formula in the United States contains plant-based DHA-omega-3 supplements is that the IQ of infants fed with it is 10 to 18 IQ points higher 6 months and 6 years later than in those who receive nonsupplemented infant formula. New mothers can reduce postpartum depression if they add 600 mg of plant-based DHA-omega-3 (or 2 grams of fish oil) to the daily diet. DHEA (which should never be taken without checking your blood levels first), SAMe, kava root, and Saint-John's-wort also have substantial data supporting their benefit for depression treatment and suppression. We favor DHA and SAMe, as Saint-John's-wort has a lot of conflicting data. You should absolutely discuss SAMe and Saint-John's-wort with your doc, because there can be some interactions with other antidepressants.

*A record that hasn't been broken in half a century.

YOU Tips!

It used to be that people who were depressed were treated with either an admonishment or a straitjacket. But depression and other emotional disorders of the brain are as much a disease as any other health problem out there, and their side effects can be as ugly as a sunken soufflé. These are some of the steps you can take to keep your mind under control.

TALK IT OUT. We're living in a world where there's too much talk—we've got talk shows, talking heads, and people who talk the talk but can't walk the walk. Funny, though, in a hypercommunicative society, many of us can't talk about anything other than sports, soaps, or why the media spends so much attention on (fill in celebrity scandal of the day). The fact is that when it comes to reducing effects of depression, the biggest cure may not be in a pill bottle, but in making sure you don't stay bottled up yourself. In treating minor depression, talk therapy over six weeks is 60 to 70 percent successful, and it's 90 percent successful when used in conjunction with drugs. How does it work? Probably through the release of those feel-good chemicals including oxytocin and learning new coping strategies. One of the more effective treatments for depression is cognitive behavioral therapy. Limited to 10 to 20 sessions, this therapy helps people learn how their thoughts contribute to their symptoms, and it suggests behavioral changes that they can make to change their environment, their response to their environment, and ultimately their thoughts. It doesn't tell you how to feel, but rather, it teaches you how to stay calm and cool when you're upset about a problem, so that you can figure out what to do and how to feel better. (It's why therapists ask a lot of questions rather than make a lot of statements.) But even just talking about your problems with your spouse, friends, or a taxi driver can help. Since women tend to speak much more than men, they may get a much larger brain chemical boost from hashing things out.

GO BANANAS. Eating a banana every day facilitates both cross talk among your brain cells and the effect of certain neurotransmitters (such as serotonin and its precursors). These two effects may mean that eating a banana a day helps keep the therapist away by preventing recurring minor depression. Plus, besides coffee, bananas are our largest dietary source of antioxidants. You read that right.

SWEAT IT OUT. If you haven't exercised in a while, the thought of slipping into a pair of tight pants and a sports bra might seem depressing in itself. Exercise, however, has been shown to be more effective than many antidepressants in reducing major depression. Part of that may be attributed to the endorphin effect of exercise; we feel that the sense of purpose and accomplishment that comes with regular exercise also helps. Sometimes action has to come before motivation, and depressed folks need to act to prime their motivational engine. For some ideas, see our band workout and yoga toolboxes on pages 351 and 361. Yoga, in fact, is specifically associated with decreased depressive symptoms and increased mood—perhaps partly because of the deep breathing that's done during the practice. In a similar way, spirituality is also associated with less depression; much more on spirituality in chapter 11.

RUB ALCOHOL FROM THE SCENE. While some people medicate their emotions with something from the freezer, others do it with something from the bottle. Make sure you or someone you love doesn't have an alcohol problem that's masking a depression problem (or is an addiction in and of itself). You can do so by asking these questions. Answering yes to any of them is a red flag.

- Have you tried to cut down on drinking but failed?
- Have you ever been annoyed by someone criticizing your drinking?
- Have you ever felt guilty about drinking?
- Have you ever taken a morning eye-opener (tailgating parties excluded)?
- Have you ever had a problem with drinking?

USE GUIDED IMAGERY. Guided imagery isn't the screen of your car's GPS; it's actually a way of making you feel better. The technique has been shown to improve the ability to cope with depression, improve mood, and decrease stress. How do you do it? Go to a quiet place (the bathroom often works well, since privacy is usually respected there). Start by relaxing and breathing deeply, then visualize yourself in different scenarios. Some variations include visualizing yourself in a pleasant place (the beach), fighting disease (seeing your good immune cells fighting off bad germs), or practicing for a big performance (doing well in your job). An example of how guided imagery can cure aches and pains: If you're in pain, visualize the spot of pain. Follow the nerve from that spot to the center of your mind. Ask your body if you can take control of that pain, and visualize the way that would happen.

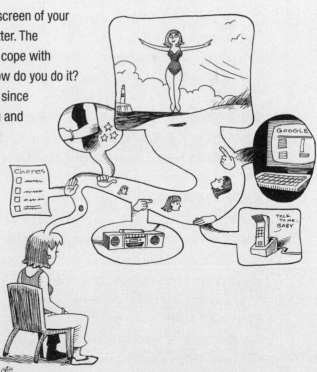

SEE THE LIGHT. People who get seasonal affective disorder have been shown to feel better when they're exposed to specially rated UV lights for the home for 20 minutes a day. Any bright light will serve the purpose, and halogen lights emit the same frequency as those made to treat SAD. Another option: Go to sports events or arenas where there are a lot of bright lights. Anecdotally, these lights seem to have the same effect.

GIVE YOURSELF TIME. Docs are taught that the normal time period to grieve for the loss of a loved one is six months to a year after the death. So it may be natural to experience depressive symptoms during that time. But we also want to make it clear that you should never feel pressure to shake the pain after a certain time period. Illusions are also a part of normal grief. An illusion is a misperception of an actual external stimulus. Delusions or hallucinations are never normal. The key is getting to the point where you can weather the discomfort enough to carry on with other aspects of your life.

TEST YOURSELF. You say he's got a problem; he says there's nothing wrong with brushing every tooth individually 24 times a day. How do you know the difference between nuance and annoyance? These criteria will help you judge whether someone has a personality disorder. They likely do if their behavior . . .

- Is inflexible, no matter what situation the person is in.
- Leads to problems in their work or social life.
- Is not part of some other mental disorder.
- Is not a direct effect of a medical condition, drug, or medication.

GET A COMMUNITY AND A BUDDY. Whether on the Internet or in person, talking to someone helps. In fact, talking and walking 30 minutes a day are the most effective strategies for treating and preventing depression. See more on our buddy plan in the next chapter.

WRITE AT BEDTIME. Approach every day with an attitude of thankfulness. Impossible expectations lead to sadness. Try to write a gratitude journal daily—writing three thank-you notes a day really does make it less likely you will suffer depression. While you're at it, put some music on in the background: research suggests that music can improve moderately depressed moods (one study also showed improved heart rate and blood pressure).

DON'T SAY DON'T. You'd think that repeatedly telling someone not to drink, not to smoke, or not to download pictures of naked women to their work computer would be enough. But your brain can do very funny things. Your brain—specifically the part of the brain that influences cravings, your insula—

hears "don't smoke" and reacts as if it hears "smoke." And that stimulates the craving for smoking. A much better approach when you want to help someone get rid of an addiction: Flip the message. Instead of saying "Don't smoke," say, "Breathe free." Instead of "Don't eat doughnuts," say, "Have a handful of nuts." Instead of saying "Don't look at naked pictures," say, "Want to get naked?"

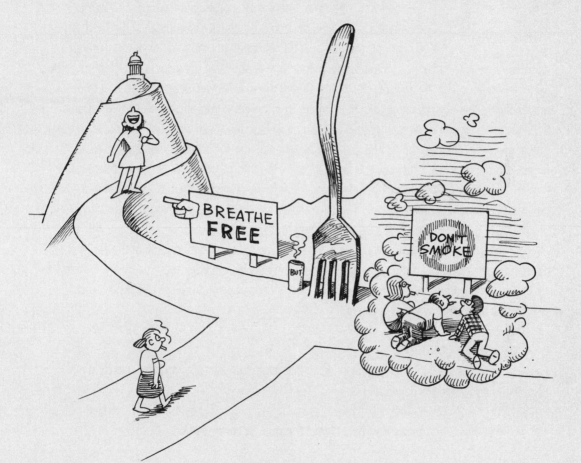

YOU Tool: Breathe-Free Program

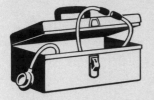

Wait, wait, wait. Before you flip the page as a nonsmoker (good work, by the way), understand that this breathe-free program isn't just an anti-smoking plan. It serves as a prototype for the way you can address any kind of addictive behavior or substance. So read on, subbing in you own addictions to get the idea for how you can address them. After all, stopping the runaway train that is addictive behavior is really about getting rational people to stop doing irrational things. One of the most powerful addictions isn't bridal reality shows; it's cigarette smoking. Here, in our Breathe-Free Program, developed with Daniel Seidman from New York–Presbyterian/Columbia as well as the Cleveland Clinic team, we're going to teach you how to stop the addiction (in our experience, the majority of smokers also have underlying depression). That way, you can gain back the 8 to 13 years you've taken off your life (half in length and half in disability and illness) through those nasty sticks. Yes, you get a do-over here and can make yourself younger even if you've burned your fingers with 20 cigarettes every day. While many addiction-busting attempts come from fear or even insults (to people who may already be suffering from low self-esteem), we want you to reprogram to think of the process as coming from a place of passion and love—where the people who care about you want to help you.

Our four-step program can change a lot of lives, so copy and share pages, or send loved ones to www.oprah.com or www.realage.com.

Step 1: ASSESS YOURSELF
Answer the following questions to see if you've lost control of your smoking behavior and it's turned into a full-fledged dependence.

1. **Have you smoked every day for at least the past several weeks?**

2. **Do you experience any of the following withdrawal symptoms after you stop or reduce your amount of smoking (withdrawal symptoms can begin within a few hours of cessation)?**

   Depressed mood
   Insomnia
   Irritability, frustration, or anger
   Anxiety

Difficulty concentrating

Restlessness

Decreased heart rate

Increased appetite or weight gain

3. **Do you experience significant distress due to the symptoms in question 2? Do you avoid social or work obligations, or leave in the middle of these obligations, due to significant distress or discomfort from not smoking?**

If you answered yes to question 1, yes to at least four of the symptoms in question 2, and/or yes to question 3, then you have a problem and may even meet the psychiatric definition for nicotine addiction. Knowing this can help build your commitment to learning to breathe free.

4. **In the past year, was there a day you didn't smoke at all—not even a puff?**

If you answered yes, think about how you did it and how you then went back to smoking. Try to learn from your experience.

If you answered no, don't despair. The movie in your head about how impossible it is to break free of smoking is greatly exaggerated. With proper use of medicines and a good behavioral plan, it's possible to break free of smoking. We know, because we've helped more than 700 people individually and more than 80,000 using our web-based programs (see oprah.com or realage.com). If you follow our plan and have a buddy to help, we believe your chance of success is over 60 percent each time you try—so three tries will get you to over a 90 percent chance of success.

5. **Do you continue to smoke despite having a tobacco-related medical problem such as bronchitis or COPD (chronic obstructive pulmonary disease)?**

Smokers are well aware of the medical problems associated with smoking. After all, they are listed on every pack you smoke. Even when told it is a matter of life and death, many continue to smoke after having a heart attack, lung surgery, or oral cancer. This behavior mystifies your loved ones and even leaves you, the smoker, bewildered, yet it is a hallmark of addiction and distinguishes it from "bad habits," which also involve automatic behavior. The difference is that bad habits don't predictably put your life in jeopardy—a 20-can-a-day diet cola habit doesn't invariably result in troubles, nor does picking your nose.

6. **Do you get less of an effect than you once did—of pleasure or satisfaction—from the same number of cigarettes each day?**

7. **Do you continue to smoke, even though you enjoy only 10 to 20 percent of the cigarettes you light up?**

   If you answered yes to questions 6 and 7, know that many people get sick of their addiction over time, especially after age 40. What was social and fun becomes rote habit with less pleasure than advertised. Keeping this in mind can motivate you to move forward with breathing free.

8. **Do you still enjoy smoking most or all of the time?**

   If you answered yes, ask yourself if it would be nice to shed the burden of guilt and shame you carry from smoking. Remember, this is your body, and there is only one available for each customer. So even with all the new replacement parts available, you still can't protect your body from the pollution in cigarette smoke.

9. **Do you feel anxious and nervous, and has this continued every day for the past two weeks?**

   If you answered yes, you may have more anxiety about getting through your breathe-free day (the first day without cigarettes). In that case, you may need to pay extra attention to the next step—working on preparation, confidence building, and motivation.

10. **Do you feel sad and blue, and has this continued every day for the past two weeks?**

    If you answered yes, you may have more emotional discomfort after getting through your breathe-free day. Your nicotine withdrawal symptoms might be harder so work out your strategies with an expert.

Step 2: DO THE PREP WORK

You're about to make a big change, one that requires some planning. Give yourself a month (31 days) to do all the prep work.

* **Promise yourself:** Make a personal pact with yourself to quit.
* **Set a quit date:** Make it at least a month from today.
* **Think of the three biggest reasons why you're quitting:** Write them on a card that you can carry with you and look at several times each day.
* **Be assertive:** Eliminate smoking in two or three situations that usually prompt you to smoke.
* **Cut back:** Reduce the number of cigarettes you smoke to one pack a day or less.
* **Go cheap:** Change to a less desirable brand of cigarettes.

- **Need a light:** Discard your lighter and matches.
- **Misplace your cigarettes:** Carry them in a different place than you usually do.
- **Role-play:** Spend a little time each day imagining yourself in stressful situations in which you are not smoking.
- **Take the Breathe-Free Pledge:** See below.

As of _____, my official quit date, I pledge to commit to breathing free!

My reasons for quitting smoking: _____

I have found a buddy I will call daily: _____. I recognize that this may be one of the greatest challenges of my life, but I also know that breathing free is the best decision I can make to protect and improve my health. Upon signing this contract, I make a commitment to myself to breathe free and free myself from the limitations placed on me by my addiction.

I don't know what will happen or how difficult it will be, but I can get help from _____ _____, and I have decided to tell my buddy about my decision to choose one of these (check one):

___ 1. Walk for 30 days and then add nicotine patches (21 or 22 mg if I smoke a pack a day or so) and bupropion (100 mg twice a day—a reduced dose of Zyban)

___ 2. Walk for 30 days and then use nicotine patches (or nicotine gum or nicotine oral inhaler) alone

___ 3. Walk for 30 days and then use varenicline (Chantix) alone

I also know that staying smoke free (not having "just one") after the initial breathe-free period is important, and I have asked my friends and family to support me and not smoke around me. I will also continue to talk daily to my buddy for at least six months, and then I'll become a buddy to others.

By committing to a life of breathing free, I will ensure a healthier future for myself, and I will protect the well-being of my loved ones and everyone around me, who will no longer be exposed to the dangers of secondhand smoke. I know that I am not only motivated but also committed and willing to make the effort to become a nonsmoker.

I deserve to give myself the healthiest life possible and breathe free!

Do these four things (A–D), which will make quitting easier and could be the keys to your success.

A. Start walking 30 minutes a day—every day.

Before you actually stop smoking, you have to establish another behavior—walking 30 minutes a day, every day—in its place. No excuses—you miss a day, you reset the clock to day 1. That is because another behavior takes at least 30 days to form. But after a month of walking, you'll have two of the things you need to stick with our plan: more physical stamina and greater mental discipline.

B. Find a quitting buddy.

Don't quit alone. We know from experience that everyone needs to be encouraged by someone. And your buddy is that someone. But you shouldn't be the only one relying on other people; try to find a support partner who needs you as much as you need him or her.

C. See if you're covered.

More and more insurance plans are offering some level of coverage for quit-smoking efforts. Ask your insurance company about its coverage. And if you aren't insured, ask your HR department—many cover the cost (about $600 for six months; it really is cheaper than a pack a day, but we know dollars spent for medical expenses and smoking are usually segregated in smokers' minds and hearts).

D. Schedule a checkup.

Quitting smoking is physically and mentally stressful, and you want to be sure you have no conditions that might interfere with the tools, techniques, and medications suggested in this program. And talk to your doctor about the following prescriptions to help you stop smoking:

1. Bupropion (Wellbutrin) in 100 mg tablets—one twice a day: Bupropion is an anticraving drug (it's also an antidepressant at higher doses) that can help you make the transition from smoker to quitter. It can interact with other medications, so make sure your doctor's aware of any drugs you're taking, particularly for high blood pressure or seizure disorders.
2. Nicotine patches: Talk with your doctor to figure out what strength would be best for you— for a one-pack-a-day habit it's usually 21 or 22 mg.

Quitting day is almost here—it's time to start getting your body ready to fight future cravings.

- **Start taking bupropion:** On day 30, two days before you'll actually stop smoking, take one tablet in the morning.
- **Keep taking bupropion.** On day 31, take one bupropion tablet in the morning.

Step 3: BREAK THE HABIT

Today's the day you stop smoking. If you've done the prep work, you're ready.

- **On day 32, QUIT:** Throw away *all* your cigarettes, and get rid of all ashtrays and any other smoking-related objects.
- **Put on a nicotine patch.** Place one on your arm, chest, or thigh (you'll be doing this daily for a while).
- **Take your bupropion:** One in the morning and one at night.

Here are your daily to-dos for days 33 through 61.

- **Take two:** Increase your bupropion to two tablets a day—one in the morning and another in the evening.
- **Patch up:** Put on a new one every day. (And don't forget to take the old one off.)
- **Keep walking:** Every day for 30 minutes.
- **Reach out:** Check in with your buddy.
- **Drink up:** Have as much coffee, tea, or water as you wish.

Step 4: ENJOY LIFE AS AN EX-SMOKER

Making it through a month without smoking is a huge accomplishment. It's time to celebrate the new YOU! Here are some to-dos for day 62 and beyond.

- **Breathe in:** Enjoy how quitting has made your lungs happier.
- **Push yourself:** Use your newfound vitality to start a strength-building routine. But take it slowly; don't increase your physical activity by more than 10 percent a week.
- **Love life without the patch:** Every two months, decrease the dose of your nicotine patch by one-third. Your goal is to be patch free after six months.
- **Say bye-bye, bupropion:** But make it a slow good-bye. At five months, decrease your bupropion to one tablet in the evening, and aim to be off it entirely by your eight-month anniversary. Tip: Just in case you feel a craving, for the rest of your life carry one bupropion tablet with you at all times, so you can take it if you need to.

YOU Tool: Finding Your Personality

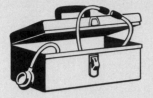 Maybe the only time you ever hear the question "Who are you?" is at a Halloween party. But let's stop for a second so you can ask yourself that question. Who are you? What kind of person are you? Unlike the YOU-Q score, which you can change, this personality test will help you identify some of your personality traits, which really aren't changeable. It's essential information that will help you better interact with the world.

Of course, if somebody were to ask you to describe yourself, you could probably come up with a few words—funny, smart, addicted to *Dancing with the Stars*. But the truth is, many of the deepest aspects of yourself are things that are hard to put a finger on. What makes you unique and complex is the stuff that everyone takes for granted about you. After a while, you take it for granted as well. So let's shine a mirror on the deepest aspects of your personality so you can learn a little more about yourself.

STEP 1: Look at the list below and rank yourself on the scale.

Authentic YOU Worksheet

CATEGORY					Moderate									
A Introvert	2	3	4	5	6	7	8	9	10	11	12	13	14	Extrovert
B Critical	2	3	4	5	6	7	8	9	10	11	12	13	14	Agreeable
C Careless	2	3	4	5	6	7	8	9	10	11	12	13	14	Conscientious
D Unstable	2	3	4	5	6	7	8	9	10	11	12	13	14	Stable
E Closed-minded	2	3	4	5	6	7	8	9	10	11	12	13	14	Open to Experience

STEP 2: Take a look at this chart, and find the columns that list where you identify yourself for: Stability, Extroversion, and Openness. For example, if you're Stable, Introverted, and Closed, we give you the label "Homebody." If you're in the middle on one of these dimensions, look at the labels that describe the values you have on the other two dimensions.

A Extroversion	D Stability	E Openness	Label
Extroverted	Stable	Open	Teacher—You like to learn new things and help others to see the way.
Extroverted	Stable	Closed	Guide—You know a lot about the areas you have experienced and like to share that with others.
Introverted	Stable	Open	Explorer—You are interested in new things and will go off by yourself to find them.
Introverted	Stable	Closed	Homebody—A great day is a great day spent at home.
Extroverted	Unstable	Open	Sensation Seeker—Bring it on! The bigger the rush, the higher the high.
Extroverted	Unstable	Closed	Blogger—You like to let the world know about what you're thinking. There are rights and wrongs in the world, and people need to know. (These are often disruptive people.)
Introverted	Unstable	Open	Lurker—There is a lot to discover in the world, though it can be a scary place. You'll check things out, but you prefer to do it alone.
Introverted	Unstable	Closed	Grumbler—Life has real ups and downs, though you tend to keep that opinion to yourself.

STEP 3: Check out four common patterns for the combinations of the agreeableness and conscientiousness dimensions.

B Agreeableness	C Conscientiousness	Label
Agreeable	Conscientious	Old Reliable—Everyone can count on you, through thick and thin.
Agreeable	Careless	Easygoing—Life goes on.
Critical	Conscientious	Nitpicker—You have high and exacting standards. You live up to them, and you expect others to as well.
Critical	Careless	Curmudgeon—You have high standards, and others don't often measure up, though you may not either.

WHAT DID YOU FIND? As you take some time to really think about who you are, you may find these labels helpful for thinking about patterns of behaviors. Though you may never have taken the time to really think about who you are, your personality characteristics are important, because they are deeply part of you.

9

The Worry War

Solve Your Most Troubling Job and
Money Issues

YOU Test: Burnout

Answer the following questions with a yes or no, considering how you feel today only.

- Do you feel as worn down as 100,000-mile tires?
- When you think about your boss, your kids, your food-begging parrot, or anyone else in your life making demands, do you feel primarily anger?
- Do you feel overwhelmed or besieged by work?
- Do you explode easily—even at trivial issues?
- Do you suffer from headaches, gastrointestinal distress, or insomnia?
- Are you considered the resident Evel Knievel, taking unnecessary risks?
- Are you stressed out by money issues more than once a month?

Answer: Ideally, we want you to answer no to all of these questions. If you nodded in the affirmative to any, it's a sign you may be suffering from burnout and stress. The more yes answers you have, the faster you're on your way to a total meltdown.

We all know at least one person who frets about everything—the weather, the plug on the coffee machine, who's going to make the *American Idol* finale. We have a name for these chronic fretters: worrywarts. (Notice that we don't call them worry whizzes. The "wart" imagery seems about right; worrying is definitely not an attractive quality.) Although none of us actively aspires to be a worrier, worrying does serve an important purpose. From an evolutionary standpoint, worry signals a lack of confidence, knowledge, or control. Where are we going to sleep tonight? What's for dinner? Was that rustling in the bushes coming from the wind or a big-toothed mammal that's thinking we're what's for dinner?

When we don't know the answers to our questions, we feel anxious, stressed, and under duress. Today's big questions are a little bit different. We worry about paying our bills, we worry about our career path, and we worry about the health of ourselves and our families. Fundamentally, this also serves some purpose: Worry helps us take some action—to ease our stress and anxiety.

FACTOID

Looking for something to do with a few saved pennies? Give them away. MRIs reveal that making a donation activates the brain's reward center—giving you a boost of dopamine. When you help others, the primitive part of your brain lights up to experience pleasure. More on helping others in chapter 11.

When you think about it, beauty is often about managing all the different kinds of stresses in your life. Some of those stresses come from bad relationships (which we will handle in the next chapters). And some of those stresses come from being sidelined with aches and pains (which we outlined in chapter 7). Some of those stresses are intensely personal (like the stress of not having the body, face, or skin you desire). Whatever the case, stress is essentially about a lack of control—or rather, your feelings about things not in your control.

Since we've covered many of the major stressors through the book (as well as previous YOU books), we want to tackle the two other big stressors in people's

Too Much Noise

Here's an underappreciated source of work stress: loud noise. In fact, the incidence of heart attacks rises by 30 percent in people who work in loud places (and can increase to 300 percent in women if the home is very noisy, too). By the way, loud noise is defined as your needing to raise your voice to be heard. If your work is louder than 85 decibels, you need ear protection in the form of earmuffs or molded earplugs. Most office gossips are much lower, though they can be just as annoying; we're talking jackhammers, dental drills, DJs, even crying babies in day care. Plugs can reduce the noise by more than 30 decibels.

lives: money and work. The truth is that of the ten identified major stressors, six of them involve money or work (such as changing jobs or having mountainous debt).* Money issues constitute more than 40 percent of the major stresses each person experiences. So, while there's a lot to cover relating to stress, we want to break through to you first on these issues. Unfortunately, many folks are frequently intimidated about bringing life lessons and stress-busting techniques into the workplace. As we'll explore throughout this chapter, stress can work for you in many ways (after all, the only time you're not stressed is when you're in that pine box). Stress helps you meet deadlines and make tough decisions under pressure. What we don't want, however, is for work- and finance-related stress to adversely affect your health or for it to control you, suffocate you, and make you feel about as vibrant as muddy socks.

As is the case with your medical health, there are more factors and situations to assess your financial health than there are Wal-Mart stores. But there are also plenty of principles that apply to lots of people—no matter the nuances of your career, your company, or your savings accounts. Too often we think about the destination when it comes to careers and money—having the ideal job or the fat bank account—and we lose sight of the journey that takes us there. If you manage the journey, the job and bank account will take care of themselves.

Just as there's no single magic pill or medicine that will melt fat or guarantee

---

*The major stressors are serious illness of a family member, serious concern about a family member, death of a family member, divorce or separation, being forced to move, being sued, being forced to change jobs, being made redundant at work, feelings of insecurity at work, and serious financial trouble.

longevity, there's no single stock or investment or plan that will predictably make you a massive amount of money overnight. Rather, developing a system of strategies and attitudes is what will help you relieve some of your financial and job-related stress.

Your Work: Frazzled or Dazzled?

There's no question that our society has a collective career crisis. Work is killing us. Just consider these facts, lest you think it's not a big deal for you: A third of all new illnesses are due to work-related stresses, and each case of work-related major stress, depression, or anxiety leads to an average of 30 working days lost a year (that's six weeks of work!). Work-related stress is second only to back pain in terms of work-related health problems (and stress causes some of the back pain). Yikes.

More specifically, you don't have to be an M.D. to know that stress can cause headaches, sleep problems, appetite problems (usually too much, but too little, too), and other psychological problems such as depression and anxiety. And that's not even considering the fact that work stress has been linked to gastrointestinal problems, hormonal problems, immune problems, an increased risk of metabolic syndrome (that's omental obesity, high blood pressure, high lousy and low healthy cholesterol levels, high triglyceride levels, and high blood sugar), as well as a six-fold higher risk of having a heart attack. Double yikes.

Here's how it works in your body: You have a stress circuit that loops between your nervous system and your stress hormones called the hypothalamic-pituitary-adrenal (HPA) axis (see Figure 9.1). When you're faced with a major stressor, the hypothalamus releases a hormone called CRH, which then causes your pituitary gland to release another hormone called ACTH into your bloodstream. That's the hormone that signals your adrenal glands to release the stress hormone cortisol, which in turn gets your adrenaline cranked up (adrenaline is the fight-or-flight hormone). All of this is fine and good for a while (the increased heart rate and blood pressure get you away from any predator), but if the stress doesn't stop, this

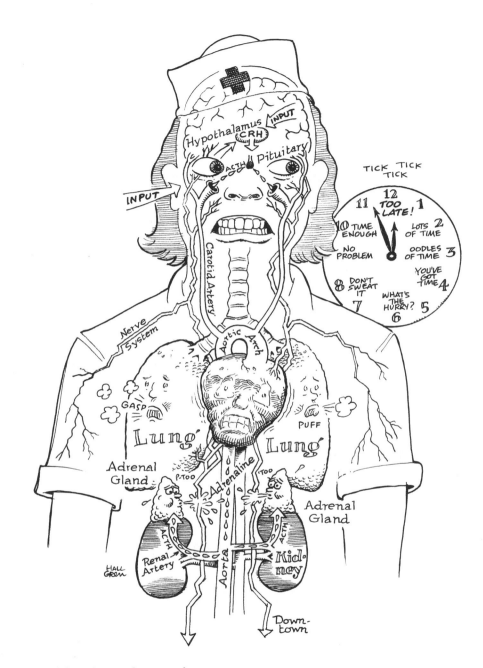

Figure 9.1 **Under Attack** When we're stressed, our brain goes through a cascade of chemical reactions through a circuit called the hypothalamic-pituitary-adrenal axis. Those secreted hormones are designed to help us in the short term (think adrenaline), but if we can't shut off those stressors, the flood of chemicals is detrimental to our health.

flood of chemicals turns against you—compromising your immune system, exhausting your adrenal glands, throwing your cholesterol levels out of whack, and causing you to crave sugar and syrups that age you. And your prefrontal cortex, which, if you had listened to it, would have prevented you from getting into the problem in the first place, is bypassed again. And guess what? Financial stresses and work stresses aren't onetime muggers; they're constantly battling you—meaning that chronic stress has real potential for pummeling your insides.

What's really fascinating from a scientific perspective is the bridge between good stress and bad stress. While many of us would typically say that life would be just grand if you could work from a hammock, the truth is that some amount of stress can be good for you and your job performance (which ultimately relieves stress, right?). Just take a look at this quick chart to see how your body reacts to stress. On the left, see the difference between being relaxed and being stressed. More important, look at the change between the acute kind (like a monthly deadline) and the chronic kind (like a nagging boss who hovers over you like a well-planted beach umbrella).

Relaxed State	Stressed State	Body Part/ Function	Acute Stress	Chronic Stress
Normal blood supply	Blood supply increases	Brain	Think more clearly	Headaches, migraines, tremors
Happy	Serious	Mood	Increased concentration	Anxiety
Normal heart rate and blood pressure	Increased heart rate	Heart	Improved performance	High blood pressure, chest pains

So where's the line between acute stress that works in your favor and chronic stress that makes you feel like retreating to the couch for the next three weeks? Good question, tough answer. It varies for everyone, but certainly some patterns

YOU Test

Do You Have a Money Problem?

We know this sounds like the start of a bad joke, but it's a pretty good indication that you have a money problem if . . .

- You rank money ahead of health, love, family, and friendship.
- You buy things just to impress others.
- You can't stand to save, so you spend any extra money at the end of the month.
- You feel guilty for spending money on necessities.
- You believe money can solve all problems.
- You can tell us—to the penny—how much you're carrying in your purse or pocket.
- You constantly pick up the bill at restaurants or bars just to be appreciated.

FACTOID People are saving at the lowest level since the Great Depression—the nation's personal savings rate for all of 2007 was less than zero (i.e., we spend more than we make as a nation), the worst showing in 73 years. Worse, consumer debt in the United States has more than doubled over the last decade, reaching more than $2 trillion. Credit card debt for the average household that carries a balance is $12,000.

emerge. Chronic stress typically develops because your job includes one (or more) of these factors:

- boring and repetitive tasks
- low level of control in your job
- annoying coworkers (and lack of a buddy or friends as coworkers)
- low level of job security (being made redundant, in HR terminology)
- working the night shift or rotating shifts
- being exposed to loud noise

Having a job with one of those characteristics makes you susceptible to the negative effects of stress and not feel beautiful; being exposed to all makes you a walking volcano.

The tactics we'll outline at the end of the chapter can help you manage these nagging things, but, perhaps more important, they'll help you look at the bigger picture—whether you're even at the right place at the right time in your career.

Your Finances: Money Matters

Without money, we have no food, no shelter, no iPods. We use it for necessities; we crave it for luxuries. And no matter how much we make, spend, save, or donate, we can't deny that money is as important to our overall well-being as almost anything else. Why?

In today's material world, net worth is often confused with self-worth. And this faulty leap of logic has created a heap of problems. For many, more money means having more power, more control, more confidence, and thus, more to worry about. And many of us get caught up in a "keeping up with the Joneses" mentality where we need to spend money whenever others do (this is likely due to our having mirror neurons, which drive us to mimic others and which we'll cover in depth on page 315).

To further worsen the worry potential, men and women have decidedly different views about money. These gender differences are probably rooted in our evolutionary past, when men did the hunting and women the gathering. Today's modern man, like his Stone Age cousin, doesn't think twice about going out and bagging a new car, then proudly coming home with his trophy, yelling, "Honey, come down here and look at the new SUV I got you." To which his wife might respond, "Why didn't you ask me what I wanted? I thought we were a team." Which might trigger him to ask, "What, are you my mother?" It's no wonder, then, that financial problems are among the most common reasons for divorce. Though nearly 60 percent of couples say they rarely disagree about money and are doing just fine with their finances, some research shows that one-quarter of all married couples divorce because of financial issues.

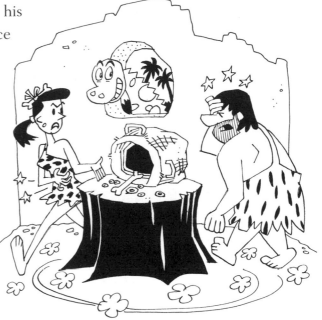

The X factor (or XX and XY factor, if you will) in financial issues is that many of us have bank accounts that are fused together with another person's. No longer can you make decisions about (and be responsible for) how your money is spent. Many times, *your* money becomes *our* money, and that money is also responsible for taking care of the milk-needing and Wii-wanting rugrats.

That, to say the least, complicates things. He may be a saver; she may be a spender. He may like to spend money on a big-screen TV; she may like to spend on a Starbucks habit. He may like season tickets to the Roller Derby; she may like a spa vacation (or vice versa). It should be no surprise that people often rank personal finance issues as the number one source of stress. Concerns about personal finance are five times greater than those about health. And to tie the health and money issues together, people have been shown to be more likely to deal with financial stressors by engaging in unhealthy behaviors.*

As so many other health issues do, this one also starts in the brain—and how specifically we're hardwired to react about money. For our Stone Age ancestors, survival belonged to the strongest and the fastest. He who grabbed the honey got the honey. He who killed the beast ate the beast. He who flexed his pecs got the woman and the kids to propagate the family name and traditions. Thus, we didn't inhibit our risk-taking behavior with the guidance of our risk-balancing prefrontal cortex. Instead, we reacted—that allowed us to survive. In today's world, that means (especially when you are young) that when you see a $150 pair of designer jeans you think you'd like to wear, you grab it without the prefrontal cortex restraining you.

Today the means of survival—food, clothing, and shelter—don't stem from the size of your muscles but rather the fatness (or thinness) of your bank account. Because of that, money has come to have many uses and meanings. We want money, for example, for security, power, love, and freedom. We also use it for such things as comfort, knowledge, even sexuality. In fact, we think it makes us more beautiful, and that's how we act. More important is that the lesson we learned about money from our ancestors is part of the very reason why we have money problems today—we didn't use our prefrontal cortices to survive and thrive.

Homo Economicus:
Financial Decision Making

We like to think of ourselves as rational decision makers—dispassionate information processors, coolly, calmly, and logically evaluating the costs and benefits of each alternative we encounter. But we're much more primitive than most of us realize. We may look like a Wall Street type on the outside, but there's still a good

* Such as smoking, drinking, or going on the fried chocolate doughnut diet.

deal of Fred Flintstone on the inside. Remember the emotions we talked about in reference to anxiety, how we're hardwired through the amygdala to react to emotions, not intellect? That's the very reason why we can have financial troubles. Just consider this example:

Recently a team of Ivy League economists looked at how consumers reacted to various pitches by banks to take out a loan. A purely rational view would have predicted that interest rates would be the only factor that had an impact—the lower the rate, the more people will borrow money from that bank. But the scientists varied more than just the interest rate; they also tested how persuasive other approaches might be. For instance, some letters offered a chance to win a cell phone in a lottery if the customer came in to inquire about a loan. The researchers found that many nonfinancial factors had an effect equal to one to five percentage points of interest. An offer of a free cell phone increased demand among men as much as dropping the interest rate five points. For a $50,000 loan, this meant some men were in essence willing to pay $16,000 more in interest to receive a $100 cell phone. So much for logical decision making.

This study highlights what is perhaps the single greatest barrier to mastering our money problems: our near-universal tendency to grab small short-term gains to our long-term disadvantage. So why do so many of us make these apparently irrational decisions? From an evolutionary standpoint, our near obsession with the short term at the expense of long makes perfect sense—at least it did 100,000 years ago. Our Stone Age ancestors lived at a time when there was a reasonable chance of dying during the course of any given day (back then, hearing the phrase "Honey, I'm home" really meant something). Your decisions didn't make it to your frontal cortex, where risk and gains are balanced. It seems clear, and with good reason, that humans in that older era began to equate delayed benefits with a significant degree of risk since there was such a reasonable chance that future benefits would never be realized. So for the average Stone Ager the decision to go with the smaller, surer, instant reward was hardly irrational. To do anything else, now, that would have been crazy. Our problem is that what was Mensa-brilliant back in the old days doesn't work quite as well today.

We see evidence of our shortsighted tendencies all the time in today's society.

YOU Test

Your Job: For Love or Money?

Why do you do what you do? Is it because you love it? Or because you've been successful and make a good salary and, well, it would be a darn shame to give it all up to write Irish poetry for a living? That's essentially the difference between intrinsic motivators—doing something for love, genuine interest, and satisfaction—and external motivators—doing something because some outside influence such as salary influences you. In general, intrinsic factors are more important and more stable—and they will help you not only in job situations but also in things such as quitting smoking (better to quit when you're ready, not because somebody nags you to do so).

Intrinsic motivations are also self-reinforcing because of our built-in desire to attribute causes to our actions. If we perform a task for an extrinsic reward, we reason that we did the task because of the reward, and not because of something inherently interesting or important in it. But if we perform the task without an extrinsic reward, then we reason that the task itself must be inherently enjoyable or important for us to continue to engage in it. If you work hard on a project for a particular boss and then the boss moves on (or your feelings about that boss change), you will not keep working hard. But if you work hard because you enjoy the job, this motivation becomes self-reinforcing. You stay engaged in the work because it's enjoyable, and that supports the belief that the work was fun. This quiz, adapted from one by researcher Teresa Amabile, will help you determine whether you lean more toward internal or external motivators.

Answer yes or no to the following statements:

When you're faced with a difficult problem, is your response "Bring it on, baby"?
Do you prefer to figure out challenges at work by yourself?
Even if you fail at a new project, are you happy that you had a new experience?
Do you feel ambivalent about whether you get recognized for your accomplishments?
Does work feel more like recess than work?
Are you able to offer up new ideas and not care what others might think of you?

Results: The more often you answer yes to these questions, the more likely it is that you're motivated by internal factors. And if not, maybe it's time for you to look for another job or at least revisit your motivation.

People won't spend more money on a more expensive air conditioner even if it means that they'll pay smaller energy bills for years down the line. Today (the immediate responses of your reptilian brain) tends to win out over tomorrow (the prefrontal cortex), even though not having enough for tomorrow is the source of stress that sits like a three-ton boulder on your shoulders. It's the same concept that derails most diets: The pleasures of nutritional sins today (hot dog! cheesecake!) win out over the benefits of the way nutritional foods will take care of us tomorrow (more energy and less pain tomorrow if you eat blueberries and walnuts today!). Most likely your prefrontal cortex often doesn't get consulted in the mall or the food court; you rely on your reptilian brain. That evolutionary problem wouldn't be a problem if credit cards and leverage didn't exist now. But they do, and your not consulting your prefrontal cortex often causes you to overspend and thus be burdened with financial stress. Unfortunately, shortsightedness isn't the only force that pushes our financial instincts in irrational directions that ultimately make us feel less beautiful.

Mental Accounting

Another psychological phenomenon that tends to suppress our more rational tendencies is called mental accounting, and here's how it works. Ten dollars should be ten dollars should be ten dollars—all ten-dollar bills are created equal, right? Not so. People tend to compartmentalize their money—mentally allocating what certain money should be used for, typically depending on where it came from. Fifty bucks from your paycheck goes to the water bill, while fifty bucks tucked in a birthday card would never go to the bill, but rather to a slew of new iTunes.* Here's a classic test that will help put the concept into perspective: After buying a $10 movie ticket, you discover that there is a hole in your pocket and the ticket is

---

* In case you're wondering, Mike's iPod playlist includes "Celebration," "Yesterday," *Chicago,* "I Left My Heart in San Francisco," "Candle in the Wind," and "9 to 5." Mehmet's has "The Promised Land" by Springsteen, "Hey Yah!" by OutKast, and "Standing Outside a Broken Phone Booth with Money in My Hand" by Primitive Radio Gods.

gone. Do you buy another ticket? Less than half (46 percent) would. Then let's say, while waiting in line to buy the ticket, you discover the same hole and that you lost a $10 bill. Do you still buy the ticket? Almost nine out of ten people (88 percent) would. It's $10 either way, but people don't view it that way.

In essence, this example tells us we hate losing $10 about twice as much as we like finding it. Psychologists call this loss aversion, a psychological phenomenon whereby people feel the pain of a loss more acutely than the joy of a gain. But rather than let this effect steamroll you into perpetually bad decisions, you need to flip it around to your advantage (like turning New Year's resolutions to through-year's resolutions; see tips below).

Outsmart Your Instincts

All our shortsighted bad habits are, at least theoretically, reversible. The newer areas of our brains, the frontal lobes, can moderate or even shut down our instinctual behaviors. In fact, as you get older, you seem to get smarter by relying more on your prefrontal or frontal cortex before you make decisions. It may take a little longer, but you make more rational and less-instinctual and less-risky decisions. Nearly alone among animals, we can delay our gratification and choose not to give into a strong, short-term urge. Our tips below outline some of those strategies. But the big-picture strategy is to look at these two factors in yourself.

YOUR LOCUS OF CONTROL: Basically, locus of control refers to whether you're the kind of person who believes either that the oncoming bus was destined to pluck you from the sidewalk or that you had the power to make a decision about whether you were going to put a foot out before the sign blinked "walk." Do you believe that your behavior controls fate or fate controls you? Interesting question, eh?

People who have a strong internal locus see themselves as being in control of their lives. They're highly motivated, they have the power to steer their career and familial paths, and they make decisions that can change the course of their lives. They can influence, even employ, many productive people. They are those who follow their dreams and change the world, handle stress, and are really happy with their careers. Those with an external locus? You got it. They blame the weather, they blame their bosses, they blame whatever supernatural power they believe in for dealing them a bad hand in life. Bad thoughts make your brain focus on negatives rather than your passion in life. So, no matter what locus of control you now have, get ready to shift to positive thoughts only.

FACTOID We can get a lot of insight into how we respond to money by looking at how certain parts of our brains light up when exposed to certain stimuli. For example, we know that in some patients who took Parkinson's medication that increased dopamine levels, it also stimulated shopping and gambling compulsions (the reward center at it again). We also know that certain areas of the brain kick into high gear when we see people who are above us in the social hierarchy, further indicating that our response to certain issues of money and status are more hardwired than they are personality quirks.

Of course, most of us exhibit both kinds of loci; it's just that one may be more dominant. To decrease work stress and feel more beautiful, start thinking with the scales tipped more toward an internal locus: that you have the power to love your job, to create a better world, and to handle tough tasks; that you have the ability to make more money; and that you have the authority to determine that a lousy career isn't just some hand you've been dealt through a series of unfortunate incidents.

YOUR EMOTIONAL INTELLIGENCE: Since stress certainly has a heavy emotional component (any work-related freak-out is evidence of that), it stands to reason that your ability to *think* with your emotions can help you manage them. Huh? Think with your emotions? We know—it sounds more oxymoronic than nonalcoholic beer. But let us explain. In fact, you don't think with emotions; you are hardwired to react with emotions. Since that's what got you here (that's how your ancestors survived), that's generally a good thing. In patients who have strokes that knock out the emotional center, they can no longer make rational decisions, so ironically, humans need that emotional center to make rational decisions. Stress-related emotions don't have to be automatically classified as yelling at interns, punching the wall, or rushing off to the restroom to cry with the velocity of the faucet. Emotional intelligence can actually be thought of as a form of problem-solving in times of stress. How so? Well, emotional intelligence can really be broken down into four abilities or skills that can help you cope with stress:

- ID-ing emotions: Tangibly identify what you're feeling—making sure to look deeper than surface-level reactions. Let's say you're jealous over someone else's successes. Ask yourself if you're truly jealous or maybe upset that you haven't achieved what you wanted to.

- Facilitating emotions: When you're feeling multiple emotions, think about different points of view to help you solve problems. In our jealousy example, identify your obstacles and figure out ways around them, rather than letting jealousy get you off track.
- Understanding emotions: Understand that emotions aren't as black and white as salt and pepper, and that we all experience complex chains of emotions. And we can learn to understand and even change the emotions of others, be they bosses, coworkers, or customers.

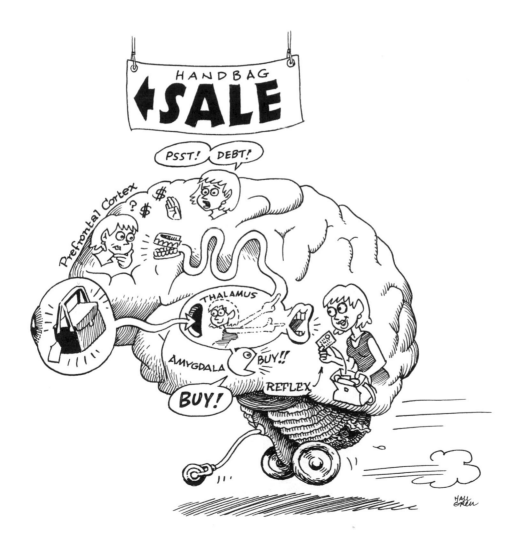

- Managing emotions: This skill doesn't mean being able to hide your crying until you get to the restroom; rather, it's what lets you determine whether an emotion is appropriate, so you can solve problems that are emotionally based. Next time you're feeling jealous, for example, you'll be able to harness that emotion more quickly and better manage your feelings and subsequent behaviors.

Once you establish this foundation of control over your stressors, you're better equipped to tackle the problems more specifically.

It's useful to distinguish between the two decision-making processes: controlled/thoughtful vs. automatic/emotional/impulsive. That's because many decision-making problems (especially with money) occur because of a tug-of-war between the two. While some decisions are clearly impulsive (great purse!), more often than not, financial decisions are a mix between the two. For example, you probably bought your house using the controlled and thoughtful process, but the reason why you fell in love with it was because of the emotional and automatic part of your brain. Some of the main problems when it comes to bad money decisions happen because of the push-pull between thinking and feeling.

YOU Tips!

While we're not career coaches or financial advisers, you should know that doctors (often the Ph.D. kind) spend a lot of time evaluating work performance and things that influence it (happy people are better performers, after all). So there are significant data that show us ways to make our work environments better and decrease stress levels. When it comes to money, of course, we're not going to tell you what your stock portfolio should look like, but we are going to try to steer you to make choices that will help you feel better and live longer, by learning how to work past the biology of decision making that gets you into trouble. After all, lavender baths and hourlong massages are great stress relievers, no doubt, but the way to truly eliminate some of your major worries is to change your behavior, not escape your problems.

SCORE A PERFECT 10. We're not going to get into the nitty-gritty of telling you whether we believe that investing in international stock is smarter than investing your life savings in some newfangled company that makes silk pencils. But of all the financial decisions you will make over your life, this one is a no-brainer. Every time you get paid, take 10 percent of that check and put it into an emergency account. It doesn't count for retirement, it's not used for bills, and it's not something you tap into when you decide that you really really really really need an automatic lollipop maker. It's something that will give you peace of mind. Having an emergency backup account to use if the car dies, or your spouse needs an extra hand to help with an illness, or you need to go to a different job, or the roof leaks, while still being able to pay bills, save for retirement, and make investments, is *the* thing that will relieve your day-to-day financial stress as much as anything short of winning the Super Six.

TAKE YOUR FINANCIAL TEMPERATURE. While we know that financial burdens can weigh us down, a lot of us would like to ignore the issues until a crisis happens—simply because we don't know all that much about it. As you know with your body, the smartest approach is to think about your health all the time—not a few minutes before the ambulance arrives. So, instead of burying your head, apply some standards of health to your financial attitudes. Overspending is like overeating—in both cases there's a serious price to pay with no easy answer if it gets out of control. Day trading is like binge eating sugar- and saturated-fat-laden foods (feels good at the time but not so great over the long haul). A retirement account is like exercise (do a little bit along the way, and the long-term benefits are exponentially greater than the investment). The simple fact is, if you treat your money with the same respect and care with which you ought to treat your body, there's a decreased chance you're going to need financial CPR.

HUDDLE UP. Too often, it seems that we treat money issues as some taboo topic. We don't talk about our financial philosophies until hubby comes home with a brand-new motorboat (and then all hell breaks loose). Since financial styles affect a marriage as much as parenting styles and sexual styles do, it's only smart to talk about the coin well before your wedding vows. Considering the staggering statistic of how many couples break up over the almighty dollar, you need a conversation about long-term goals, about short-term needs, about budgets, about emergency plans, and about an overall financial strategy that will keep your account (and marriage) intact.

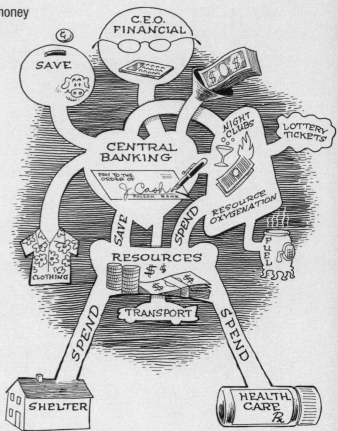

SHIFT YOUR THINKING. Some examples to help put money issues into perspective:

- Turn January's gym memberships, yoga classes, etc. into *through*-year's resolutions. Ask your workout facility to remind you with daily e-mails alerting you of just how much money you've thrown down the drain in the 77 days since you last worked out.
- Many companies are now offering "auto-enrollment" programs whereby a certain percentage of each paycheck is directly routed to the employee's 401(k) plan. Should you opt out of this plan, ask your company for daily e-mails that could alert you exactly how many dollars would be absent from future wallets/purses.
- Opt for rational decision making rather than wishful thinking. Emotions can distort our decisions. For example, emotions affect our perceptions of risks. People are good at persuading themselves that what they would *like* to happen is what *will* happen. Wishful thinking can help explain high rates of new business failure, trading in financial markets, undersaving, and low rates of investment in education.

WRITE IT DOWN. Carry a small notebook or diary with you in your purse or bag and record your daily purchases for one month. At the end of the month, sit down and look at your purchases and consider how to cut back or improve by 10 percent. You'll likely be amazed at what you can live without.

ALIGN YOUR MISSIONS. So often, we get caught up in the minutiae of our jobs—tedious annoyances and struggles that may be temporary roadblocks but feel more like concrete mountains. While there's plenty of research that shows that people who work with the muscles above their neck create all kinds of stresses for themselves, it's the people who focus on the *why* of their jobs (as opposed to the *what* and the *how*) who can manage the day-to-day problems more easily. That is, if you can define the purpose of your career or feel passionate about the mission of your company, you can much more easily handle the occasional server maintenance that disrupts your in-box. The flip side is that if you're working in any area (or company) that doesn't align with your own values, all the little stuff snowballs into a big ole ball of daily disasters.

SHIFT TO ENERGY MANAGEMENT. You know what we hear all the time from people who feel more overworked than a Buffalo snowplow driver? "I have no time." No time to think, no time to work, no time to tell people I have no time. So what we all think we have in today's day and age is a time management problem. We're overburdened and undermanned. You know what we think? It actually has little to do with time at all. Our problem is more of an energy management problem. If we feel energized, excited, jazzed, and ready to rock at work, then time management is no longer an issue. And you get to a somewhat cosmic point (like "the zone" for athletes) where you're managing time efficiently and smartly. You can't wait to get to work, and you enjoy going home as well. So, really, your goal maybe shouldn't be to delegate more or take on less; it should be to manage your health so that you feel as energized as a caffeinated puppy without having to rely on artificial and temporary means to do so. See chapter 6 for our tips for adding caffeine- and fat-free ways to add more energy to your power source.

FIND A BUDDY. The best way to enjoy your job more: Have a buddy or best friend at work. Having a buddy or close friend at work isn't an excuse to gossip; it's really a key to managing stress and consistently choosing healthy behaviors. A good buddy will help keep your blood pressure lower and the pounds off, but it has to be one with whom you share similar goals (if you choose an overweight buddy, you'll be more likely to adopt the habits that will also make you overweight). Having a friend there will help you be more productive at work, too (which will also lower stress). The Gallup organization has found we're more productive at work and don't miss as much time when we have a buddy or best friend at work. Why? Maybe we feel that obligation, that accountability to the buddy— and we enjoy our work more.

TALK TO PEOPLE. More than half of people who get jobs do it through personal connection (not necessarily friends but acquaintances, as well). Don't think you have many connections? Wrong. The theory of six degrees of separation is really true.* You're not networking to use people but to create a network of people who can support you—some may support you emotionally as you go through tough times at work, while others may be the needed contacts who will help you get a foot in the door. Ask yourself who the people are that you need to know (role models, competitors), and go out and meet them. They'll help you fulfill your dream, so why leave it to chance?

STAY PUT. Owning your home (paying off your mortgage) has more health benefits than continually switching homes. Realize that the average American sells his or her home every seven years. So if you're in a starter home, you should consider staying for a while longer than you anticipated. The benefit is twofold: Longer-term home ownership lets you accumulate financial value, as well as giving you more to spend on healthy choices: a double bonus of stress busters.

OPTIMIZE YOUR WORK ENVIRONMENT. If you can make the office an empowering place, you can improve your health and decrease your stress. Some ways to do that:

Color. The U.S. Public Health Service did a two-year study of public buildings and found that when they analyzed the room with additional lighting and additional color there was a 5.5 percent production improvement. A combination of green and red seems to be the most productive. So-called ugly colors—white, black, brown—caused a drop in performance even on IQ tests by as much as 12 points in one study.

Light. Green light and blue light increase activity slightly, but a yellow light increases activity by about 30 percent.

Artwork and greenery. Keeping plants in the office gives us the feeling of living things, growing things; they're also healing, comforting, and empowering. Artwork can be edgy in lobbies to set a tone of innovativeness but shouldn't be edgy in the workplace because you want people to focus on the work, not on the artwork. Think natural and calming pieces.

Air quality. Sick building syndrome has been reported by 23 percent of U.S. office workers, manifesting itself in such problems as respiratory ailments, allergies, and asthma. Push your bosses to make sure the office has proper ventilation and clean air.

Temperature. Optimal productivity performance appears to be at 72 degrees, and going too much colder is associated with making more mistakes at work.

* Researchers found this out by asking 100 people to send something to a specific person in Boston, but it could be sent only via personal acquaintances, and it took only six passes before the original reached the target person in Boston.

Humor. One of the secrets of a good office environment is having people who can laugh and have fun. Now, we're not saying you should be practicing your best Chris Rock on your cube-mates (after all, everyone's sensibilities are different), but maybe you should embrace, not scorn, the office clown. He's just trying to make you happier and healthier.

PICK YOUR PASSION FIRST, PAYCHECK SECOND. When it comes to careers, a lot of people have it backward. They pick a career because they think they may make a lot of money in it. Maybe they will, and maybe they won't. But if you pick something you don't like and end up not making money, then your brain can feel more fizzed than shaken-up soda. So what we tell young people all the time is for them to find a career that they're passionate about. Do that and you'll naturally excel because you'll love what you're doing, and, in many cases, the money will follow.

YOU BE THE PUPPETEER. Too often, we let the boss steer us, strong-arm us, scare us, and bleep us over to this side of Saturday. And while we surely have to answer to our superiors, there are also ways that you can handle a boss who's difficult to work with. First tactic: Stop thinking about your boss in the principal model—that is, you're the student and she's the principal (and the only way you end up in the office is if you do something very, very bad). Second tactic: Strip the hierarchy of some of the perceived power at the top. You can never have a bad discussion with a boss if you start with the exact same premise and goals—that you're both out to help customers and clients. To help your boss is to help the company. With some dialogue that evens the playing field ("We both want what's best for the customer, so let's figure out the best path"), there's less backstabbing and more back patting.

CONTROL YOUR FLOW. While it would be a mistake for us to assume there's only one way to work, we do think there are some traits and behaviors that can make time and energy management a whole lot easier. Some things you should consciously try to integrate into your workday if you don't already:

- **Map your day:** Though you don't have to stick to an exact schedule, you can get some stress relief if you can organize your tasks and not leave your day to total chance. Don't work off the in-box . . . work off your plan for the day. (Manage the in-box only after you've done what you desire to do.)
- **Break often:** Take a walk, have a bottle of water, clear your head. It's all part of energy management. The few minutes you spend away from your desk will make you more efficient when you get back.
- **Enlist troops:** We know that people are pretty stubborn when it comes to trying to accomplish goals on their own; they think it's a sign of failure if they show weakness or an inability to do a job. But you'll reduce stress (and save time) by asking for help when you need it.

REPURPOSE YOUR LISTS. Whether you work for a company or your family, we bet that you live and die by the list. Doesn't matter whether you use Post-its, a notebook, a wipe board, a PDA, or scraps of tissues—we want you to keep not only a to-do list but also an I-hate list. That is, when something bothers you in your job, write it down. Revisit the list in a week. If it's still bothering you, maybe it's time to aggressively pursue a solution (or another job). Our guess: Most of the time, those annoyances will be as fleeting as a one-hit wonder. And that should help you realize that it's the big picture, not the little one, that counts. For times when that list grows too fast, well, it's always smart to keep your résumé handy. After all, you're now going to follow an internal locus of control, correct?

ASK FOR IT. Face it. Your boss doesn't want to give you a raise. It's more money away from his bottom line. But does that mean you ought to roll up into a ball of dough when talking about making more dough? No way. The truth is that women earn about 11 percent less than men with equivalent education and experience. In one interesting study, researchers told participants that they'd be paid anywhere from $3 to $10 to play Boggle. At the end, they were paid $3. And guess what happened. Eight times more men than women asked for more money. Similarly, four times as many men as women report that they negotiate for more money during a job offer. The message: Ask, ask, ask.

NEVER HANG IT UP. Every five-year increase in age at retirement is associated with a 10 percent decrease in mortality, especially from the heart (perhaps because when you retire you lose a reason for the heart to keep beating). Even if you quit your lifelong day job, pick up another responsibility, so you have to get up in the morning and fulfill a purpose.

BUT PLAN FOR RETIREMENT ANYWAY. Even though we advocate that you never really retire from working (in the sense that you instead would watch bad TV all day long), you still need to plan for the time when you step away from your main source of income. Start your 401(k) plan with as much money as you can afford and can contribute without pain. We advise putting 10 percent of your salary in a retirement account. By the end of two years, you will love your foresight. Have the option to contribute that much or more every year, as well as to increase the percentage contributed with every pay increase. You can survive on what you were making, so each increase that goes to financial security that decreases money stress and the large number of illnesses that it causes. Plus, nothing gives you freedom to follow your passions and relieve stress than having a retirement fund.

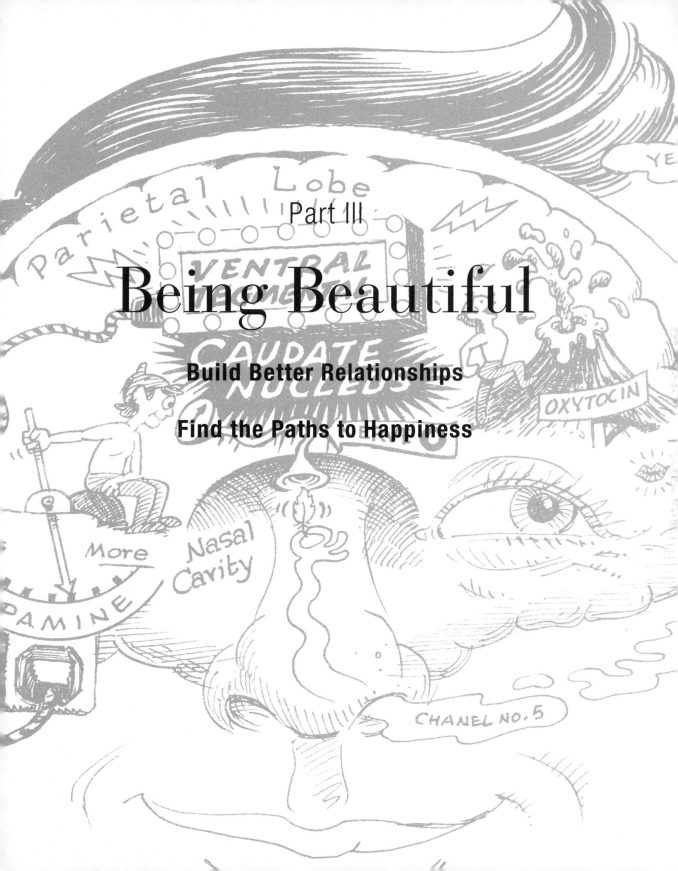

Part III

Being Beautiful

Build Better Relationships

Find the Paths to Happiness

For some, happiness is a bottle of wine shared with your romantic interest. For others, happiness is a silent walk on the beach in a light rain. Whatever your particular definition of happiness may be, we believe that the idea of being beautiful really comes down to two big, umbrella concepts: First, love the people in your life and practice trusting and forgiving them. Second, and equally important, love yourself and all of your imperfections (many of which you're working to correct, right?).

Now, "be happy with yourself" may seem as simple an instruction as "fold your underwear." The point, however, isn't that many of us don't even wear, much less fold, underwear; it's that most of us wrestle with this simple ideal. Why? Because often we find ourselves at odds as we try to balance between two opposing forces. In one corner, we all have a strong hardwired drive for uniqueness and individuality. And in the other corner, we have a biological need and craving for social conformity and belonging. Sometimes, that can be quite a challenge: Be different, but be the same. Stand out from the crowd, but fit in. Get a tattoo, but not on your forehead.

Why does this even matter? Because being beautiful and finding happiness with ourselves and through our interactions with other people has tremendous health implications: Good relationships with other people (and having a real buddy) can help stave off depression and add years to your life, especially if you're trying to weather the storms of stress. Having internal struggles about your own self-value and purpose in life can increase your chance of developing both physical and mental ailments—and influence your overall feeling of happiness (not to mention longevity).

One of the reasons why finding this balance is so darn hard is the fact that there can be a canyon-like gap between reality and perception—that is, how you really exist and how others perceive you (and that's really the foundation of the YOU-Q Test you took at the beginning of the book; remember to take the test again to see what you've learned).

Solving this conundrum—and opening your world up to look beyond cursory perceptions—is what really gives you the inner strength and beauty to find happiness. Ask yourself:

- Do you have relationships that are strong and healthy and contribute to your happiness?
- Have you found ways to give to others and show gratitude for the gifts you've been given?
- And are you able to go beyond the superficiality that surrounds you in your day-to-day life, to explore and connect with the deeper and more meaningful purposes in life?

Those questions really lie at the center of making "beauty" a full-circle concept. The more beautiful you look and feel, the happier you are. And the happier you are, the more beautiful you look and feel and the more you can share with others your purpose in life. And that's a beautiful thing.

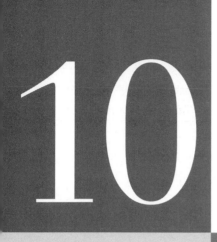

10

That Lovin' Feeling

Improve Your Relationships with
the People Close to You

YOU Test: Quite a Pair

How would you describe your current romantic relationship?

a. Great, nirvana, I've found the love of my life

b. Strong and steady but could use more sparks

c. Rocky, bumpy, I'd rather be at work than at home

d. My only relationship is with the washing machine

Results: Clearly, the ideal relationship is one that is categorized more like A than any other answer. This chapter hopes to help get you there if you're not—and make sure you stay there if you are.

One of the amazing things about people is that we all have different goals in our lives. Some of us want to be rock stars and some of us want to study stars; some of us want to cook fish and some of us want to catch them. While our interests, goals, and careers are as different as our facial features, the biggest drive of all is applicable to nearly everyone: finding that special some-body to call honey, to snuggle with in bed, and to argue with about the best *Idol* contestant.

That feeling—of love, of bliss, of emotional connection, of physical fireworks—lies at the heart of how happy we are. We need other people, love other people, crave other people. Without that singular bond on a romantic level (and multiple ones at the family and friend level), it's very hard for most of us to be happy. That said, we should also be clear that our feelings of happiness in relationships extend beyond just the ro-mantic sort. Strong social networks with friends, fam-ily, and our pets are strong contributors to our happi-ness (and the converse is also true: bad relationships can be a trigger for stress and bad health). While the health benefits of a safe monogamous sexual rela-tionship are extremely important, research also indicates that strong social ties, such as having a best buddy, are pretty good substitutes for most of the health benefits of a spousal relationship. And they are much better than having an unsatisfied or un-happy spousal arrangement.

FACTOID Do you think the concept of "opposites attract" is just a way to explain how Type As end up with Type Bs? In one study, women were given smelly T-shirts of men (nice experiment, eh?) and told to pick the ones they found most attractive. You know what they picked? Not the Iron Maiden Ts, but the ones of people whose genes were most different from theirs, indicating that we're hardwired to diversify the gene pool. This also keeps siblings from being attracted to each other, which (besides being weird) increases the chances of genetic defects in offspring.

Here we're going to explore the biology of our romantic relationships—how we find the right person and how we continue to love that person. What's especially interesting about this particular topic is that it encapsulates all three components of beauty: You need to look beautiful—at least if you hope to continue the species—because it's used to attract a mate. You need to feel beautiful to signal that you are healthy and worthy of parenting a potential mate's offspring. And when someone indicates that he or she is attracted to you and interested in what it takes to perpetuate the species, it naturally gives you the joy and confidence you need to be beautiful. On every level, love, not to mention the intimate/exciting/body-melting sexual relationship that goes with it, is the biggest beauty boost of them all.

The Biology of Attraction

Before we get into the biology of love and maintaining a happy, healthy (and sexual) relationship, we should take a step back and explore what it is that attracts you to your mate in the first place. You might be thinking that you need information about attraction as much as you need a hole in the heart. That's because you already know what you like in a mate—be it in body parts, in personality traits, or in styles of facial hair. While it's true that you and your senses can be attracted to many different people and be repulsed by as many others, there is some science to the process of finding the perfect mate. How? With the body part that gets about as much sexual attention as the popliteal fossa:* your nose.

While your initial attraction to someone may be physical, one of the true messengers of love is chemical. We're attracted to people who have good smells (like flowers) and repulsed by those who have bad smells (like Dumpsters). Though we tend to spend a lot of time and money disguising our smells with perfume, deodorant, shampoo, and detergents, our brain helps us cut through all that gunk to

---

*That's the squishy area behind the knee. We'd venture to guess that while probably uncommon, there surely are a few people out there who do have a fossa fetish.

How Do the Blind Find Love?

Seems as though attraction would be a bit difficult if you couldn't visually size up a mate's face, muscles, or curves. Sexually, blind people rely even more on their senses of smell and touch than others do. Chubby partners are more attractive to those without sight because they have more texture to their body. To form an image of the other person's body, blind people touch their partner's complete body, an intensely erotic experience in itself. While scientists have also found that voices are a major erotic stimulator for blind people, the key components during sex are touching, smelling, and licking.

detect the unique smells of different people. Now, we're not talking about the kinds of major odors that should send you straight to the bath; we're talking about microsmells—called pheromones—that are like dog whistles of the body. They're so subtle that you can't detect them consciously, but they're powerful enough to influence decisions about attraction.

Pheromones—sometimes odorless steroids that can be detected at picogram concentration (that's one-trillionth of a gram, sort of like a single molecule dancing along)—float through the air and stimulate nerves in your nose. The nerve signals are carried to your brain and trigger complicated chemical reactions that ultimately end with a question such as "Can I buy you a drink?" (They're also important because they help animals distinguish one another—so that father doesn't breed with daughter and thus increase the chance of genetic mutations.)

In the past five years, scientists have become extremely interested in this "accessory olfactory system"—that is, it's just starting to be understood, which causes some skepticism in scientific circles. But this is how the theory goes: The pheromone system starts with nerve cells in a pair of tiny, cigar-shaped sacs called the vomeronasal organ (VNO), where the signals are first picked up (see Figure 10.1). Located just behind the nostrils in the nose's dividing wall, the VNO is a pretty primitive structure. The nerve fiber attached to these organs—specifically called cranial nerve zero because all the other numbers were already taken before it was discovered—responds specifically to scents from potential mates.

Nerve zero begins in the nose and ends in the brain area that deals with sex.

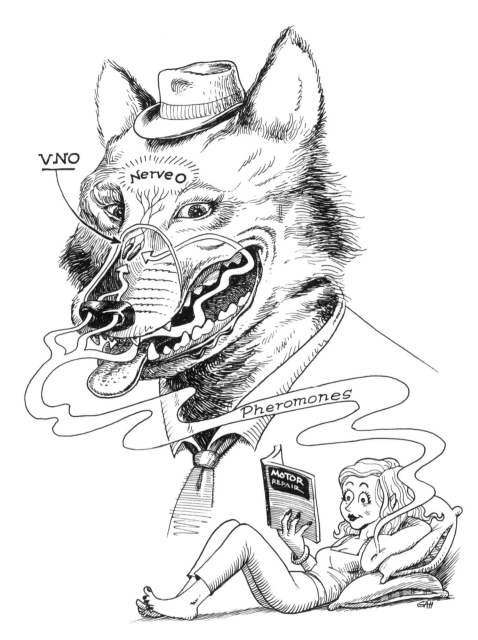

Figure 10.1 Scent of a Woman (and Man) We all know when our mates smell really good (or really bad), but our sense of smell actually kicks in at a much more subtle level. We all react to other people's scents through pheromones, which work through a specific nerve in the brain called the vomeronasal organ, or VNO. Those scents seem to go a long way in determining who we're attracted to.

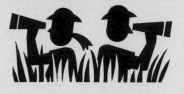

Safari Secrets:
Lessons from the Animal Kingdom

Many male animals, from hippos to horses, grimace—flaring their nostrils (this is called Flehmen response) when they're in heat so they can sense the females who might be receptive. The grimace also opens glands in the back of the throat near the tonsils that are designed to sense the female pheromone and bring a couple together—once the bull proves himself against other bulls and is accepted by the female. Men almost certainly have those glands in the roof of the mouth as well.

Because this nerve is important in the sex drive of other animals,* people theorize that it plays a big role in our sex drive, too. Why? Pheromones and testosterone both seem to be direct drivers of sexual desire and activity in long-term relationships. Even after we find a mate, we can respond to all kinds of pheromones from different people; some attract us and some repel us. Some research even indicates that specific pheromones applied to the skin increase the amount of sex we have.

The Biology of Love

We've all heard the clichés to describe being in love: butterflies in the stomach, goo-goo-ga-ga eyes, heart going pitter-patter, loins raging like 300 hungry wolves. And for good reason: Our bodies change when we're in love. And those biological changes are more than just the intangible tugs and tingles we may feel inside. They're real changes that our bodies go through when we're feeling connected with someone—when we're feeling happy. So, for the sake of science, we'd like to disband the poetic clichés to describe love and come up with a new one. Next time you're in love, try a new line: Tell that special someone that your caudate nucleus is on fire.

It's true: MRIs show that two parts of your brain—the caudate nucleus and the ventral tegmental area—light up like a movie marquee when you're in the romantic phase of love (see Figure 10.2). Why? Because of the love potion ingredient called dopamine (it's also the addictive substance that sugar, sleep, thirst, and tobacco release). When you're in love and nurture that relationship, your brain

---

* Whales, in case you're wondering.

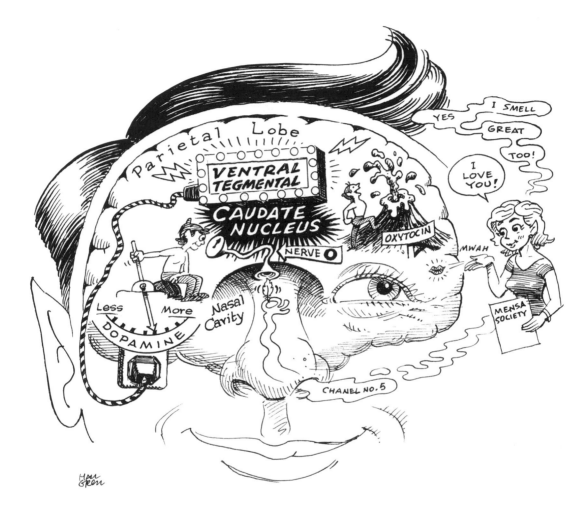

Figure 10.2 Love Potion The real aphrodisiacs aren't oysters; they're the chemicals swirling around inside our brains. While levels of dopamine surge when we're in love, we also get a surge of oxytocin (which promotes a feeling of togetherness). These chemical levels decrease over time, which is why it's vital for couples to reinvent their relationships every few years.

pumps out this feel-good chemical. Dopamine drives reward-seeking behavior or craving and increases your brain cells' release of the euphoria hormone serotonin, so the better you feel, the more you want. And because that dopamine pathway increases with risk taking, we often seek what's new and exciting.

Dopamine and serotonin are high when in "romantic" love, and when you're without your loved one, you become lovesick for chemical reasons. (The poets are just conjuring up lines to describe a reproducible biologic phenomenon.) Being lovesick actually makes serotonin levels drop 40 percent—down to the same level as people with obsessive-compulsive disorder. Being in love triggers the increase of happy chemicals, serving as the chemical reason for why we feel happy when we're in a good relationship.

Unfortunately, you develop a tolerance to dopamine over time; your brain cells release the same amount, but your receptors turn inward so they don't get the dopamine message, which is why relationships can lose some of their luster after a few years. One way to continue this chemical high is to try new (and sometimes even exotic) behaviors to increase dopamine levels and stimulate some more receptors (that's why new sex positions and sex in different rooms seem exciting, especially for men). But don't worry, because another hormone, oxytocin—the powerful chemical that makes you feel intimacy and community—comes to the rescue. When apparently unromantic researchers blocked oxytocin in prairie voles (animals that mate for life), those little buggers got right out of their holes, gathered up their music collections, and moved on out. No oxytocin, no intimacy, no lifelong love. Oxytocin, by the way, is also increased by talking, perhaps explaining why communication is so important in relationships.

This increase in oxytocin—and really the entire symphony of brain chemicals that influences love—is one reason why 99 percent of humans live in pair bonds. That's not only marriage, but any intimate relationship with one strong partner, be it a spouse, a significant other, a parent, a sibling, a close friend, or a cat or dog (women desire this community feeling more than men). From a survival-of-the-species point of view, it's important that we live in communities—hence the evolution of these biochemical effects. Nevertheless, after around four years in a relationship, the chemical tide that drives humans to stick together starts to recede. The timing isn't a coincidence, since by that time offspring, if there are any, will no longer be entirely dependent on the mother, leaving her better able to provide for herself and her children. Without chemical handcuffs, fathers are more prone to leave, which is why relationships need to move from being purely romantic to a deeper level of beauty and create a fertile field for lifelong pair bonding.

FACTOID

There's a biological reason why humans are hornier during the summer (and it has nothing to do with the dramatic seasonal increase in tank tops). Here goes: We all have a third eye called the pineal gland located in the middle of the brain, which secretes melatonin. That's what helps us sleep. Melatonin blocks our sex hormones, and the long and bright days of summer cause a decrease in melatonin production (which is what stimulates breeding in some animals—and vice versa when days are shorter and nights are longer). So our pineal gland senses the length of the day and increases our sexual drive in relation to it. What's the upside? The child is born in the following spring and has the summer to grow before enduring the challenges of winter.

The Biology of Sex

Humans are the most sexual species around. How do we know? (The answer is not from National Geographic specials.) One example: Women are sexually active for almost their entire lives and throughout all times of their menstrual cycle—meaning that they can choose to have sex even during times when they are physiologically unable to produce offspring. That means that sex must have some higher purpose and function than simply reproduction. Another: Sex drive does not need to decrease with age, meaning that we strongly desire the physical connection even after we're unable to bear children.

The Pet Connection

We all know all the good things that pets can bring to our homes (stained carpets aside). But they can also improve your health: Owning a dog, for example, lowers blood pressure of hypertensive people, and it does encourage walking. Although an hour of walking a dog by our patients provides the equivalent of eight minutes of fast-walking steps on the pedometer—so make sure you really do walk and not just watch the dog. Does it relieve stress in the way that having a romantic relationship does? It's hard to tell for sure, but a couple of studies indicate that it may. (Sorry, but cats have failed the few tests they have been used in to date.) And that's why pets are such a good source of healthy relationships, especially for people without mates, as well as widows and widowers. These pets can very much serve a buddy role that we talked about in the chapter about stress.

What's that higher purpose? For one, sex can serve as that nirvana moment between couples—a time when you feel complete happiness and intimacy, a time when you express your love to your mate. In other words, sex is designed to make you feel good. Real, real good. How good? For starters, consider that:

- Men who have sex three times a week can decrease their risk of heart attack and stroke by 50 percent.
- Women who enjoy sex tend to live longer than those who don't. Great sex makes your body feel and be the equivalent of two to eight years younger—same for men who have 150 to 350 orgasms a year, compared to the average of once per week.
- Having orgasms seems also to help decrease general pain.
- Increasing sex from once a month to once a week, according to researchers, is the happiness equivalent of an additional $50,000 in income for the typical American.

It's also interesting to look at the gender-based evolutionary functions of sex. Thousands of years ago, the woman felt that it was her job to grow the species and raise the children, so she needed someone who could protect the family. Her body responded better to intimacy (she provided that intimacy so that men could help her reach orgasm). A man had different intentions. When he saw a bunch of marauders marching through camp, he would get aroused by the threat to his family and mate—a signal that his sperm needed to beat out other men's sperm. So a man responds sexually to anxiety, risk, and excitement, in contrast to a woman's desire for intimacy.

That hard-wired difference is one way to explain the different ways that men and women feel aroused—and it's the basis for helping you figure out how to better mesh the sexual preferences and differences in your own relationships so that you don't only go through the motions when it comes to sex but also experience the emotions.

While you may think that the biggest sex organ of all is one that's covered up by the latest style from Jockey or Victoria's Secret, your brain is actually your biggest sex organ. Some researchers have said that sexual thoughts, for example, go through a man's brain once every

52 seconds and through a woman's only once a day. And even conservative researchers say that men have many more sexual thoughts than women do. Perhaps that's because men have 2.5 times the amount of brain space devoted to sexual drive that women do (or because women have more important things to think about).

Sex, of course, is more than just thinking about it; it's also about craving it. That craving originates in a part of the brain called the insula. Blocking messages to the insula is one of the ways that cigarette cessation techniques work—good news for many, they don't block sexual craving messages; in fact, bupropion, the drug we most often use in our breathe-free program with nicotine, actually in-

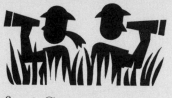

Safari Secrets:
Lessons from the Animal Kingdom

The leopard and lion actually hurt the female during intercourse. The leopard will have sex every 15 minutes for four days and has a barblike protuberance on its penis that hurts the female upon removal. He also bites her neck, and this demonstration of stamina as well as the pain it causes in his partner prompts her release of a ripe egg for fertilization. Sex isn't always sensual; the pain aspect helps dissuade the female from mating with others.

creases libido in most people. The insula (remember it from chapter 8?), a primitive area of the brain, is especially active in women who have more frequent orgasms.

Let's now look at the way men and women biologically work when it come to sex:

WOMEN: During sex, your pupils dilate, nostrils flare, heart rate increases, oxytocin level increases, sweat glands open for cooling, breasts enlarge by 25 percent, and nipples increase in height by half an inch. Infrared cameras also show increased blood flow to the lips, nose, and labia. All of these things happen as the sexual stimuli build up to the almighty orgasm (see Figure 10.3).

A good question to ask right about now: Why do women have orgasms? Evolutionarily, it was one of the ways that women could tell whether a man would be a good lifelong partner, because it could help women distinguish between a caring, patient male and a selfish or impatient one. Nevertheless, female orgasm can be so subtle that some women don't even know when they've had one. Here's what happens:

During intercourse, your vaginal walls make fluids that let your partner's penis slide with just the right amount of friction. Together with the sights, sounds, and smells of sex, the stimulation to the clitoris, labia, and breasts all builds up a crescendo of intense physical sensation. This is about the time when your brain tells your vagina and nearby muscles to contract. Why? To bring his penis in deeper and increase the chance of his sperm hitting its target—the egg. In the process, some women even ejaculate. During orgasm, the uterus dips in like an anteater and sucks up the semen into the uterus to further increase the chance of fertilization. The female orgasm also causes hormones to increase contractions in the vagina and uterus and help move semen into the uterus (women

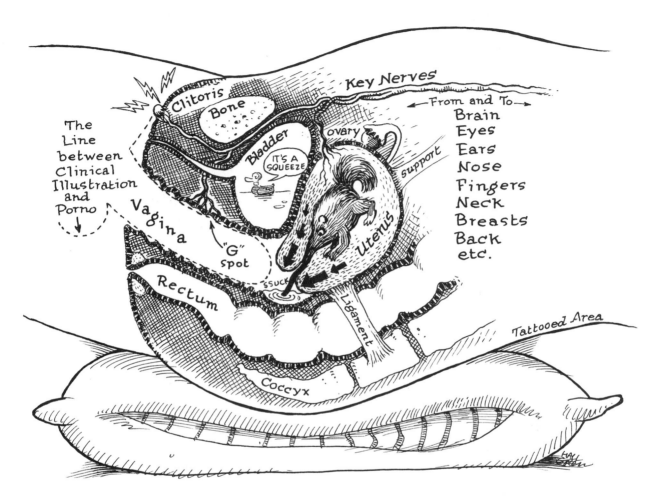

Figure 10.3 Oh, My One of the most important functions of the female orgasm (besides making her feel happy) is so her uterus can vacuum up a man's sperm to enhance fertilization. The evolutionary message: A man who can make a woman feel good through orgasm is symbolically someone who will care for her and be unselfish enough to protect her.

Frisky Food

As if there weren't enough reasons to shop for good food, here's one more: good sex. This sex-slanted shopping list will spice up your kitchen, as well as your bedroom. These are the anecdotal reports that keep recurring enough to probably have some validity:

Apples (sweet breath)

Asparagus (rich in Vitamin E, which helps hormone building)

Bananas (contain bromelain enzyme, believed to improve male libido; you also can't beat the shape)

Celery (contains androsterone, a hormone released by male sweat that turns women on)

Figs (high in amino acids to increase libido)

Garlic (contains allicin, an ingredient that increases blood flow to the sexual organs)

Nutmeg (significantly increases sexual activity in rats)

Oysters (high in zinc, which helps produce testosterone)

Wild yams (may increase genital sensitivity)

who orgasm between 1 minute before and 45 minutes after their partner's ejaculation have a higher tendency to retain sperm compared to those who don't have an orgasm).

The female orgasm, of course, isn't an easy thing to describe. The brain serves as the main conductor in this symphony, but it might involve many different instruments, sometimes including the area known as the G-spot, which is parallel to a gathering of nerves on the male prostate. Women usually do not have a single spot like some magic sex-me-here button but rather a region of nerves like those spread over the surface of the male prostate. That's because as a woman's reproductive organs develop in utero, her rudimentary prostate moves away so these nerves end up on the vaginal wall. So if you insert your index finger upward into the vagina and make the "come here" movement, you will touch the G-spot region that exists in some women. The region is often not that sensitive either, but you

GEE!

This Nerve Serves Both Sexes

Uterus
Spine
Blad.
Colon
G

never know until you try. The fact that women can be stimulated to orgasm through not only the genitals but also the mouth, nipples, and other parts of the body points to the complexity of the system—and reinforces the fact that the true biology of sex really evolves within the brain. (One theory is that sexual stimuli are carried from the cervix and uterus to the brain through the vagus nerve—one of the nerves stimulated during deep breathing and meditation.)

MEN: If you allow us a few moments to talk about the male anatomy, we think you'll be pretty amazed. Biologically, men's sexual organs are much different than those of other species. For one, a man's penis doesn't have a bone, unlike those of other species. Why? The bone makes for easy and fast access for males in the animal kingdom (to inseminate their partners quickly); men give up the bone but gain a disproportionately large penis for their body size in return. The evolutionary implications: One, men use the penis as a tool of attraction, implying that women do place some value in using it as a diagnostic for evaluating potential mates (not so overtly these days). And two, the lack of bone implies that men do equate emotions with sex, since they must be aroused for an erection; instead of easy and fast access, which can be painful to the females, it takes more care to have a sexual relationship between two people.

Another interesting observation: Humans have proportionally smaller testicles than males in other species; that's because other species need to ejaculate more semen to fertilize partners who are in heat prior to other males of the tribe and ensure propagation of their genes. Human males don't need the size because of the biological drive to be monogamous (at least serially).

Now, it doesn't take a sexologist to know the purpose of the male orgasm: Find the egg, fertilize the egg, begin shopping for Barbies. But what's interesting is that this mad dash to the egg isn't some New York City marathon where all the starter sperm strap on their Nikes with the goal

FACTOID

The sources of sperm and testosterone—the testes—are filled with tubules that look like cooked spaghetti. If these seminiferous tubules from each testicle were stretched out, they'd create a string three feet long. At age 50, tubules begin to narrow due to thickening of the connective tissue within tubules, and sperm production decreases. Sperm never lose viability (the oldest father on record was 94).

Talk to Each Other

We live in a world that gives us feedback. Our bodies give us feedback when we eat something we don't like (burps). Our computers give us feedback when we boot up. And our stereo speakers give us feedback if we point the mike in the wrong direction (the piercing sound that makes it feel as if blood is coming from your ears!). Funny thing, though: A lot of us have trouble giving feedback to each other—really good, genuine feedback—especially in our romantic relationships. Our "feedback" comes off as criticism, snarky remarks, and attacks on character. Use these strategies when you're trying to help each other—to really help them, and not hurt them.

When Giving Feedback . . .

Know the Four Qualities of Good Feedback

Specific: Feedback must be based on observable behavior, not one's feelings or the conclusions drawn from the behavior. For example, "Thanks for helping the kids build a Lego volcano." Specific compliments help.

Timely: Do it now. Don't let criticisms fester.

Actionable: Make sure it's based on something over which a person has control. "The color of your eyes scares me!" isn't helpful.

Positive: Give both positive and critical feedback, but tip the balance in the positive direction.

of making it to the finish line. Some of the sperm do that, but others are more like defensive linemen. Their job: to stop other men's sperm from scoring. Some sperm even have a dual role—blocking other sperm but allowing their own sperm with their genes to penetrate more effectively.

Now, during a man's orgasm, the brain is firing like a lit-up pinball machine, causing contractions in most muscles of the body. The purpose: Like a woman's, these contractions help increase the chance of pregnancy by enabling the penis to penetrate as deeply as possible. The glands that make semen, mostly the prostate, squeeze repeatedly, propelling sperm as deep and as far as possible. The prostate, by the way, is often referred to as the male G-spot, because it's made up of some of the same types of tissues as some of the spots identified around the nerve plexus that is the G-spot in women and can be stimulated in a similar fashion by some adventuresome couples.

When Receiving Feedback . . .

- Listen without comment, looking directly at the person. When he or she has finished, don't make any statements, but do ask questions if you want clarification. Don't accept, don't deny, and don't rationalize. Because we are rarely taught to give feedback well, you will often get feedback when the giver is angry about something in the moment. Listening should be as active a pursuit as speaking.
- Recognize the courage it took to give you the feedback and consider it a sincere gift intended to help you grow. Thank the giver for the feedback. Make it short but something you can say sincerely, such as "You've really given me something to think about, thanks." It's hard to feel real appreciation when you hear negative messages about your appearance or behavior, so it's important to have simple words of gratitude prepared ahead of time.
- Know that feedback can be tough to receive, even if we solicit it and are grateful for it. Although it's simply another's perception, feedback can shake up your feelings about yourself. Plan to do something nice for yourself when you know you're facing tough feedback. Try to do something that bolsters self-esteem—have dinner with friends or engage in an activity that you are particularly good at.

Normally, ejaculation cannons semen forward through a man's urethra and out the tip of his penis. Semen, by the way, contains hormones like oxytocin that also have a feel-good effect on women. The reason ejaculation never gets mixed up with urine is that there's a tiny muscle at the entrance of the bladder that prevents semen from slipping backward or urine from propelling forward during orgasm (it's a roadblock of sorts, so the only way for the semen to go is out). Now, some men suffer from what's called retrograde ejaculation, in which that tiny muscle doesn't work right, causing semen to backtrack into the bladder rather than to the promised land (causes for this include some side effects of surgery or medication). Retrograde ejaculation doesn't affect a man's ability to achieve an erection or ejaculate, but it may affect his fertility.

The opposite of retrograde ejaculation, of course, is when semen shoots out faster than a round from an Uzi—something that can cause angst in men and stop

The Evolution of Attraction

When it comes to sexual desire, there are biological and evolutionary reasons why our bodies (and our behaviors) work the way they do. Look at the adjacent page to learn some of the anthropology of attraction. While lust is best for finding a mate with the best genes, relationships based on love prove anthropologically to be the best for child rearing.

- Without a bone in the penis (like some other species), men need strong arousal to achieve an erection.
- White sclera (whites of eyes) and light color of iris exaggerate pupil size, which signifies that she is interested in the potential mate.
- Men prefer women with a waist-to-hip ratio of 70 percent because it's a sign of better childbearing odds.
- Women use memory stored in the hippocampus to size up men. When a woman is in love, there's more activity in the hippocampus, so she can "remember" if he'll make a good father.

a satisfying sex session in its tracks. Premature ejaculation can be caused by a number of things, including medication, hormonal changes, high blood pressure, and stress.* One of the other causes—an enlarged prostate. Since the prostate generates 95 percent of the substance that comes out during ejaculation, it's no wonder that it has a lot to say about what comes out and when. Since an enlarged prostate gets more stimulation during sex, the friction can stimulate orgasm—leading a man to ejaculate whether he wants to or not.

---

*Premature ejaculation affects one-third of men. Some treatment options include antidepressant medications (SSRIs) and behavioral techniques. Some docs suggest the man masturbate an hour or two before sex to help delay ejaculation during sex. Another technique is called the squeeze technique, in which the woman squeezes the penis at the point where the head meets the shaft for several seconds, right before a man feels like he's going to ejaculate. That should help delay orgasm; wait 30 seconds, then continue.

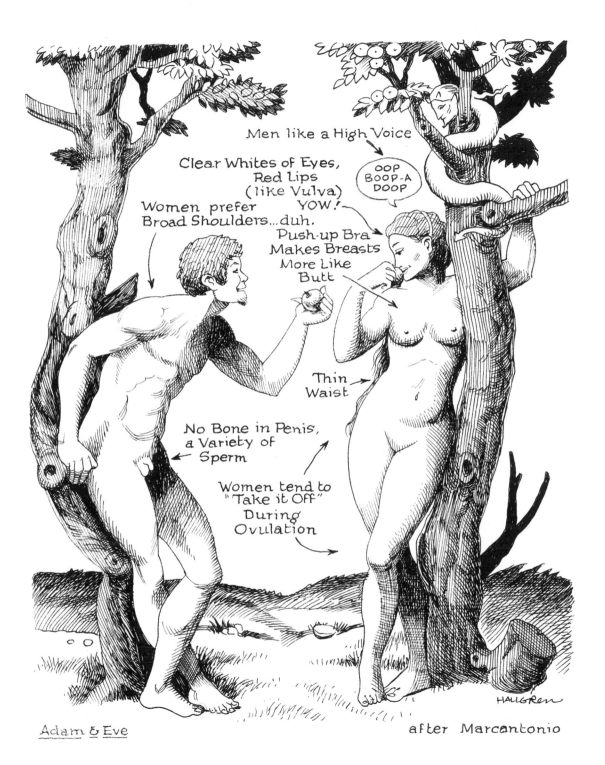

Adam & Eve

after Marcantonio

YOU Tips! Improving Your Love Life

It may seem a little odd for us to be making recommendations about how to improve your love life and your sex life. While we're not in the business of recommending battery-operated toys or suggesting that you transform your favorite yoga position into a newfangled sex position, we are certainly able to tell you how you can maximize your body's biology and chemistry to strengthen your relationships.

REINVENT YOUR RELATIONSHIP. Many couples gradually grow apart and have to reconnect. Why? A woman marries a man because she appreciates his potential and then tries to adjust him to fulfill this potential. Conversely, a man marries a woman who is exactly what he wants, and then she goes off and changes. So in effect, as soon as you fall in love, both of you start racing in different directions. Thankfully for you and any offspring, you are held together by chemical handcuffs such as dopamine and oxytocin. But as their levels wane and the cuffs slip off after five to seven years, you need to continually reinvent the marriage. People who have been married 30 years have really had four marriages. Next time you're not talking to each other, use this as an icebreaker.

DON'T TALK TO HIM AS IF HE'S A WOMAN. Women—typically much more in tune with relationship issues than men are—tend to have a better handle on communication, while men don't as easily pick up on subtle cues that women project in relationships. So, instead of hitting him, teach the man in your life about these insights, and don't assume he knows what you want (even if you think it should be obvious), so you can share expectations and be happier.

DO THE LITTLE THINGS. Sometimes we think that relationships are made or broken on the grand gestures, the big fights, the four-foot teddy bears won at the carnival. But we could strengthen our relationships immensely with more attention to the details (which can help keep the big problems from surfacing). Try these:

* Do something positive every day to "deposit" a good feeling in your relationship. A note on a napkin, a kiss on the cheek, a helping hand on a home project. (By the way, if you feel good about yourself, that's also a great gift to give to someone you love.)
* Make a date. As we get older, especially as we cart the kids to multiple events or work two jobs, it's harder and harder to carve out so-called sweetheart time. Plan time together for just the two of you. Share meals when possible, take a walk, hold hands, or just sit on the couch and catch up while the kids are in the other room playing Wii.

- Compliment daily. You're never too busy to give compliments. A well-timed "Great hair, honey" can prevent you and your partner from taking each other for granted.
- Reflect. Remember what your spouse was like when the two of you first started dating. Focus on the characteristics that first attracted you to each other (don't just look there, bucko).

NEGOTIATE. The only rules in a marriage are those that you both agree on. As long as no one is harmed (this is key), any "rules" or policies between partners may be negotiable. That could deal with anything from finances to parental discipline to how you decide where to go on vacation (you do go on vacation, right?). This will help you maintain a relationship filled with vitality and passion. So again, that means you need to talk through your issues—and your desires. Compromise on big issues, or at least agree to take turns taking the lead on decision making on big issues.

STAY FOCUSED. When you have kids, you are biologically driven to protect your gene pool, i.e., your world revolves around them. They cry for food, they need to be taken to T-ball practice, they request to be dropped off at the mall with their teenage friends. But even as you play protector, parent, and mentor to your children, you need to remember that what created the relationship is your partner, not your children.* And you need to remember that when it comes to both your time and your attention. Tough, we know, but it's helpful to remember that the happier the marriage, the easier it is to deal with the demands of raising children. Bonus: Tending to your marriage will give your children the opportunity to grow up in the care of a loving partnership (which will give them the good examples they need when they grow up). Plus, the kids will leave eventually, and you'll have just each other for the rest of your lives. Remember that kids will not treat themselves the way you treat them—they will treat themselves the way you treat yourself. Sacrificing all your happiness and giving up all your life aspirations for them will encourage them to do the same when their turn comes. And that's not good for their relationship with their future partner.

DEVELOP A SHARED VISION. In your prenuptial conversations you may have decided not to have children, to raise the children a certain religion, or never to buy artificially flavored drinks. All those premarriage goals and values are well and good, but you will be continually challenged by new issues and problems (kids, death, money), so an important tool is to be able to talk through and develop a shared vision—especially as your relationship evolves. In developing a shared vision, both partners must develop, grow, work with each other, and talk through problems in nonjudgmental ways. And if

---

*We know this is tough medicine to swallow with the divorce rate hovering around 50 percent, but it's important to remember this as you nurture and grow your relationships, as well as your children.

you disagree, take advantage of the different approaches to solving problems that each gender brings to the argument.

GIVE YOUR SPOUSE SPACE. A lot of us think that marriage and commitment have to come with a 24/7 contract—you're together all the time. You live together, you eat together, you vacation together. Heck, you can't even use the bathroom without knowing where your better half is. But partners in any relationship need a little space and can actually thrive on it. They need to live their own lives, as well as develop their own interests and friends. It's unrealistic to expect another person to fulfill your every need. The truth is that couples grow when individuals can remain individuals. Why? Because each of you will bring more back to the marriage if you're relaxed and refreshed.

BE UNPREDICTABLE. Can you name three things that would please your spouse right now? Yes? Then do one of them. Right now (go ahead, we'll still be here when you're done). Remember, the surprise isn't necessarily *what* you do per se, whether it's planning a surprise night out or trying out our special foot massage* on page 126: it's the fact that you unexpectedly took the time to do something special.

EMBRACE A LITTLE TENDERNESS. Pointing the finger works only on the cover of this book—not in relationships. Placing blame on or judging or analyzing your partner will only distance you from each other, so if the issue isn't all that serious (hello, toilet seat), then be playful and don't take yourself so seriously. Laugh at your own foibles, not your partner's. One of the best ways to give a little ground and prove to each other that you're in this together is actually one of the simplest (and hardest) for couples to do: Say you're sorry every once in a while. It's the relationship Band-Aid that can heal a heck of a lot of wounds.

MAKE AN APPOINTMENT. Many of our adult problems come from the fact that our parents weren't emotional with us as kids. Successful relationships require that we peel back this frustration and don't hide from the intimacy that we may sometimes fear. To communicate more effectively on big issues, make an appointment (it ensures your partner will be ready for you).† After you speak, your partner should mirror back what he heard you say by asking, "Is there more?" Next, he validates what you have said by pointing out what makes sense. By doing this, he demonstrates and starts feeling empathy toward you. Then it's his turn to speak. By focusing on love rather than being right or

---

*The area of the brain that senses the feet is right next door to the area of the brain that senses the genitals. Meaning: A foot rub is one of the most erotic forms of foreplay around.
†We know you've heard this from psychologist Harville Hendrix. We're a big fan of his, too.

controlling another's behavior, the couple sidesteps the pitfalls of typical arguments. It slows down the pace a bit but is much more effective in the end.

TRY THE YOUR WAY/HIS WAY FOUR-WEEK TRIAL. Sounds kinky, eh? Here's how it works: For two weeks, you make every major decision. All decisions big and small (except for sex, which always must be consensual) go your way. Then, for the next two weeks, your partner will make all the decisions. It goes for everything—what you're having for dinner, what time to go to bed, what you watch on TV, whether you spend Saturday at Starbucks or cleaning out the garage. While it may seem a little odd, it actually works in helping mend relationships that may have conflict. Why? First, it separates the actual issues from the power struggle over who is right. Once the couple buys into the experiment (obviously an important first step), they act according to their partner's wishes. It also works because it means you're reaffirming your trust in each other; just by agreeing to the experiment, each partner shows trust, first, by complying with the other's wishes, and second, by seeing that neither makes extreme demands (even when they have the power to do so). When they see that the other isn't power tripping them, each feels safer about hearing the other's preferences and accommodating them. The real benefit: This experiment sure helps decision making and negotiating once you reach day 28.

KNOW YOUR BODY LANGUAGE. A wink, a hair stroke, crossed arms—every nonverbal move or action goes a long way toward communicating whether we want you to hang around or get the hell out of our face. When you consider that 90 percent—*90!*—of our communication is conveyed nonverbally, you realize that how we gesture is as powerful as what we say. (The two parts of the brain that control this kind of communication are the amygdala and the cingulate gyrus, for those of you scoring at home.) Truth is, women are much better at picking up and using signals than men, so women, help your man read your signals better. Reading body language correctly can help head off problems and help you better communicate verbally rather than letting issues fester.

The way you talk. Roughly 40 percent of what you communicate is achieved through the components of what's called paralinguistics, the part of nonverbal communication that conveys emotions and attitudes through tone, pitch, volume, pauses, and throat clears. What's even more amazing is that these signals have five times more communicative value than the actual spoken words. Specifically, these are some of the messages that can be conveyed about personality traits:

- An increased rate of speaking generally implies that the individual is more animated and extroverted.
- Flatness in the tone of voice indicates more withdrawn and masculine characteristics.

- A nasal sound is considered undesirable.
- A person with a weak voice is usually perceived as lacking confidence, which lowers credibility. A strong voice, on the other hand, shows great confidence.
- A deeper voice in men means more testosterone at time of puberty, so more able to defend his spouse.
- A higher-pitched voice in females means more estrogen at puberty, so more able to birth viable children.

The way you move. Here's a stat that will blow every neuron in your mind: The human body is capable of making more than 700,000 unique movements (Cirque du Soleil performers, closer to 800,000) and more than 10,000 separate facial configurations (the face and hands being the most expressive parts of our bodies). But the really interesting thing is that all humans make at least a few of the same faces when expressing basic emotions—namely happiness, sadness, surprise, fear, anger, and disgust. In the 1960s, before TV made it to some distant Pacific islands, these expressions were discovered to be the same on that otherwise isolated island as in populated countries. These basic expressions are virtually identical in every culture on Earth, and in fact we don't have the ability to control them. But we do have the intrinsic ability to pick out fakes and imposters. Take the smile. A genuine smile—where the corners of your mouth turn up and the skin around your eyes crinkles—can be produced only as an involuntary response to genuine emotion. A nongenuine smile is when the lips part and the corners of the mouth are stretched to the sides.

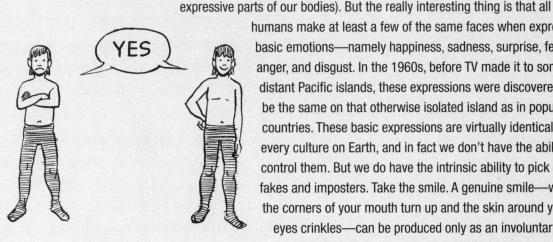

The way you touch. One of the most common ways touch is used to communicate is through the handshake. At its most basic level, the handshake communicates trust, goodwill, or agreement with a common decision. A firm handshake conveys confidence, but one that is too firm can seem threatening, while a person with a dead-fish handshake can appear ineffectual. A handshake that uses two hands or extends to the elbow can convey care or condolence. But we also use tons of other "touching" signals—a pat on the back to show support or a stroke of the arm to show sexual interest.

YOU Tips!

TRY TANTRIC. When you hear the term *tantric sex,* you may assume that we're talking about the ability to have a sexual interlude that lasts longer than a transcontinental flight. But that's not really the goal of tantric sex. The goal stems from the desire and ability to have more of a physical and spiritual connection during sex. Physically, for men, that means developing the ability to, as tantrics say, "retain the seed"—that is, having the ability to control ejaculation to allow sexual energy to flow. But the essence of that practice—and of the tactics below—is really about mindfulness, or being deeply aware of yourself, your partner, your life, and what's called the sacred life force. These tips can help you maximize your sexual experience—and bring deeper emotional levels to your relationship.

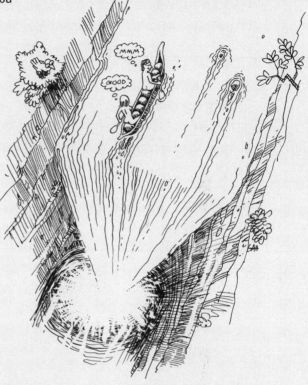

- Change your mind-set: Stop thinking that your sexual satisfaction is the responsibility of your partner. We're all responsible for our own experience. Be open to discussions about sex with your partner, and be open in exploring your own body to help your partner help you.
- Men, when you're by yourself, you can practice increasing your sexual energy. Bring yourself to two or three peaks at a time—ejaculating only after you've come close to the edge a few times. (Deep breathing can help you teeter on the edge without falling over.) What you're doing is priming your prostate gland like a pump to help improve sexual performance.
- Challenge yourself. You give yourself goals at work and in life, so why not create some for the bedroom? It can be anything—practicing Kegel exercises during the day or working to locate your G-spot if you haven't.

- Be softer. One of the main tenets here is to slow things down. Don't be in such a rush to get to bed or to finish up. Carve out time to have a marathon lovemaking session in which the final goal isn't necessarily an orgasm but simply the journey itself.

PLAY TO YOUR PARTNER'S STRENGTHS. We all know the whole Mars and Venus debate. Men are different sexual creatures than women. Men respond to new visual cues; women respond to friendly emotional ones. Go a little deeper, and you understand that it's more that men respond to fear and excitement, and women respond to intimacy. Instead of agreeing to disagree, couples should capitalize on their differences to help make their partners more comfortable in bed. So what does that mean? A man should make it a habit to look into his partner's eyes during sex: That eye lock is a way to increase intimacy (and oxytocin). And a woman should acknowledge that her partner's arousal may be based more on urgency, meaning that it's not so bad to have the lights on during sex, crave a quickie, or meet up for a lunch hour that involves absolutely no lunch at all.

GO CRAZY. There's a reason why bungee jumping, river rafting, and sneaking into the supply closet can make the perfect first date. Doing novel things with another person stimulates dopamine—the feel-good chemical that's elevated when you're in love. Also, since men are aroused by fear and anxiety and heart rates are elevated during both attraction and danger, it increases the likelihood that a man will find his partner more attractive during a daredevil date. The dopamine is actually firing high when you first get together but not necessarily on the 80th date, so it's even better to make special new adventures or variations more common the longer you're together. Novel choices are especially great for couples whose libido has diminished or whose sex life has gone stale.

MIX IT UP. Guys, listen up. While men have orgasms in 95 percent of sexual encounters, some reports have women having orgasms in 69 percent of encounters.* Interestingly, the more varied the sexual activity, the more likely a woman is to have an orgasm. That means mixing it up among manual, oral, and genital stimulation. Oral sex, by the way, increases a woman's chance of having an orgasm.

OPEN THE FRIDGE. While you're probably thinking that we're going to tell you to get some chocolate sauce and whipped cream, the truth is that food plays a vital role in our sexual desire—some because of the smell, some because of the shape, and some because they alter your body chemistry to make you a more desirable mate. Our choices:

*We couldn't have made up a better number for this statistic if we tried, eh? Of course, getting these numbers is hard to do, and some reports have much lower numbers.

- Take advantage of pheromones: Capitalize on those scents by exposing yourself to them: Research shows that the scents of lemons, doughnuts, and licorice increase penile blood flow (necessary for men to achieve an erection). Don't eat the doughnuts (that slows blood flow dilation down); just smell. For women, it's licorice and cucumbers. Why? For women, the phallic shape subconsciously plays a large part in that. Another good one to smell for its pheromone effect: baby powder. It makes the female partner think of the evolutionary goal of sex, at least subconsciously.

- Strengthen the sperm: If your goal is to consummate your attraction with reproduction, then you should also supplement yourself with zinc, selenium, folic acid, and vitamins C and E, which have been shown to increase sperm count. But most important is DHA-omega-3 fats—the active ingredient in fish oil that can be obtained in even more purified form from the algae they eat.

- Go back to that sauce: Chocolate has long been considered a love drug, because some of the ingredients* have a feel-good effect. One study also shows that caffeine may have a positive effect on female libido.

GET YOUR DRIVE BACK. If you feel as if you've lost some of your sex drive, try these tactics for restoring some of your long-lost libido:

- Check out our battery of tests from chapter 6. A change in hormones or energy levels could be a primary driver.
- Ask yourself what happened in your relationship when you noticed your sex drive changing. If you can ID the out-of-bed problem, it can help lead to an in-bed solution.
- If you're suffering from some kind of vaginal pain (see chapter 7), some strengthening exercises (called Kegels) may help, depending on the issue.
- Experiment with more oral sex, fantasies, or watching each other in videos or in real life. Change things up to charge things up.

* Phenylethylamine, tryptophan, and anandamide.

- Get comfortable with yourself. You can try to reboot your system by experimenting with your body and finding what brings you joy (for instance, many women like the shaft of their clitorises stimulated, rather than the tip, so you need to be able to communicate that to your partner). Get comfortable with the fact that a mirror, sex toys, and locked doors can be a healthy part of a solo experience that can energize your sex life with your partner.

CHECK YOUR WAIST. Fat doesn't just make it hard for you to see your organs. It also makes it hard for them to function, which is why increasing waist size means decreasing libido. One of the reasons why men lose libido: omental fat (fat around the belly). That omental fat converts testosterone to estrogen and thus diminishes sex drive. So if you're experiencing a loss of sex drive, a doc may first check the size of your testes (they should be roughly a ratio of 1¹/₂ inches height to 1 inch width, or three finger widths by two finger widths). If they're normal size, it could mean that omental fat is causing the testosterone drop. While you're losing the belly fat, a medication called clomiphene, which blocks the conversion from testosterone to estrogen, may help. If you want to keep your libido (or get it back), get your waist size to less than half your height.

GO ALL LOMBARDI ON HIM. When it comes to sex, some women are as silent as a 1920s movie. They fear that they can't tell their men what they want in bed—maybe because they're shy, maybe because they're embarrassed, or maybe because their partner's ego is as delicate as a silk blouse. But the best thing you can do with your mouth to improve your sex life has nothing to do with the X-rated thoughts crossing your mind right about now; it's talking. Women need to teach, coach, and encourage their men to give them what they want—and how they want it. Believe us, it's much more of an ego boost for men to know they're pleasing their women than not to know something was wrong in the first place.

KEEP IT PUMPING. Good sex isn't just about blindfolds and finger paints. It's really about good blood flow. That ensures you're getting the right nutrients to your brain, as well as the right stimuli to your sex organs. So improving your sex life means avoiding the things that decrease blood flow (nicotine, drugs, saturated fat, trans fats, sugar, syrups, diabetes, high BP) and embracing the things that increase blood flow (exercise, avocados, fruits, vegetables, 100 percent whole grains, ginseng, ginkgo biloba, L-arginine, lemon, citriulline).

11

That's the Spirit

How to Find True Happiness

YOU Test: Awe, Shucks

Answer yes or no to the following questions. Have you ever had an experience when . . .

- You had no sense of time or space?
- You couldn't express it in words?
- It felt like pure perfection?
- Something greater than yourself seemed to absorb you?
- Everything seemed to disappear from your mind?
- Everything in the world seemed to be part of the same whole?

Results: If you answered yes to at least four of the questions, it's very likely that you had some kind of awe-inspiring experience. As you're about to find out, that sense of awe is a big part of what helps make us happy.

Today the word *awe* gets thrown around like a dishrag. LeBron James, awesome player. What an awesome skirt you just picked up at the sale. That wave? Totally awesome, dude.

For now, let's break away from the word's informal and loose definition of awesome and dissect it a little. Awe—a relatively unstudied emotion that exists somewhere along the boundary line between pleasure and fear—can come from a variety of stimuli. We can be in true awe of Tahitian sunsets, an artist's masterpiece, a tear-inducing symphony, a hero's actions, or a heavenly piece of tiramisù. When we experience awe, we react by engaging all of our attention, thoughts, hopes, and needs. It consumes us, primarily because it's an experience in which we feel—really feel, deep in our solar plexus—as if the world is bigger than us. Why? More likely than not, it's because an awe-inspiring experience is both unexpected (we couldn't see it coming) and mysterious (we have no idea how it came to be).

In many ways, that's exactly what happiness is all about: finding our path to happiness through things in our lives that help us experience feelings of awe. That feeling certainly can come in the form of a knee-shaking romantic relationship, and it can come in many other forms, as well—like your relationship with others, or coming to realize your true purpose in life, using spirituality to think about the big things in life that have the power to truly make you happy.

The big secret of finding happiness: living simply enough that you can recognize and experience these awe moments. Now, if we were to ask a thousand people for their secret to happiness, we'd surely hear two thousand different answers.* The responses would run the gamut of wants and desires—owning a 40-foot sailboat, living in good health, working in a no-stress job, having sex three times every day, watching sunsets along the beach, spending quality time with the family, winning an Oscar, winning the Super Bowl, winning the lottery. All may be

* We're always changing our mind, after all.

perfectly fine answers. But the kind of happiness we mean when we talk about the looking beautiful, feeling beautiful, being beautiful trilogy lies at a much deeper level.

In this chapter we're going to explore six paths to happiness through deeper meanings and purpose in life—the things that make you truly unique and truly beautiful. Some of these ways have a clear biological and evolutionary basis, while others are just beginning to be understood. And many of them are starting to gain scientific support for their healing powers. Here you'll find us talking about things that are extremely personal—things that we'd share and talk about with our own family and friends. We're not backing a particular religion or saying there's one spiritual prescription to heal all problems, but we do believe that this area of health—that which addresses deep issues of the soul—is absolutely worth exploring and talking about with those close to you. In any case, it's clear that a "beautiful being" isn't about just what you can do for yourself but what gifts you can pass to others.

The Six Paths to Happiness

1: Being Positive—and Generous

We all have friends or family who fit the polar ends of personality—the cheerleader types who can smile even after getting puddle-pummeled by a bus and the negative types who frown at butterflies. Positive emotions play a crucial role in developing the enduring relationships that are critical for our happiness. (One example: the boomerang smile—that is, a shared smile between mother and baby.)

We know negative emotions change our brain function to increase stress, which increases the risk of things such as cancer and heart disease. Since we also know positive emotions change the way brains function to reduce stress, they can help cancel out those health risks. The best evidence comes from studies on meditation and relaxation therapies, which show their ability to calm a jumpy heart. Other studies have found a strong correlation between positive moods and the improvement of physical symptoms such as listlessness and weakened immune function. All are clearly contributors to happiness (or lack thereof).

Part of the reason happiness is an important part of the beautiful triumvirate is that you can't really feel happy unless your body feels tuned and your mind feels sharp. Without a sound body, you can't form a sound mind. One of the strongest correlates of happiness is having the health to accomplish your purposes in life.

Almost every study of longevity indicates one secret that makes people healthier and happier: helping others. Some research shows a 60 percent decrease in mortality figures among those who help others; they're aided by what's called the "helper's high." Specifically, it's the dignity, the joy, the passion, and the purpose of helping others—whether it's helping another person quit smoking, building a home for a person in need, or mentoring a child at school—that have these beneficial effects. Research shows that people who donate money are happier than people with the same amount of money who don't donate to others.

Helping others inspires gratitude for what life has given you, and this is what really turbocharges your happiness—and helps you define your own purpose in life. After all, the real secret may be realizing that true peace isn't about being happy, giddy, and feeling as if you're charged up on Red Bull all the time. It's about slowing down enough to realize that you have a lot of gifts—gifts that you should be passing along to others.

2: Feeling Empathy

In the same way we know people with extremist personalities, we all know people at both ends of the empathy spectrum: the ones who will rush right over with a freshly baked lasagna when your cat dies and the ones who make you work until 9 p.m. on the night your kid has the solo in the seventh-grade choral concert. Typically, we'd call the latter Scrooge "coldhearted." But the biology's all wrong. Ain't the heart that's cold; it's the brain.

As with virtually every one of our biological functions, there's a survival value in feeling empathy for others; teaming up with a community to get a job done or fend off an attack is more advantageous than doing it alone. It's more than just adaptation at play, though. It's brain function. Our moral system is largely dependent on how connected we feel with others; the more connected we feel, the higher our degree of generosity and compassion.

Part of the biology comes from a phenomenon involving what are called mirror neurons (see Figure 11.1). Someone does something around you (yawns or crosses her arms), and you pick up on it and reflect the same action back. Mirror neurons—like tiny, neurological video cameras—record life as it happens. They're how children learn and why you may pick up a southern accent after living a year in Louisiana. These neurons are found in various areas of the brain, and they fire in response to people's actions. When you see a person performing an action, you automatically want to simulate the action with the brain (certain circuits in the brain may actually prevent you from doing it, though). This applies to watching someone dance on *Dancing with the Stars* or serve an ace at the U.S. Open, which is why we can perform better after a real pro shows us the way. Mirror neurons enabled the brains of our ancestors to increase dramatically in size, because their learning (and survival) ability grew so dramatically.

The cool thing is that mirror neurons don't fire only with yawning and other inconsequential bodily blurts; your mirror neurons also react to emotions, generating empathy. When you see someone touched in a painful way, your own pain areas are activated; when you see a spider crawl up someone's leg, you feel a creepy sensation because your mirror neurons are firing. Social emotions such as guilt, shame, embarrassment, and lust are based on a uniquely human mirror neuron system found in the part of your brain called the insula (remember, the part of the brain associated with addictions). It's why you feel sad in the face of tragedy; you can empathize with the people who experience it. It's what allows you to connect with other humans—and transcend your differences. It's also one of the reasons why church services and rituals can be so effective in helping people stay happy; they help teach you how you're supposed to feel and how powerful it can be to help others.

We also know that different parts of the brain react depending on the morality

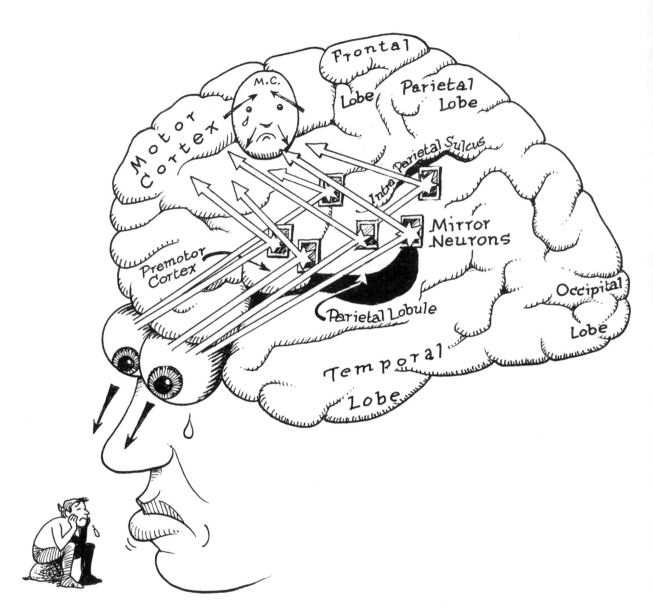

Figure 11.1 **Mirror, Mirror** Mirror neurons allow us to copy others when they influence the motor cortex (MC), like making us yawn when other people do. They're also responsible for making us feel empathy in our parietal lobe when other people are in pain. They may go a long way in explaining why helping others contributes so much to our own happiness.

What You Can Learn from Buddhism

When some people think about meditation, the first association that pops into their minds is Buddhism. But most people know as much about Buddhism as they know about supernova nucleosynthesis. The goal of Buddhist meditation isn't to suppress emotions that are harmful (as many might expect) but rather to identify how they arise, how they are experienced, and how they influence us over the long run. For Buddhists, the good life isn't achieved by transcending an emotion—not even hatred—but by effectively managing it. The three mental processes that are most toxic to the mind (and that lead to all kinds of mental suffering):

- **Craving.** Me, mine, mmmm. Cravings happen when a person exaggerates the good qualities of an object (icing!) while ignoring the bad ones (calories!). Therefore, cravings can disrupt the balance of the mind, easily leading to anxiety, misery, fear, and anger.
- **Hatred.** The reverse of craving, hatred exaggerates the bad qualities and deemphasizes the good ones. It's driven by the wish to harm or destroy anything that gets in your way. The impression is that the dissatisfaction belongs to the object, when the true source of it is in the mind alone.
- **Delusion.** According to Buddhism, the self is constantly in a state of dynamic flux and is profoundly interdependent with other people and the environment. However, people habitually delude themselves about the actual nature of the self by superimposing the interpretations of their own reality.

Try this to help channel negative emotions: Wear some kind of wristband or rubber band on your wrist, and every time you find yourself doing something positive (such as resisting bad cravings or feeling empathy rather than hatred), switch the band to the other wrist. That ritual of positive reinforcement helps reinforce good behavior—and can act as a warning against bad behavior. (If you're too good a person, try to avoid abrasion of the skin on your wrists from passing it back and forth too much.)*

*Modified for positive feedback from Pastor Will Bowen.

of the decisions you make. In some MRI tests, researchers found that the left frontal lobe and temporal lobes were activated when making moral judgments, and it seems that when some of that neural circuitry is injured, morality can also be impaired. Cats have very small frontal lobes so they tend to not be as compassionate. Women appear to access this part of the brain (not the cat's, their own) more than men, especially during childbearing years.*

3: Finding Authenticity

With all due respect to our brethren in the animal kingdom, there's no question that human beings sit atop the earthly hierarchy. After all, it's not as if ants developed the space shuttle or a leopard penned *Macbeth* or northern birds text-message each other about their final Florida destination. While it would be nice to sit back, thump our chests, and extol the many virtues of mind and body, the true human experience—that which serves as one foundation for *being* beautiful—happens not necessarily because we're smarter. It happens because we're deeper. That, folks, begs a pretty big question: Where does the *being* in *human being* come from?

Let's think of "being" as existing on three levels—ranging from automatic, instinctual actions to highly developed spiritual and contemplative ones. Who we are and what we feel represent a highly fluid meshing of multiple forces in all three of the following levels:

- **Level 1:** Automatic being. The most primitive of the levels, this one is essentially categorized by our animal within. We hungry, we eat. We tired, we sleep. We tingle, we make babies. Simply, the emotional center in your brain decides how you feel, and your mental motherboard tells you not to overthink. Just act.

- **Level 2:** Educated being. If level 1 is primal, then level 2 is cultural or social. We learn how to feel or behave in certain situations and then act accordingly. Much of these actions are based on routines of how we've learned to do things (such as how we argue or how we drive to work using the same path) and aren't instinctual. Here, our brains take the information we receive, process it for a moment (but just for a moment), and move on.

---

* In this regard, female brains become more like male brains after menopause.

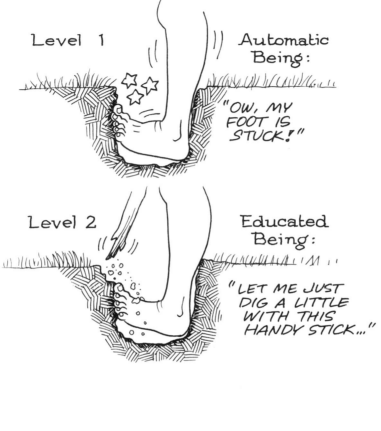

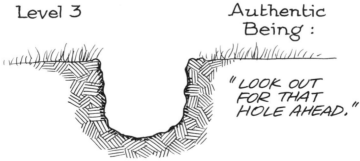

Figure 11.2 Deep Thoughts Thinking about your own existence and how you operate on many different levels—from the very basic to the extremely spiritual—will help you come closer to meeting the expectation of your potential you.

- **Level 3:** Authentic being. This third level is what separates man from meerkat. It involves the uniquely human capacity to enlarge our attention, to contemplate the big picture, and to be open-minded enough to think beyond primal instincts and learned, habitual behaviors. Perhaps the best way to describe this level is through the image of a wheel with a hub and spokes. In essence, authenticity happens when you can shift your thinking to realize that you're not the hub in the center of the wheel but are connected to the center at all times, and the world works together elegantly. You're just one of many nodes in a highly interconnected world of relationships.

Most of our lives are spent driven by external factors and motivators (striving for that pay raise, promotion, or Hummer limo) as opposed to intrinsic ones with a higher ideal (a love of the work you do and your purpose). So to find our true, authentic self and be happy about what we find, we must know how we exist in relationship to other things—specifically to other people and to the world at large (one of the reasons why finding and being a good buddy are so important). When we break through the instincts and the habits, we break through a level of superficiality that many people typically tend to live with. And that's when we break through to a deeper experience in life.

This takes some time, some practice, and some energy; in fact, our brains can dramatically increase their energy consumption levels when we focus. Since the brain consumes 20 to 25 percent of our calories when we're at rest, augmenting its activity can be an important change in the status quo.

4: Embracing Emotion

If you understand the magnificent machinery that is the human brain, you'll better understand why some of us bounce around with great joy and others slouch through life like Eeyore (from *Winnie-the-Pooh*). That three-pound bugger is more powerful than our strongest computer, more artistic than a Renaissance painter, and often more mysterious than our entire universe.

Every day, we're pummeled with thousands upon thousands of pieces of information. And it's not just information per se, like the kind you read in the paper or an e-mail; sometimes it's informational stimuli that you take for granted as part of your everyday routines, such as traffic lights or coffee shop menus. Frankly, your brain is pretty darn good at inputting all that info (red equals stop, venti is the extra-large cup). But because of that influx and onslaught of sensory information, we need some kind of prioritizing system to help manage the inflow.

Remember from our chapter on stress that our neurological gatekeeper is the amygdala—which instantly assigns emotional meaning to this type of information. Often, we suppress those emotions—even though they're automatic. Our goal here shouldn't be to ignore emotions when they come up—whether we are reacting painfully to a loss of a loved one or getting angry when we're mad at our boss or kids.

In fact, we're biologically hardwired to pay attention to emotions and use them intelligently. For example, we recommend that you use empathy to help harness anger (for example, thinking that maybe the jerk at work has some home stresses that are causing him to be a jerk). Our goal should be to observe emotions—and even learn to *think* with these emotions to help give our lives even deeper meaning. That is why meditation is not the emptying out of our brains so they are devoid of ideas, but rather a technique to gently nudge out ideas that enter, without your becoming emotionally attached.

Now more than ever, we're understanding the biology behind this sense of transcendence beyond our typical reality. For example, we're now able to explain how out-of-body experiences happen, at least physically. The primary senses of sight, smell, hearing, and touch have great blood supply, but the part of the temporal lobe that integrates these senses together is in a watershed area that suffers from inadequate oxygen when your blood pressure drops too low. When this happens, the sensory input becomes disconnected; many people who have had near-death experiences report "leaving" their bodies. Transcendent experiences are also associated with things such as hallucinogenic drugs and even orgasms—when you experience the feeling that nothing else matters. Thankfully, humans have healthy ways of achieving these states of disconnect (like meditation). As we search for meaning in life, we're moved by these experiences that reveal the big picture.

5: Exploring Spirituality

For some, being spiritual means going to church every day. For others, it means finding a silent place (you're less likely to be disturbed in the bathroom) to meditate and think about the bigger picture in life. And for a few, it means closing your eyes and looking to the sky when the field goal kicker is looking at a 50-yarder with time running out.

There is some hotly disputed evidence suggesting a genetic influence in the amount or degree of spirituality a person can have—that people who are more spiritual than others actually have a gene that's linked to a specific spirituality receptor in the brain. Which would mean that people have various dispositions for feeling spiritual, just the same way they have predispositions for heart disease. Of course, we also have the ability to tweak, modify, and change those predispositions with the choices we make (just as in people with predispositions for heart disease). You may remember from YOU: *Staying Young* that the telomere caps on the tips of our chromosomes are a way of judging your rate of aging—the longer your telomeres, the more your stem cells can reproduce and repair damage elsewhere in your body and the younger you are. People with purposes in life (ones that don't stress them) have much longer telomeres (almost eight years' worth longer) than their chronological age and other health behaviors would justify—the telomeres seem to be elongated by having that purpose.

Scientists have long speculated that religious feelings can be tied to a specific place in the brain. They found this out by studying a form of epilepsy in which seizures originate as electrical misfirings within the temporal lobes. Epileptics who have this form of the disorder often report intense religious experiences, leading researchers to speculate that localized electrical storms in the brain's temporal lobe might sometimes be related to religious experience. These feelings may be connected to the limbic system, which comprises interior regions of the brain that govern emotion (amygdala) and emotional memory (hypothalamus). It's also possible that different religious feelings arise from distinct locations in the brain (and individual differences might also exist).

So now the question is: How can you learn to be spiritual? Well, primarily through training your brain with transcendent experiences such as meditation or prayer—that is, altering your state of consciousness to focus on a sacred image or thought.

Maybe you got your first taste of prayer before meals or before going to bed. Maybe you pray every Sunday or every day. Or maybe the only time you ever prayed was in the half second that your car hydroplaned on the highway. Clearly, we all have different perceptions of what praying means—and what it does. And, like many other things, prayer works for some people and doesn't do diddly for others. (There are a lot of conflicting data to do with the effects of prayer, proving just that.) For us, prayer isn't asking for a specific answer or outcome (give us rain!) but rather gaining the ability to cope with a desperate situation (a drought). The purpose of prayer isn't to change the Divine or alter what your god is thinking but to change you—to give you the strength to manage tough times. Prayer, to us, is somewhat interchangeable with meditation in that it's silent contemplation.

Few people would say that prayer gets the medical and scientific attention that, say, Alzheimer's research gets, but that doesn't mean that there isn't some impressive scientific evidence about the power of prayer. For example, we know that prayer and meditation change neurological structure. Meditation leads to a thicker cortex (any kind of regular mental activity builds new brain connections). And we know that meditation works for relaxation, at least partially by soothing the vagus nerve—a nerve that carries a truckload of information to the brain.

So you can build up your brain just like your biceps if you do the correct exercises. Some studies have also shown that the frontal lobe (which deals with concentration) lights up like a campfire during prayer and meditation. Still other researchers used EEG tests to show that meditating monks had higher than normal gamma waves, which are thought to be helpful in synchronizing separate forms of brain function to help form a unified perception of the world (the purpose of prayer and meditation, after all, right?).*

And believe it or not, though your body is not spending energy during such meditation, your brain can almost double its activity level.

Regardless of what motivates people to pray, there's no denying that a lot of people do it. One study shows that 36 percent of people use complementary and alternative medicine, but that number almost doubles when prayer is included in the definition. Those respondents say they use prayer for their own health and to help others. Even more telling: Of those people who said they prayed for health reasons, 70 percent said that prayer was helpful. Why? Seems as though it may work through several different mechanisms:

- **It relaxes.** A form of meditation (no matter what your religious preferences), prayer helps to slow breathing and brain activity, and reduces heart rate and blood pressure. All relaxing, all good.
- **It's positive.** Let's face it: When you pray, you typically don't finish feeling as though you want to rap somebody's ankles with a wooden spoon. Afterward you're filled with peace, joy, and other emotions that are worthy of being printed on holiday cocktail napkins. There's some evidence that these emotions lead to positive physiological responses throughout the entire body. Our stress hormone levels prepare for a peaceful existence. Perhaps more important, our immune system

*Buddhist monks hypertrophy the meditation centers of their brain on MRI scanning and can selectively increase blood flow to these areas within minutes of entering a meditative state, proving that we can retrain our brains.

becomes less agitated so that chemicals such as pro-inflammatory cytokines, which act like kerosene on a fire, are not driving our joints and arteries to overreact to every biologic stress inside us. The result: a less inflamed, more beautiful place to live.

- **It's better than nothing (i.e., the placebo effect).** We'd be remiss in our reporting if we didn't say that some of the benefits derived from prayer can be accounted for simply because the person feels as if it's helping, whether it's helping physiologically or not. (Placebo responses account for as much as 70 percent of the beneficial effect of some medical procedures and drugs. Our stance here is that thinking you're doing something to help yourself is a big part of prayer anyway.)

- **It's supernatural.** Perhaps the hardest reason to quantify, it's also one of the most powerful. Praying people believe in supernatural forces and in a god's ability to heal, and that seems to have a strong effect on their health—even if the real mechanism of effectiveness is through one of the three previous reasons. Now, no two mystics describe their otherworldly experiences in the same way, and it can be difficult to distinguish among the various types of mystical experiences, be they spiritual, traditionally religious, or simply awe-inspiring moments. If you're an atheist and you live a certain kind of experience, you will relate it to the magnificence of the universe. If you're a Christian, you'll associate it with God. The point, for us, isn't the differences between the spiritual experiences but rather the similarities—and that we can get to that place in lots of different ways.

We think it's likely that future tests and studies will continue to show the relationships between health and silent meditation. In fact, we feel that understanding these mysterious energies is the next big frontier in medicine. That is, we define life at the level of the cell. As long as the membrane maintains an energy gradient between the inside and outside world, our cells are alive. When you aggregate cells into organs and then put them in the right spot to make a human, you have life. That's why we're interested in adjusting energy in the body through such vehicles as acupuncture, homeopathy, pulsed electromagnetic fields (which can reduce pain by 90 percent through nitric oxide), and hard-to-explain methods like Reiki and prayer. After all, the things that matter in life—like love—can't always be measured with blood, machines, and complex calculations. They're measured in the way you live.

6: Understanding Unhappiness

Here's a surprise for you: Being happy means that you realize that there are times you will be unhappy and recognize that life sometimes stinks. What's uplifting in those times is appreciating life and facing the challenges that come with it, realizing that you're facing challenges fellow humans have also faced.* Now, let's be clear that we're not saying you should lower your expectations for your so-called perfect life or downsize your goals; we just believe that if you can align your expectations with reality a little more by expecting to face challenges, you'll be better off in the end. There's an interesting biological reinforcement for this notion, too: Your levels of C-reactive protein (a marker of damaging inflammation) have been shown to be higher when you have expectations that are unattainable. Makes sense: You worry when you're not hitting goals, so that makes your body more vulnerable to stress. We need to start learning how to be comfortable being uncomfortable.

Depending on who you live with, work with, or share poker chips with, you've probably heard every lament there is. Unhappy with the job, unhappy with the spouse, unhappy that the TV remote is lost again.† These unhappy moments stress us and cause inflammation in the rest of the body and less focus for our brain. While our goal here is certainly to find a steady level of peace and happiness in our lives, we also know that we can't expect our euphoria to last as long as a Wal-Mart week: 24/7. There's actually some benefit to experiencing some un-

---

*That's the proverbial joy of knowing you've run the marathon, even if it's occasionally painful while you're doing so.
† It's wedged into the side of the couch and under the pillow.

happiness.* The original survival value of unhappiness: When you were unhappy and pessimistic, you were better prepared for problems that might arise. Today, though, unhappiness still serves an important purpose. Unhappiness forces you to think through problems to help you gain wisdom and perspective, to think about what gives you happiness so you can set new directions and develop new ideas that may actually change your life.

Let's take smokers as an example. Part of the reason smokers have such difficulty quitting is that they have developed a misaligned coping mechanism (you're stressed by that boss, so you go out to smoke; but the boss is still there when you return). Smokers often feel that they're locked into a cycle of unhappiness: When they quit, they're unhappy, and they feel as if they're the only people in the world who are, so they get even unhappier, which makes them want to smoke again to feel happy again. But realizing that this cycle of unhappiness is natural could actually help smokers (and others facing challenges) get through tough times.

But remember, happiness also correlates with having the health to achieve your goals—so getting rid of maladaptive coping mechanisms (like smoking or other unhealthy habits) is important, too. If you can't align your expectations with your reality, you're more likely to experience an inner conflict that gently (and often subconsciously) tugs, gnaws, and claws at you because something doesn't feel quite right. Seems so simple, yet most of us are confounded by even the simplest behavioral modifications needed to course-correct. Why? Because most of our perceptions and actions are subconscious and automated, which has tremendous survival value for each of us but does not offer the autonomy we crave to bring our expectations and reality into sync.

So much of our life is lived with a veneer crafted around us—to protect us, to shield us, to keep our true selves away from the world. Very few times do we get to experience a true, deep reality when the veneer's gone and we see the bigger picture of what's out there in the world, how we fit into it, and how we can help others. We obsess over our day-to-day responsibilities, we fret about making mis-

---

* Let's also be clear that there's a big difference between day-to-day unhappiness and true clinical depression, which is destructive and unhealthy.

takes at work, and we taunt and nag and snip at people we dislike (and sometimes people we love); in essence, we're often shackled by the superficiality of our world. You might live too much in the past and future when you should be bathing in the present, when you could be thinking about relationships, about new ideas, and about all the deeper truths of the world—your world—and how you fit into it.

YOU Tips!

We wear scrubs, not collars. We deliver medicine, not sermons. And our specialty is biology, not theology. So we're not going to stand at a pulpit and try to deliver ten commandments for moral living. However, to dismiss the very distinct link between looking, feeling, and being a beautiful being would be a great mistake. So we are going to stand here and offer our prescription for doing the right thing, embracing spirituality, and finding a happier you.

GIVE, THEN PASS. There are few feelings in the world that surpass that of knowing you've helped someone—whether it's through a financial donation or a mentoring program or giving up your seat on a crowded bus. It feels good—and is good. So good, in fact, that some researchers have found that the effect of giving, of altruisms small and big, is similar to the so-called runner's high (the rush of endorphins). But unlike exercise euphoria, this rush can last a long time. The evidence: Ninety percent of people who experience this high give their health condition a better grade than those who don't. The reason: It seems that charity might really start at home. Your thoughts about helping others help you. They seem to be able to do things that strengthen your immune system, boost positive emotions, decrease pain, and provide stress relief. Separate studies show that charitable heart attack patients recover faster than those who aren't, and those who do volunteer work have death rates 60 percent lower than those who don't. But here's the catch. When you give something to somebody, we want you to find a way to allow them to have the dignity to pass it along to someone else. Though people very often need help, they also don't want to feel like charity cases. They want to feel that they can also pass something along to others. This also makes giving more attractive, since you are really priming the pump of a chain reaction that will help many more people than the one group you targeted with your kindness. So be explicit in your giving and ask how the recipient will pass it forward. Try to pick situations where this expectation is clear.

PASS THE PASSION. While many people think they should give to charity or do something to give back, that's not the only concept that's important. It's not the obligation to give back but the privilege of doing something bigger than yourself. You don't have to donate money, just time and passion. You don't have an obligation to society to find a bigger purpose—you have an obligation to your own health and happiness. And the more you value what you are doing with your mind, the more you'll do healthier things with your body.

CREATE RITUALS. One of the reasons why church, music, and prayer can be such an uplifting experience is that the weekly rituals reinforce a sense of community (remember the idea of being individual *and* connected to others?). You can experience those spiritual highs by attending church, but you can also do it through other rituals—such as nature walks with a group of people in your neighborhood or an annual trip with your family or a nightly dinnertime routine in which each person shares one wonderful thing that happened to him or her that day. Rituals also reinforce behaviors (smokers are reminded of this every time someone taps the top of a pack of cigarettes).

SAY THANKS. Any parent raising a child knows how much time is spent teaching that child some manners. Say thank you when someone gives you a present. Say thank you when somebody holds the door. Say thank you when the server notices you left your child's favorite toy under the booth and rushes out of the restaurant to give it to you. As adults, we surely don't need reminders for the typical thank-you moments. But many of us may need reminders to do so beyond the typical door openings and gift receiving; after all, part of our purpose here is to get a little deeper, right? Once a week (or more often as you enjoy it more), think of someone who has had an effect on your life—big or small—and write that person a note of gratitude (not via e-mail either; be personal). Gratitude is one of the gifts you can give others that also has some selfish benefits: Some research shows that fifteen minutes of daily gratitude can dramatically decrease stress hormones in your body. Another cool practice used by some friends: Keep a gratitude bell in the house, and when one member of the family does something nice for another, ring the bell. It's a great way to teach kids that helping others really matters.

USE SPIRITUALITY AS A TOOL. Some people say they're spiritual; some go to church regularly. But the real test of your spirituality is to apply it skillfully when you need it to solve real-life issues. That is, can you think before you act? Can you use things such as deep breathing, meditation, and prayer to help you be humble, compassionate, and empathetic when you're under high stress or when you have a family crisis? That ability and skill is really at the heart of what transcendence is all about. So what do you do? It means doing things like counting to ten before overreacting with emotion in an argument with a spouse or family member. It means slowing down the thought process so you're really thinking through problems and conflicts and using your authentic being to address issues. It means asking yourself not what your spiritual leader of choice would do about a conflict but what he or she would *feel* about this challenge. You want to tap into your heart more than control a behavior. And it means taking an issue one step further than its surface-level solution. So, for example, if a child is starting to get bad grades at school, find out what else is going on in the child's life.

BE A BETTER BELIEVER. Funny to hear it said that way—you can be a better believer in the same way you can be a better chef. Yet you can. While you may think your beliefs are all set, the truth is that you might simply be being more stubborn than a stereotypical in-law. The problem with that? A closed mind often doesn't allow you to see, understand, and experience other belief systems to give you a better picture of the entire world. These are five ways that can help you become more open and aware:

- Be curious, ask questions, and try to distinguish between facts and opinion.
- Know that beliefs are different from knowledge, which is often different from reality. You can't live your life totally blinded by a system of beliefs; you have to integrate them with the world around you. That is, belief is one part of life—but it's not the only thing.
- Learn from others, and ask about their beliefs—to open yourself up to new possibilities.
- Manage stress to avoid damage to the hippocampus, which helps regulate emotion, memory, and other systems needed for maintaining healthy beliefs. Say only positive thoughts out loud.
- Fill your glass up if it's half empty. Optimism, simply, is healthier than pessimism. In a study, nuns judged optimistic by their essay answers 40 years prior to death lived about eight years younger (longer and with less disability) than the nuns whose essays were judged to reflect pessimism.
- Don't judge others too harshly. After all, as long as no one is being hurt, if they derive joy from their beliefs and you don't, who is better off?

IF FOR NOTHING ELSE, DO IT TO BUILD A BETTER BRAIN. It's a myth that we use only 10 percent of our brains. The truth is that we're actively using our whole brain even if not all of the time. Every cell in the brain is alive and potentially stimulating the parts of the brain that we are using. Research shows that spiritual thought can make your brain more interactive and stimulate more brain activity. So even if you find no other reason to meditate for a few minutes every day, think of it as a gift to yourself—the five minutes you can spend in silent contemplation are working to build your brain to take on bigger and better things.

DON'T ALWAYS THINK SO MUCH. In general, emotions are hardwired, so they are very predictable despite their reputation of being irrational. Emotions have actions associated closely with them. In fact, they exist to cause action, but thinking is *not* about taking action unless it helps you override an emotional decision to act. Now, here's the catch. Wisdom must be transformed into insights that are fired up by our emotions for it to become subconscious and part of our innate behavior. Theoretical knowledge without practical application is not enough. In other words, your love and wisdom must be combined into an action such as doing a good deed for all your thinking to matter. And unless you get emotional about the task, it won't become part of your natural instinct.

STAY SIMPLE. Happiness is really rooted in simplicity. Excessive thoughts and actions diminish it. Excesses cloud basic values. One reason is that motivation is about removing extraneous stimuli so you can focus emotionally on the important task at hand. In the end, happiness comes from filling one's heart with love while practicing charity and dispensing kindness. Pretty simple, huh?

IT'S ALL ABOUT YOU. We paraphrase one of our heroes, C. S. Lewis. You *have* a body, but you don't *have* a soul; you *are* a soul. No matter what anyone tells you that might upset you, your essence is beautiful and has been inside you the whole time. We're just trying to help you shine like the gemstone you really are.

YOU Tool: Green Living

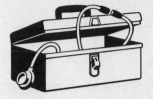

While you're showing your respect for your family, friends, and colleagues, there's a substantial gift you can give by helping save the planet and showing respect for all future generations. This is more than just acting smart; we believe it's a moral obligation. This toolbox will show you the little ways you can not only avoid harming the environment but help restore some of it, as well. After all, how can you feel beautiful if your surroundings are trashed? You want to create your own personal sanctuaries around you—and that should be an incentive to live as green as you can.

AT THE STORE

Stop the plastic water bottle habit. Besides causing environmental pollution, plastic bottles may be toxic to your health. The chemical called bisphenol A may be responsible for birth defects, cancer, heart disease, diabetes, and even Attention Deficit Disorder. Bisphenol is present in hard plastic bottles, lines tin cans, and is present in plastic food containers and some plastic wraps. Instead, use reusable glass thermoses for water storage, or you can even reuse an old glass pop bottle for carrying water. Drink real tap water in a glass, not specially bottled just for you at a special price of $2.50 per bottle. You can easily measure contaminants in your tap water with simple kits available from hardware stores. And every water company has to post its most recent test results on its website and send them to each home once a year (look for them in June and July). If the levels are greater in any sample for any contaminant or if your water isn't crystal clear, choose from dozens of tap water filters and then test your water again. We prefer a charcoal filter, but remember you need some of the trace minerals that come from tap water. In addition, next time you drink a bottle of water, remember that you could fill a third of the bottle with the oil it took to produce the bottle. You'll also save enough money to purchase organic food at the expensive places (at inexpensive outlets such as Wal-Mart, Costco, and Trader Joe's, organic food can cost no more than nonorganic). And you'll save landfills from filling with mountains of plastic. While you're at it, get rid of the paper cups and plates. Switch to the ol' china and glasses.

Bag it, baby. We use 500 billion (that's billion) plastic bags a year around the world. Use them for ten minutes, and then it's into the landfill they go, staying there long enough to greet your descendants 500 years from now. Instead, use reusable cloth bags (keep them in the car or kitchen). Or choose paper bags, since paper is a renewable resource and easily recyclable.

AT HOME

Switch lights. Of course, you know you're supposed to turn them off when you're not using them. But you can also help by going with compact fluorescents. A 23-watt compact fluorescent will give you as much light as a 100-watt incandescent—and last ten times as long and use a quarter of the energy. (The downside: They contain about 5 mg of mercury, so they need to be recycled properly. Check with your municipality for drop-off sites for items containing mercury. Different states have different regulations; you can get more info on your state's recycling laws by checking www.lamprecycle.org.)

Save water. In the best of all possible worlds, everyone would collect shower or sink water to nourish their plants. Barring this, you can still help the environment by not running your shower when you're not in it (what are you doing anyway?) and by turning off the sink water when you brush your teeth, shave, or wash your hands. Running hot water for five minutes uses as much energy as it takes to light a 400-foot room for a year. Install low-flow showerheads that will save two and a half gallons of water each minute (with air infusion, it feels as if you are getting the full amount of water and water pressure) and use those low-flush toilets—power flush makes them more efficient. Seventy percent of office water use can be saved by this alone. Other water-saving opportunities: do only full loads of laundry, and water your lawn once every three days at the most. If you install a sub-surface irrigation system, you can save 80 percent of your water use and have a perfect-looking lawn.

Insulate, insulate, insulate. And then insulate. Reduce heat loss in your walls and attic. Consider installing R-49 fiberglass insulation in the attic. This will save money and oil. Use R-15 fiberglass insulation in walls or R-21 if your walls are deeper than 2X6.

Take your hangers back to the cleaners. Don't throw them out. When you take your shirts in to be cleaned, take back your old hangers. Your cleaner will save 8 cents a hanger, and you'll prevent them from winding up in the landfill. Creative cleaners should put a nickel deposit on the hangers. Or they can switch to the new recycled paper hangers.

Recycle. Not just glass, paper, and plastic but batteries, fluorescent lightbulbs, and electronic devices. More than 60 million tons of materials are now recycled, which is about a third of our waste. A good start, but this percentage needs to double.

Remember the broom. You really don't have to plug in the vacuum cleaner (one of the most wasteful uses of energy) for every dog hair on the floor. For smooth surfaces, consider rubber-bristle brooms and a dustpan or a Swiffer, which works with electrostatic energy to attract dust.* After you use them, you'll wonder why you traded in brooms for vacuums in the first

---

*Coauthor Craig Wynett, who introduced the YOU docs to each other, was also instrumental in inventing the Swiffer.

place. (If you really want to save time and energy, a dog with a long tongue will keep your kitchen floor clean.)

Skip the wood fire. Though heating your home with a wood fire seems more romantic than a Shakespearean poem, wood smoke is much more carcinogenic than cigarette smoke and a contributor to particle pollution in neighborhoods.

Turn down the heat. On your water heater, that is. A setting of 120 degrees is comfortable for most, even though factory settings may be higher. Wash your clothes in cold water to help save on electricity. And turn down the heat at night and when you're out during the day.

IN YOUR YARD

Plant a tree. Sounds trite, doesn't it? But by replacing grass with bushes and trees, you're reducing the need for gas-guzzling and polluting mowers, providing oxygen to the environment, and removing carbon dioxide. Add to that the habitats you provide for birds and small animals, and you can't beat the tree plan.

Compost. You can do your own personal recycling of all your vegetable debris, leaves, old cut flowers, grass clippings, and newspapers. You really don't need the wheelbarrow, hoses, sprayers, pitchforks, shovels, rakes, and screens that some "experts" tell you to buy. In fact, nature will take care of itself quite nicely. You can put the plant material in a hole in your backyard, or you can buy or build a box. Throw in a little dirt and let the rain and your neighborhood worms do the work. After a few months, your compost will be the perfect material to nourish your newly planted Christmas tree.

FOR YOUR ELECTRONICS

Save energy. Unplug unused appliances. The newer computers are great at saving energy in the "sleep" mode, but make sure yours has an EPA Energy Star label. This tells you your trusty old computer isn't burning unnecessary fuel. If you have a less efficient model, turn it off after using it. And think about buying an energy-saving Smart Strip by BITS 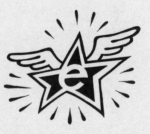 Limited. This gem automatically shuts off your printer and other devices when you turn off your computer. Your printer is among the most wasteful appliances in your home.

Use rechargeable batteries. Save money and keep landfills clear of toxic batteries. Today's chargers are more powerful and faster than the old ones. And don't forget to recycle dead batteries.

WITH YOUR CAR

Be efficient. You may not be in the market for a hybrid, but you can save some energy with the wheels you have in more subtle ways. Keep your tires properly inflated to improve your gas mileage. And ease up on the road rage, wouldya? Not only will it hurt your heart, but it will also hurt your gas mileage. Hard braking, fast acceleration, and speeding can cut gas mileage by a third. On the flip side, cruise control can help you save gas.

The Be-YOU-tiful Plan

Live the Ultimate Beautiful Day (and Improve Your YOU-Q)

Throughout this book, you've read all kinds of tips and tricks that will absolutely help you become even more beautiful than you already are, but you may be thinking that following some kind of two-week ugly-to-knockout makeover would be like trying to put toothpaste back into the tube.

The reality is that you can make small changes that will lead to big results in just 24 hours. That is, by slipping little behaviors into your regular routines (the devil is in the details, after all), you'll reengineer your life to become aware of the subtle places where you lose momentum in achieving your most beautiful and happiest life.

With these new insights and a plan that you can follow no matter what your lifestyle, you'll automate your life by trial and error to see what really works for you. Take the knowledge that we offer and apply "news you can use" so you can close the gap in your YOU-Q (go ahead and retake the test after doing our perfect day for two weeks, and find the area you want to work on).

Here we'll outline the Ultimate Beautiful Day—the perfect 24 hours. While it's true that you already know to wash your face and brush your teeth, you can achieve long-lasting beauty by paying attention to those details every day to help you achieve and maintain total beauty. Use these tips throughout your day, and you'll find yourself walking taller, feeling better, looking great. And smiling more.

The Ultimate Beautiful Day:
Daily Care and Maintenance Day

We all know the classic definitions of a beautiful day. Some may say it's spent at the beach. Others may say it's spent in the sack. Some may say it must involve some sweat or a salmon dinner or a round of 18 at Pebble Beach. Others may say that the minimum requirements for a beautiful day should include the word *pedicure*. Any of those things may very well fit your criteria for a beautiful day. Now, however, we're going to present you with a different kind of beautiful day—a day in which the things you do reflect on the core of improving your inner and outer beauty. Remember, if you've made it this far, your ancestors (and you) have already made the major leagues when it comes to beauty. Now your choices can make each day better for you. A beautiful day doesn't have to be a day in which you're removed from reality; it can be a day in which you're immersed in it.

That's why we've built this beautiful day around a typical weekday in most people's lives; we left time for you to do your job, whether it's at an office or running a family, and we snuck in those tactics that you can seamlessly include while you're working your job or shuttling your kids. After all, improving yourself and your health shouldn't overwhelm your life; it should be integrated as a vital part of it.

So what you'll find here is a sample day with some sample times—a day that includes some of our favorite tips and tricks. After all, routines are good because they're automatic—ensuring that you'll integrate good habits into your daily life, rather than struggling to do so. Most of the tips are supported by first-rate medical research, while others are yet to be studied extensively, but they're the recommendations that we'd give our family and friends. You'll find hundreds of pieces of advice throughout the first 11 chapters and the nearly 20 toolboxes throughout the book. In this perfect day, we condense some of the best of them to help guide you through a 24-hour period that will make you see yourself—and the world around you—in a way that you may never have before.

6:00 a.m.*

WAKE UP BEFORE YOUR ALARM CLOCK AFTER SEVEN TO EIGHT HOURS OF SLEEP. This is the amount of time your body needs to recharge; plus, sleep is the major stimulant for your own growth hormone (there's something special about it not being from a vial). Your own growth hormone helps keep skin taut and vibrant. After all, nobody looks all that beautiful with bags† under the eyes. When you wake up, take a few minutes for an inventory of the way your body feels—specifically the minor aches and pains that may subconsciously distract you from the focus of your life. Our tool kits will help you address the most common of these. When you wake up, perform a few light stretches (like those from our yoga workout on page 361). Take just a few minutes to get your blood going, think about your breathing, and prepare yourself for your day. While you meditate to the sensations of your body, dream about one big idea you want to pursue today.

6:20 a.m.

PERFORM YOUR MORNING BEAUTY ROUTINE. These are some guidelines:

- In the shower, rinse your hair (you can shampoo whenever you want, but don't feel compelled to shampoo more than three times weekly) and wash your body. Blot your hair dry or use the cool setting on your hair dryer, but avoid the scorched-earth approach; heat can damage the delicate cuticles. Use a brush with smooth or rounded teeth or bristles, which will massage the hair and scalp without damaging them. Remember, hair is most fragile when wet.
- Wash your face and use a moisturizer that has vitamins B3 (niacin), B5 (pantothenic acid), Vitamin E, and alpha-hydroxy acids. You can

---

* Give or take a few hours or minutes, depending on your particular schedule, lifestyle, and whether or not baby Amelia is wailing in the crib. Adjust your times accordingly. The average wake-up time in America is 5:47 a.m., so we're giving you an extra 13 minutes for your, uh, beauty sleep.
† Paper or plastic.

also include various small-molecule antioxidants such as ubiquinone and ferulic acid. Remember to read labels on everything (see our guidelines in Chapter 1). Use a moisturizer that has UV protection. You want to protect your face during the day and feed it with nutrients at night.

- Use deodorant, not antiperspirant.* We believe you don't need to stop the natural bodily function of sweat†; simply use a deodorant to mask any unpleasant smells.

6:40 a.m.

BRUSH YOUR TEETH—FOR A FULL TWO MINUTES. Periodontal disease is one of the leading causes of heart problems (not to mention the fact that the only thing most people want to see toothless is an approaching shark). Use a soft brush, and rub the bristles up toward the gums. We also like sonic brushes, because they spray into the crevices of teeth to have a cleaning effect beyond where the tips of the bristles actually touch. Floss between all teeth so that the strand gently touches the gums. Brush your tongue (or use a tongue scraper) to help control bad breath. Use a neti pot to clean your sinuses, especially if you have chronic sinus problems.

7:00 a.m.

HAVE A BREAKFAST that may include 100 percent whole grains, healthy fat, fresh fruit, or a little healthy protein—such as egg whites, which contain skin-nourishing biotin. Some of our favorite options include steel-cut Irish oatmeal, Total with 2 percent fat yogurt without added sugar but with fresh berries, or 100 percent whole grain cereal with low-fat or hemp milk. And don't ever think about fast food at breakfast time, since we find that most breakfast fast food violates every good nutritional guideline.

---

* Some clothes that require dry cleaning can be ruined by sweat, so men might want to wear undergarments and women use antiperspirants when wearing delicate clothes.
† Unless you're trying to protect your dress shirt from becoming classified as the next Great Lake.

7:10 a.m.

POP THESE PILLS. Your morning supplements should include: half of a multivitamin (with at least 500 IU of vitamin D, 600 mg of calcium, and 200 mg of magnesium), 600 mg of DHA (omega-3 fatty acids, either by itself or in 2 grams of fish/cod liver oil), and 162 mg of aspirin (if you're over 40 years old and have checked with your doc). Take with a full glass of water. These will help you with heart health, and keep this in mind as well: What's good for your heart and arteries is also good for your brain, sexual function, and skin (prevents wrinkles).

7:15 a.m.

WHETHER YOU'RE GETTING TO WORK OR GETTING YOUR KIDS TO SCHOOL, we know you'll be spending a little travel time during the day, stuck in your car or a bus or, if possible, on your two legs. Take the opportunity to practice some stealth Kegel exercises (squeezing the muscles that control your urine flow; you can identify these muscles by starting and stopping urination midstream).* The more they're developed, the better your sex life.

Or, if you're in line for your favorite morning caffeine-infused beverage (you're going with the green tea, right?), try something different from eavesdropping on the two customers on the couches. Instead, spend a minute focusing on proper posture. Back straight, butt in, chest out, shoulders back, head high, jaw aligned, making sure your top and bottom teeth aren't touching each other. Focus. Focus. Feel good? We thought so. Practice good posture every day (sitting and standing), and you'll be amazed at the changes in how you look and feel. Slow, deep belly breaths go great with excellent posture. The air should move like a wave through the body, starting with the belly while you inhale and eventually puffing out your chest, reversing the actions when you exhale until you're pulling your belly button toward your spine.

* First practice in the privacy of your home, not in the car!

8:30 a.m.

ATTACK YOUR DAY, BE IT AT HOME OR AT WORK. One of the most important things you can do: create a clear game plan for what you want to (realistically) accomplish. Don't overwhelm yourself; just systematically tackle what you can today and save what you can't for tomorrow. The ubiquitous to-do list works because it takes the pressure off of you from forgetting the things you need to take care of but that may slip through the cracks. And be where you need to be on time so you can control the agenda. Maintaining the locus of control helps us cope with and reduce stress.

9:00 a.m.

MAKE A NOTE TO GREET EVERYONE YOU MEET WITH OR TALK TO WITH A HEARTY SMILE—A GENUINE ONE.* Upbeat people excel. Upbeat people have good relationships. Upbeat people feel good.

10:00 a.m.

TAKE A QUICK AUDIT OF YOUR ENVIRONMENT, WHETHER IT'S AT HOME OR WORK. A couple of things to note: The optimum work environment includes yellow light, lots of greenery, high air quality, and even a cube-mate who's unafraid to crack a joke every now and then (more details on page 276). While you're making a list of how you want to redecorate, you can fiddle with the thermostat. Research shows that optimal productivity occurs when the environment you're working in is 72 degrees Fahrenheit.

10:45 a.m.

TAKE A FIVE- TO SEVEN-MINUTE WALK, AND CLEAR YOUR HEAD. Remember, the key to successfully managing stress and accomplishing tasks isn't about time management as much as energy management; it's about having the vitality to move fast, move efficiently, and move smartly.

* You remember that illustration of the smiles, don't ya?

10:50 a.m.

HAVE A MIDMORNING SNACK OF NUTS OR GREEN TEA (the polyphenols can help thicken the epidermis). Besides helping you stay satisfied, they contain biotin, which helps you metabolize fat and carbs. Add an apple or carrot—nature's teeth whiteners.

12:30 p.m.

LUNCH BREAK. Two good choices: an oil and vinegar–dressed salad topped with veggies and salmon, which contains carotenoids that improve skin elasticity so you don't wrinkle. Or have a soup (not cream-based), which can help slow the time it takes food to travel through your system—keeping you fuller longer and helping protect against waist and weight gain. Even if you're rushed, practice slow and deliberate eating.

1:00 p.m.

FOR THE OTHER 30 MINUTES OF YOUR BREAK, TAKE A WALK. Put UVA and UVB sunblock on your face and the backs of your hands before you go. A little sun on your arms and legs helps generate vitamin D. While you're walking, make a mental list of three to five things that you can purchase over the weekend that can help you achieve your goals for inner and outer beauty. Some suggestions:

- Water purifier, not only for drinking water but also for your shower (chlorine in shower/bath water can dry out your hair and skin).
- Decent shoes (even for guys). High heels are the most destructive piece of clothing you can own. Find shoes that have a big toe box and heels that are less than two inches. And make sure you have comfortable sneakers by trying on at least five pairs before choosing.
- Home kit to test for radon in the house and new air filters to make sure you're breathing easy.

Or, instead of walking: If time (and the environment) allows and your body needs it, take a power nap of no more than 30 minutes. It's the ultimate biological battery recharger.

2:00 p.m.

WHETHER YOU'RE AT HOME OR AT WORK, take a moment and notice the greenery around you (you do have some plants around, don't you?). The feeling of living things (other than the next-door neighbor or backstabbing cubicle mate) can be healing, comforting, and empowering (which is especially nice in times of stress). Plus, they add oxygen to the environment.

3:30 p.m.

HAVE A MIDAFTERNOON SNACK, SUCH AS A PIECE OF FRUIT. Meanwhile, if someone tries to derail your beautiful day with a snarky comment or an unwarranted outburst, try to manage your anger by understanding why they're angry (problems at home, they too are stressed). It doesn't excuse them from lashing out and it doesn't mean you shouldn't stand up for yourself, but it helps you channel your anger so you can respond constructively.

6:00 p.m.

HAVE ONE GLASS OF ALCOHOL WITH DINNER. Our favorite is red wine; the alcohol has tremendous cardiovascular benefits, and the resveratrol (from the grape skins that give the wine its color) helps cells live longer. Lean toward a meal with healthy fat, protein, and fiber, and use small plates to help control portion size. Cover half your plate with vegetables. Notice that you're eating early enough that the rich pharmacy of chemicals and calories in your food will be digested and won't interfere with your sleep (or deposit themselves on your thighs).

6:25 p.m.

HUG SOMEONE.* Make it a good one.

* Someone you know, preferably.

6:30 p.m.

POP THE OTHER HALF OF YOUR DAILY SUPPLEMENTS (including multivitamin, calcium, and magnesium), then handle any household bills and chores you need to finish. If you're doing tasks, assign everyone in the family a job and work together; the teamwork builds not only a clean home but also a close family. For bills, tuck away 10 percent of your income into an emergency account—not retirement, but rather a true financial ER that can bail you out of an emergency to help relieve one of life's biggest stressors: cash (or rather, lack of it).

7:00 p.m.

CALL, E-MAIL, OR IM A FRIEND, YOUR PARENTS, OR YOUR GROWN CHILDREN. This isn't necessarily your buddy, but if it is, lengthen the time. You need to make efforts to connect socially with someone whom you care for and understands your passions and can help you hit your goals and passions; that's one of the elements that will help you grow and develop a more spiritual side. Nobody home? Then write a note of thanks to someone who's influenced your life. Pick anyone: a middle school teacher, your first boss, the volleyball coach who instilled in you that practice is just as important as the game.

7:15 p.m.

DO THE TWENTY-MINUTE BAND WORKOUT (see page 351) to help you increase your lean muscle—which will help you burn fat, add tone, and change your body shape (of course, if your schedule or preference steers you to doing it in the morning or at lunch hour, by all means, do it then). Or, if you prefer, do a yoga workout (both are on the DVDs) to strengthen and lengthen your muscles. The added flexibility, balance, and muscle tone will make you look and feel strong, energetic, and ready to take on and face the frenetic world around you. Add ten minutes of focused work on your core (mainly your abdominals and lower back) to develop your biological back brace. Not only will it help you develop a show-stopping belly, but it will also protect you from injuries that will send you squealing for the ibuprofen.

8:00 p.m.
YOU'RE JUST IN TIME FOR YOUR FAVORITE SHOWS OR ENJOYING YOUR HOBBY, BUT STAY ACTIVE. Put a stationary bike or elliptical cross-trainer or rowing machine or treadmill in front of the tube so you can pedal or do other physical activity during your favorite shows, or do the plank position (see page 181) during commercials. Be demanding of folks who are entertaining you; don't fizz out in front of the tube unless the material really warrants your attention.

8:30 p.m.
PLAY WITH YOUR KIDS. It's a great way to teach each other, and you learn a lot from their behavior. When you're done, lie down with them when putting them to sleep, since they're tired and let their guard down. They'll speak more honestly and will listen better. It's the opportunity to pass along your wisdom—one of the greatest gifts you have to offer.* You can also read to them or just make up stories to stretch your mind and their imagination.

9:00 p.m.
LOCK YOURSELF IN THE BATHROOM, take a seat, and get into a meditative state (the bathroom, because it's less likely you'll be bothered in there).† Spend five minutes humming the word *yummmmm.* That will help you clear your mind, destress, and start thinking of higher purposes—and meanings of life beyond just getting the kids' lunches ready for the next day.

* Besides the keys to the car.
† Unless your teenage daughter shares the same bathroom.

9:10 p.m.

NOW THAT YOUR MIND IS CLEAR OF MINUTIAE, take the opportunity to jot down a few ideas about how you want to live large and find a purpose bigger than you. Some ideas to get you going:

- Ask yourself the best way you can help others—be it with your time, talents, money, or emotions. Giving to others is also a heck of a high that you can give yourself (plus, you'll live longer to keep doing good). Prove to yourself that you are something more than you thought you were.
- Assess your career situation and make sure that you're following a passion more than a paycheck, and that the company you work for has the same values that you do.
- Figure out some rituals that you can instill into your own family—be it a regular dinner or Saturday outing or some other regular routine that keeps you close and connected.

9:15 p.m.

PREPARE TOMORROW'S BATCH OF DRINKING WATER. Fill up your bottle(s) and stick them in the fridge so that you have cold, filtered (not bottled) water to drink throughout the next day.

9:20 p.m.

PREPARE YOURSELF FOR BED WITH ANY CLEANUP DUTIES. Brush your teeth (yes, two more minutes). Wash and exfoliate your face (wash with fragrance- and residue-free soap), and use a moisturizer with vitamins A and C (remember, you're feeding your face at night, when the sun cannot denature all the restoring antioxidant vitamins). You can find all the details in Chapter 1. Make sure the lights are dim and the room is cool so you can gently slip into restorative sleep rather than attempting to abruptly "fall" asleep after sending out a few e-mail blasts while watching the late shows.

9:30 p.m.

MUTUAL MASSAGES WITH YOUR PARTNER: Start with the feet and stay there as long as you like. The benefits are more than just emotional bonding; a massage with oil (aromatherapy) has also been shown to have destressing health benefits.

9:40 p.m.

HAVE SEX. Feel beautiful. Tell your partner what you need (and ask your partner the same). On alternate days (days, not weeks!), you can read a few pages of invigorating prose.

9:42 p.m.

JUST KIDDING. Keep going, please.

10:10 p.m.

DRIFT INTO SLEEP WITH A PEACEFUL MEDITATION, thanking your higher power of choice for the beauty of the day. Remember what made you most grateful today. Please note that you have nearly eight hours before you have to awaken. The perfect day.

YOU Tools

More Strategies for Helping You Become Even More Beautiful

Workouts designed by Joel Harper, www.fitpackdvd.com

Throughout this book, we've given you hundreds of tips and tools to help you in your quest for your own desired state of beauty. Here we're going to add a few more tools to the chest—namely a strength workout using a resistance band, a yoga workout, some important health tools, and a few more surprises along the way. We hope that your body isn't a total fixer-upper, but in any case, these tools will help you improve your body—and your mind right along with it.

Index

The Band Workout   351

The Yoga Workout   361

The Perfect Gym Bag   375

Health Utensils   377

Your Eyes   383

The Biophysical Battery: Energy Blood Tests   387

YOU Tool: The Band Workout

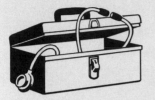

Some people use dumbbells to work out. Some use barbells. Some (including us) use their own body weight. Another great way to work and tone your muscles: a resistance band. These stretchy bands offer various amounts of resistance, so that you can push, pull, and move to test all the muscles of your body. We recommend you do the following workout, designed by trainer Joel Harper, two or three times a week.

Follow these guidelines for the workout:

1. Use a band with handles and always grip the handles firmly.
2. Choose a band you can use comfortably throughout the entire workout. As soon as that becomes easy, use a thicker band.
3. Keep the band away from your face.
4. If you find the band uncomfortable on your skin, wear a long-sleeved shirt.
5. Breathe normally and stand upright.
6. When tightening the band, wrap it around your hand, not the handle.

THE WORKOUT

WARM-UP: Figure Eight

(Warms up shoulders and arms)

Stand with your feet shoulder-width apart and circle your arms and hands together in figure eights, down, around, up, and across to the other side. Repeat eight times.

1) STANDING CHEST PRESS

(Warms up/strengthens chest and arms)

Grab both handles and place the band behind your back, just underneath your shoulder blades (wrap the band around your hands to shorten it). With your hands out to your sides at shoulder height, act as if you're hugging a tree and bring your hands together in front of you on the exhale. Inhale and bring your hands back to your sides. Do 25 times.

Advanced: Do 50 and work your calves by rising up on the balls of your feet as you bring your arms together.

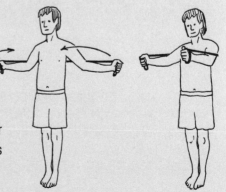

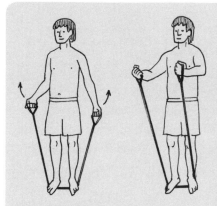

2) STANDING CHEST PULL

(Strengthens chest and arms)

Stand on the band with your feet shoulder-width apart. Hold the band down by your sides, then slowly lift your right hand (palm side up) out in front of the right side of your chest and then back down. Move your left hand up and back down; do 25 times for each arm. If this is easy for you, do both at the same time.

Advanced: After you're done, hold both hands at the highest point for 30 seconds with palms facing up.

3) CHEST OPENER

(Stretches chest and arms)

Leave the band loosely in your hands and interweave your fingers behind your head without touching your head. While standing upright, act as if there are strings on your elbows and hands, pulling them directly behind you, as you take five breaths deep into your chest.

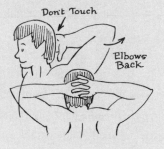

4) LATERAL RAISE

(Strengthens shoulders)

With your hands at your sides and your palms down holding the handles, lift your arms straight out to your sides 25 times, always leading with your elbows, not your wrists.

Advanced: After you're done, hold the handles up for 30 seconds.

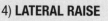

5) NECK STRETCH

(Opens neck)

With hands hanging down to sides and shoulders level, gently drop your right ear down toward your right shoulder. Let go of all the tension in your body. Hold for three deep breaths and switch sides.

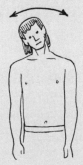

6) LATERAL CIRCLE

(Strengthens shoulders and rotator cuffs)

While standing on the band and holding the handles, reach your arms out to your sides and bring your hands as high as you can but not more than shoulder height. Rotate clockwise the size of a cantaloupe 25 times, then switch directions and do 25 times.

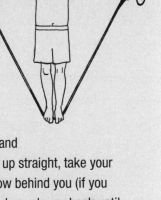

7) CHICKEN WING

(Stretches shoulder)

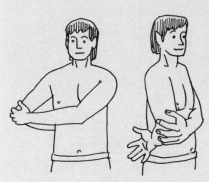

Place the back side of your right hand just above your right hip. Standing up straight, take your left hand and clasp your right elbow behind you (if you can't, slide your right hand behind your lower back until you can reach your elbow). Gently pull your elbow toward your belly button and take five deep breaths into your upper chest, opening the tightest area. Keep your chest lifted and shoulders even. Do the same on the other side.

8) LATERAL PULL-DOWN

(Strengthens upper back and arms)

With your feet together, wrap the band around each hand three times. Lift your hands above your head with your palms facing forward. With straight arms, pulse your hands away from each other 25 times, keeping the band taut the entire time.

Advanced: Do 25 times balancing on your left foot, with your right knee in line with your right hip; then switch sides and do 25 times.

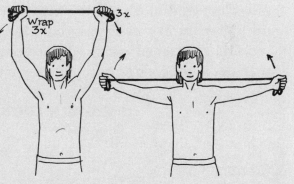

9) LATERAL HOLD

(Strengthens upper back and arms; builds stamina)

Hold the band above your head with your hands apart for 25 seconds with the band as tight as possible. Don't tighten your face or scrunch your shoulders.

Advanced: Do the exercise while balanced on your toes.

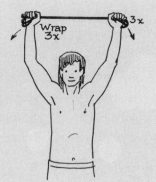

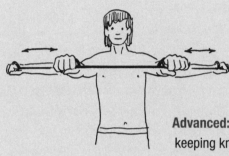

10) SHOULDER HEIGHT

(Strengthens upper back and arms)

With your hands holding the handles at shoulder height and your arms straight out in front of you, pulse your hands away from each other 25 times.

Advanced: Do the above and bring your knee to hip height. While keeping knee stationary, swing your lower leg from side to side. Do 25 times and switch sides.

11) PALMS OUT

(Opens upper back and shoulders)

Without the band, interweave your fingers and turn your palms away from your body (so you're looking at your knuckles). Reach your palms as far away from you as you can as you hunch your back and curl your tailbone under. Take five deep breaths, expanding your rib cage.

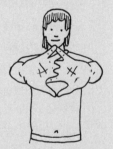

12) SIDE TRICEP EXTENSION

(Strengthens triceps)

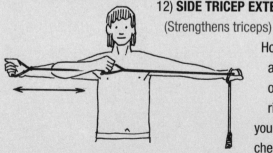

Holding the handles in both hands, wrap the band around your left hand only and reach both hands out to your sides to shoulder height. Take your right hand with palm facing forward and, leaving your elbow stationary, bring your hand toward your chest 25 times. Switch and wrap the band around right hand and do 25 more on the left side.

Advanced: Balance on one foot and wrap the band around one more time.

13) ARM CIRCLE

(Warms up biceps)

Stand with both feet on the band and hold the handles. Reach hands out to your side, palm side up, and reach your arms out as high as you can. Do 25 cantaloupe-size circles and then switch direction.

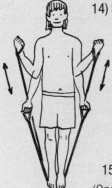

14) SIDE CURL

(Strengthens biceps)

With hands down to your sides and holding the band handles, turn your thumbs as far back as feels comfortable. Curl your arms up 25 times. Resist bringing your arms to the front.

Advanced: Do 50 in double time.

15) GOING TO JAIL

(Opens shoulders and arms)

Without the band, interweave your fingers behind your tailbone. With your chest lifted, arms straight, and shoulders down, lift your fingers toward the ceiling. Resist rolling your shoulders forward.

Advanced: Bend forward and drop your forehead down toward your shins and press your knuckles toward the ground.

16) PENGUIN

(Strengthens butt and entire leg)

Stand on the band and hold the handles. Bring your hands up to elbow height. Keep open hands facing up (don't squeeze band). Step your right foot to your right, plant it, then bring your left foot over to it. Then step your left foot to the left and bring your right foot over to it. Go back and forth 25 times.

Advanced: Lift your leading foot off the ground and tilt your body from side to side.

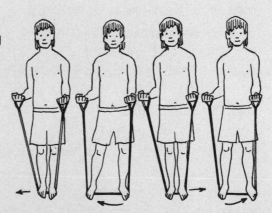

17) CROSS LEG DROP

(Stretches back and hamstrings)

Without the band, cross your left foot over your right. Ideally you want your big toes in line, but go to where you feel comfortable balancing. Slowly walk your hands down your legs as far as feels comfortable; really relax your neck, as if your head were a bowling ball elongating your spine, and take three deep breaths into your back. Switch sides and repeat.

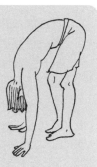

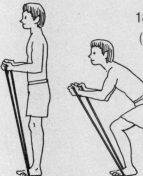

18) SQUAT

(Strengthens and tones entire leg)

With the band under both feet and feet shoulder-width apart and holding the handles in front of you, drop down as far as feels comfortable, as if you were sitting in a chair. As you squat, reach your arms straight out in front of you at shoulder height. Come all the way back up to slightly bent knees. Do 25 times. **Advanced:** In squat position, pulse 25 times.

19) BUTT BLASTER

(Burns butt)

Get on all fours and wrap the band underneath your right heel with the handles underneath both hands. Kick your right heel back 25 times and switch sides. Really focus on squeezing your butt and lifting your leg every time. Look slightly above your hands during the movement.

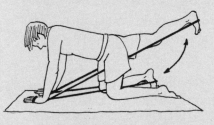

Advanced: Do 50 times each leg and pulse at the highest movement 25 times.

20) THREAD THE NEEDLE

(Stretches hips and lower back)

Without the band, lie on your back. With your knees bent, place your right leg on your left thigh just above the knee. Reach your hands up and through your legs and clasp your left leg. Pull your knees slightly toward your chin and press your tailbone back down to the mat. Resist overarching your neck; keep it straight and relax down on the mat. Take three deep breaths and switch sides.

21) CROSS-LEGGED LIFT

(Strengthens lower abs)

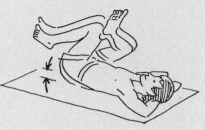

Lying on your back without the band, cross your right leg on top of your left with your right ankle against your left thigh and your interwoven hands behind your head. Slightly lift your legs up with your lower abs and set your left foot back down. Do 25 times each side.

Advanced: Really lift your tailbone off the ground and crunch your upper and lower body with your left leg going higher up in the air. Do 25 times each side.

22) CROSS-LEGGED TWIST

(Strengthens obliques and abs)

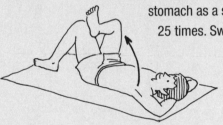

While on your back without the bands and your right leg crossed over as in Thread the Needle, place your left hand behind your head and your right hand on your stomach as a sensor to keep it from lifting. Use your core and twist 25 times. Switch sides. Focus on keeping your face relaxed, your chin away from your chest, and your elbows out of your line of vision.

Advanced: Do exercise with your left leg straight up toward the ceiling 25 times; then switch sides.

23) SPINAL TWIST

(Opens hips, back, and spine)

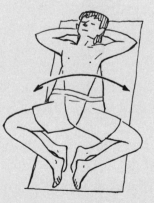

Lie on your back and interweave your hands behind your head. With your knees bent and feet flat on the ground while exhaling, slowly drop your knees to the right and look straight up at the ceiling. To increase the stretch, lift your knees a little higher. Keep your upper back and shoulders on the mat throughout entire pose. Hold for 30 seconds and switch sides.

This band workout can be found on the *YOU: Being Beautiful Workout* DVD.

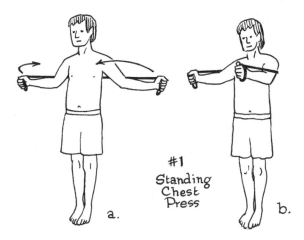

#1 Standing Chest Press

a.

b.

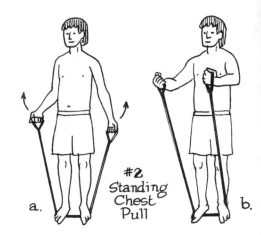

#2 Standing Chest Pull

a.

b.

#3 Chest Opener

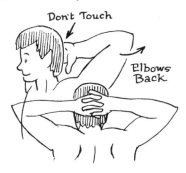

Don't Touch

Elbows Back

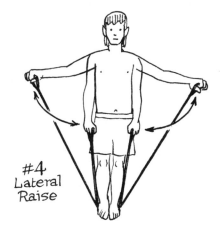

#4 Lateral Raise

#5 Neck Stretch

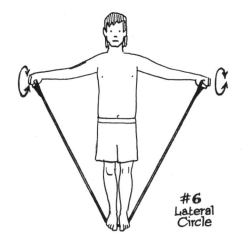

#6 Lateral Circle

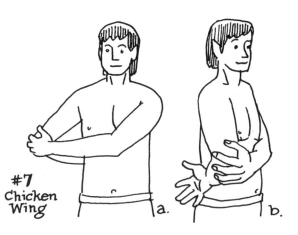

#6 Chicken Wing

a.

b.

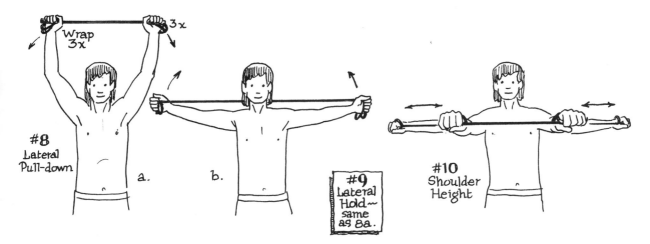

#8 Lateral Pull-down

Wrap 3x   3x

a.   b.

#9 Lateral Hold~ same as 8a.

#10 Shoulder Height

#11 Palms Out

#12 Side Tricep Extension

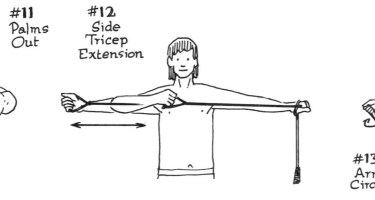

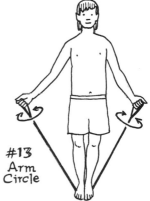

#13 Arm Circle

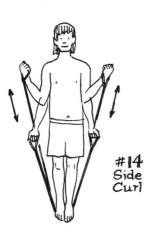

#14 Side Curl

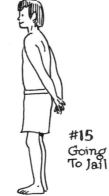

#15 Going To Jail

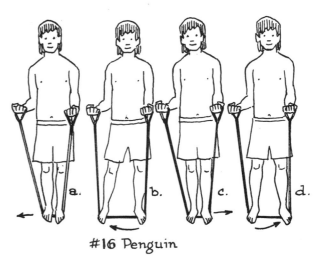

a.   b.   c.   d.

#16 Penguin

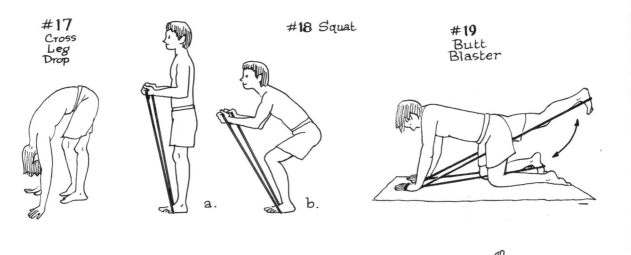

#17 Cross Leg Drop

#18 Squat

a.   b.

#19 Butt Blaster

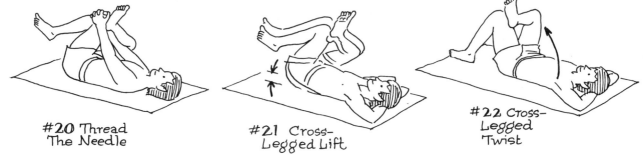

#20 Thread The Needle

#21 Cross-Legged Lift

#22 Cross-Legged Twist

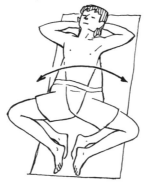

#23 Spinal Twist

YOU Tool: The Yoga Workout

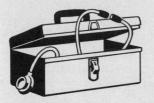

You don't have to be a human rubber band to appreciate the beauty of yoga. This ancient practice not only stretches your muscles but also allows your mind to focus and trains your brain for meditation. The beauty of this workout is that any skill level can participate; you need to move only as far into each pose as you possibly can. In fact, the only imperative you have to remember is to take deep belly breaths using your diaphragm to pull the lungs down during inspiration. (If the poses we outline below are too difficult for you to take continuous deep breaths, then back off to avoid compromising this golden rule.) That's important because most of us never take a single deep breath all day long. To exhale, suck your belly button toward your spine to push the diaphragm up and empty all the air from your lungs. Inhaling deeply brings a chemical called nitric oxide from the back of your nose and your sinuses into your lungs. This short-lived gas dilates the air passages in your lungs and the blood vessels surrounding those air passages so you can get more oxygen into your body. Nitric oxide also doubles as a neurotransmitter to help your brain function.

Other benefits of yoga:

- Yoga and the deep breathing associated with it help create a negative pressure in your lungs, acting as a vacuum cleaner to draw lymphatic drainage back into your veins. What are lymphatics? When your tissue is fed by blood, some of the waste material seeps out into spaces between cells and becomes lymph. Your lymph nodes serve as a portal to pass waste material back into your blood vessels for cleansing; these same nodes get inflamed when we are sick, which is why you can feel them getting enlarged. Yoga stimulates the flow in your lymphatic system by exercising your muscles and through the vacuum action of deep breathing.
- Yoga trains you to loosen the muscles and joints that are ignored in your day-to-day life. Routines get the blood flowing as you warm up and free your body to experience the new stresses you will inevitably face each day. The practice also helps you handle the weight of your body more effectively, which builds bone and muscle strength so you are more resilient. And it improves your balance so you don't fall.
- Yoga also helps you to focus your mind on remote parts of your body, such as tight joints and muscles, as you gently but firmly deepen into your poses. Attaining the "empty" mind called for in meditation proves difficult, especially for novices, because the mind wanders. But if you can concentrate on the tension in your hip, for example, as you focus your mind on your pose, then

you're well on your way. The goal in yoga is not really emptying your mind, but rather freeing the mind to let any and all ideas rapidly pass through it without any attachment.

THE WORKOUT

This workout is a process of self-realization and is designed to help you feel empowered and build your self-discipline. Follow these guidelines to improve your yoga experience.

- Never force any pose so you feel a painful strain. Go to where it feels comfortable.
- If your knees feel discomfort, use a rolled-up towel, pillow, or blanket as a cushion behind the knee joint (in the popliteal area, if you know where that is).
- Resist locking your elbows.
- If a pose is difficult to balance, stand against the wall. Your balance may be different from one day to the next. Imbalance during poses may mean an imbalance in other parts of life.

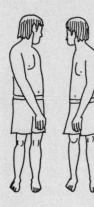

1) STANDING TWIST

(Warms up spine; loosens body)

With your feet shoulder-width apart (mountain pose) and your knees slightly bent with relaxed arms, twist your upper body loosely from side to side. Look where you are going. Breathe normally for 30 seconds.

2) STANDING LEANING STRETCH

(Opens lower back and obliques)

Interweave your hands and turn them palm side up above your head. Take a deep inhale and exhale as you stretch to the right; inhale and come back to center and exhale to the left. Do five times.

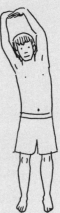

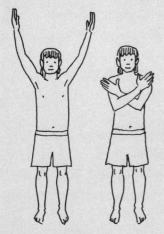

3) X

(Warms up upper body)

With your feet in the mountain pose, bring your straight arms up toward the ceiling in a V shape with the palms facing each other. Inhale, and on the exhale, cross your hands in front of your face, bringing your hands to shoulder height with the palms facing you. Inhale; then exhale and cross your arms again, switching the arm closest to you. The exhale should be sharp and come from your navel. Do continuously for 90 seconds, alternating your arms.

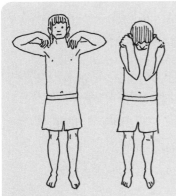

4) **LADYBUG**

(Opens upper back, neck, and lungs)

Inhale deeply and place your fingertips on your shoulders with your elbows out to your sides in line with your shoulders. Keeping your fingers on your shoulders, on the exhalation, bring your elbows out in front; keep exhaling and drop your head, bend forward at the neck, and look down to your toes. On the inhale, come back to elbows out to side. Repeat five times.

5) **TIGHTROPE**

(Helps with balance, strengthens ankles)

With your feet in the mountain pose, bring your hands, palm side up, out to your sides at shoulder height. Lift your heels off the ground and balance on your toes. Hold for 30 seconds, taking deep breaths from your navel up into your chest.

Advanced: Do it with your eyes closed.

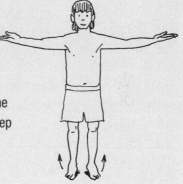

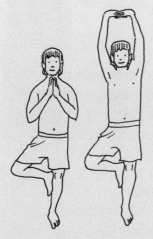

6) **TREE**

(Helps with balance)

With hands in prayer (thumbs against your chest) and your feet together, slide your right foot up your leg, placing the sole of the foot flush against the leg. Lift your foot as high as you feel comfortable, bringing your knee into line with your hip, and hold for 30 seconds. Then switch sides.

Advanced: Interweave your fingers palm side up and stretch them above your head.

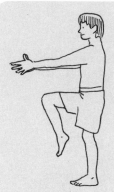

7) STORK

(Improves balance and focus; strengthens arms, shoulders, and legs)

While in the mountain pose, bring your right knee up into line with your right hip or as high as 90 degrees. With your right toes pointing toward the floor, inhale and raise your straight arms (palms facing up) in front of you, to shoulder height. Resist leaning forward; keep your standing leg pressing into the ground, stand erect, and gaze straight ahead at a fixed point. Hold the pose for 30 seconds, return to the mountain pose, and switch sides.

8) HORSE

(Strengthens quadriceps and knees)

With your feet wide and toes turned out 45 degrees, bend your knees so that they're directly above your heels; bring your hands center and into prayer. Squat down as low as feels comfortable, but with your tailbone no lower than in line with your knees. Feel the length of your spine by elongating the distance from your tailbone to the top of your head. Hold the pose for 30 seconds.

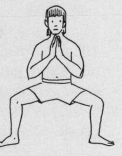

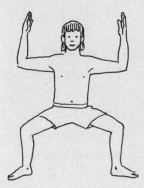

9) GODDESS

(Strengthens quadriceps and knees, opens chest, increases arm strength)

While in Horse, extend your arms out to the side with your elbows slightly below your shoulders. With your palms facing up, bend your elbows to a 90-degree angle. With your palms facing your ears, hold for 30 seconds. Relax into the pose. Don't raise your shoulders; keep them lowered and relaxed.

10) TRIANGLE

(Opens spine; helps balance the body)

Stand with your right foot pointing directly to the right and your left foot forward at a slight angle. Inhale deeply. As you exhale, move your right hand down your leg toward your right ankle, stopping wherever you feel comfortable, and simultaneously lift your left hand above your head with the palm facing forward. Look up at your left hand, keeping your shoulder parallel to your hip the entire time. Resist trying to twist your shoulders. Take five deep breaths and switch sides. Do twice.

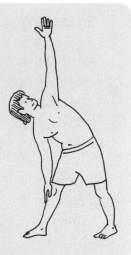

11) CAT BACK/COW

(Improves flexibility of spine and torso circulation)

Get on all fours with your weight evenly distributed; keep your knees under your hips and your wrists under your shoulders. Arms are straight but not locked, and your fingers are spread and facing forward. Start with a straight line from the top of your head to your tailbone. Exhale as you lift your upper back and tuck your tailbone underneath and look toward your belly button, tucking your chin in. Inhale as you reverse into cow and lift your tailbone up; your belly button goes toward the ground. Look straight ahead as the top of your head faces the ceiling. Use your entire spine throughout the movement. Do five times.

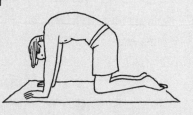

12) EXTENDED CAT STRETCH

(Warms up and awakens entire body; great for your spine)

Adding to Cat Back, lift your left knee off the ground and bring it toward your forehead while simultaneously tucking your forehead under. Then inhale and smoothly extend your right leg behind you with pointed toes. Lift your head and look forward. During the entire movement, keep your hips in line and your pelvis steady as you elongate your entire body. Do five times and then switch sides.

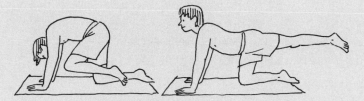

13) THREAD THE NEEDLE
(Opens upper back and shoulders)

Start on all fours; take your right hand palm side down and slide it under your left armpit. Keep extending it as you exhale and slowly lower your right ear and shoulder to the mat. Simultaneously drop your left elbow onto the mat or as low as feels comfortable. Hold for 30 seconds and switch sides.

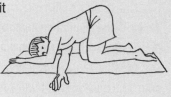

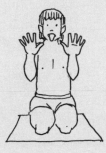

14) LION
(Awakens and simultaneously relaxes facial muscles)

While on your knees, sit erect and take a deep inhale. On the exhale, stretch all your facial muscles apart, open your mouth as wide as you can, try to touch your tongue to your chin, and open your hands as wide as you can with palms facing out. Look at the tip of your nose and make a loud "Ha" sound. Do four times.

15) WRIST EXTENSIONS
(Opens wrists; helps with carpal tunnel problems)

Bring your hands out in front of you palm side down. Interweave your fingers chest high. Relax your shoulders and gently pull your elbows apart, creating space in your joints. While keeping this space, raise your active left wrist and lower your passive right, keeping both forearms parallel to the ground. Now your right wrist is bending up and your left wrist is bending down. While keeping your fingers interlaced, gently go back and forth several times, opening up your wrists and switching your leading hand.

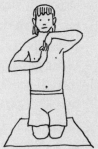

16) CAMEL
(Opens chest and the front of the body; strengthens spine)

While on your knees (use a towel if needed), place your knees and feet six inches apart. Place your hands on the back of your hips, fingers pointed down. Drop your head back completely and support yourself with your hands. Take a deep breath and exhale as you press your thighs, hips, and stomach forward, using your spine strength. While taking deep breaths, hold bend for 20 seconds and come out slowly.

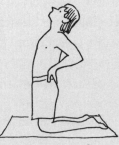

17) **LUNGES**

(Stretches your thighs and groin as well as lengthens your spine)

While on all fours with your knees below your hips and your hands below your shoulders, step your left foot forward, placing it next to your left hand. Your left shin stays perpendicular to the ground; on the inhale, bring both your hands up onto your left thigh. Keep the front of your knee behind your big toe. Don't raise your shoulders up toward your ears; keep them broad. If this is too hard, leave one hand down until it feels easy and then come up. On the exhale, gently twist your right hip toward your left heel, so that you feel a stretch along your back thigh. Inhale and exhale four times and switch sides.

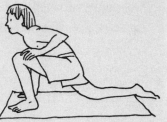

18) **DOWN DOG**

(Strengthens and stretches the legs and shoulders; energizes the whole body)

Start on all fours with your hands shoulder-width apart and your feet hip-width apart. Tuck your toes under. While inhaling, lift your knees off the ground and straighten your legs. Lift your hips back and up and spread your fingers out, pressing your palms flat to the floor. Keep your neck relaxed; your head should be in a neutral position. Lift your quadricep muscles; keep them activated. Draw your heels toward the floor. Hold for 30 seconds and release back down to the mat while exhaling.

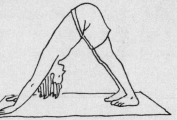

19) **COBRA**

(Develops strength and flexibility in your back)

Lie on your stomach with your hands palm side down under your shoulders, keeping your fingertips directly underneath the tops of your shoulders. Your legs are together and tight like a rock. Point your toes and put your elbows flush against your sides. While looking up at the ceiling, use your spine strength and lift your torso off the floor just to the navel. Resist pressing with your hands and arch your back as much as feels comfortable. Keep your shoulders relaxed and down away from your ears. Hold for 20 seconds.

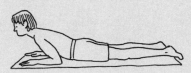

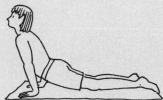

20) DIAGONAL REACH

(Strengthens your back with emphasis on your lower back and butt; improves coordination)

While lying on your stomach, place your right hand, palm down, underneath your relaxed forehead. Bring your left straight arm beside your left ear, then lift it off the ground while simultaneously lifting your right leg. Focus on stretching your left fingers as far as you can

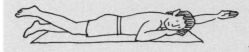

away from your right foot and feel your whole body lengthening. It is more important to elongate than to lift higher. Hold for 20 seconds and switch sides. Do two times.

21) HALF FROG POSE

(Stretches quadriceps; great for your knees)

Lie facedown and rest your forehead on the back of your left hand. Lift your right foot toward your right hip and grab your foot with your right hand. Pull the foot gently toward your outer hip. Breathe evenly and hold for 30 seconds; release and switch sides.

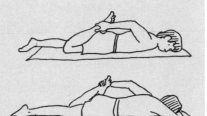

22) DOWN DOG ONE LEG

(Strengthens and stretches the legs, stretches calves, energizes the whole body)

While in Down Dog, take your right foot off the ground and wrap it around your left ankle. This added weight will open up your calf. Hold for 15 seconds and switch sides.

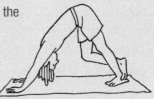

23) ROLL AND MASSAGE BACK

(Massages back and improves balance)

While lying on your back, bend your knees and clasp your hands onto your hamstrings. Curl your tailbone up and round your back. Start rocking back and forth as much as feels

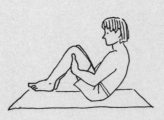 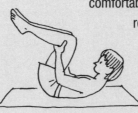

comfortable, taking notice of any skips in your roll. Try to round your body as much as possible, so it rocks smoothly back and forth. Use your lower legs to swing your body. Do for 30 seconds.

24) LITTLE BOAT POSE

(Stretches hips, lower back, and spine)

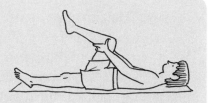

While lying on your back, hug your knees in toward your chest with your hands. Release your left leg down (either straight or bent, whichever feels more comfortable) and interweave your fingers on the outside of your right leg, just underneath the knee. Slightly pull the right knee in toward your right shoulder as you relax your neck and keep your shoulders down. Resist overextending your neck; elongate it and look straight up. Hold for 30 seconds and switch sides.

25) LITTLE BOAT TWIST

(Stretches hips, lower back, and spine)

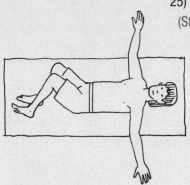

While on your back, reach your arms straight out to shoulder height, flush against the ground, palm side down. With knees bent and feet flat on the ground, exhale as you slowly drop your knees to the right and look straight up at the ceiling. To increase the stretch, lift your knees a little higher. Keep your upper back and shoulders on the mat throughout the entire pose. Hold for 30 seconds and switch sides.

26) HALF BOAT

(Tones stomach and back)

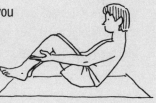

Sit on the floor. Keeping your knees bent and together out in front of you and your hands holding your legs, lean back to about a 45-degree angle. Slowly bring your feet off the ground with your calves parallel to the ground and balance. When you have your balance, release your hands to knee height.

Advanced: Straighten your legs into a V shape. Hold for 30 seconds.

27) BUTTERFLY
(Opens hips and groin)

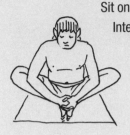

Sit on the floor with your knees bent and the soles of your feet together. Interweave your fingers on the outsides of your feet and draw your heels comfortably in toward your tailbone. If this is too hard, place your hands on your legs. With your back straight, slowly tilt your upper body forward. With time and as your hips loosen, you will ultimately be able to drop your chin down on the other side of your toes. Hold for 30 seconds.

28) HALF BUTTERFLY
(Stretches back, hamstrings, and calves)

While sitting erect with you legs out in front of you, bend your left leg back into Half Butterfly. Flex your right foot up (resist contorting your foot); keep it straight as if there were a board below it. Walk your hands down your

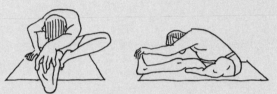

right leg, slowly lowering your forehead toward your right shin. Stop wherever it feels comfortable. Hold for ten seconds, taking deep breaths into your rib cage. Then switch sides. **Advanced:** Pull your toes back with the opposite hand.

29) CORPSE
(Relaxes entire body)

While on your back, let your arms relax down to your sides palms facing up, extend your legs out straight, and let your feet flop down. With your eyes closed, travel mentally throughout your entire body, relaxing from your toes to the crown of your head. Cover your eyes with a cloth if you like. When you are ready to come up, roll onto your side, hold for 15 seconds, and then slowly come onto all fours before standing up.

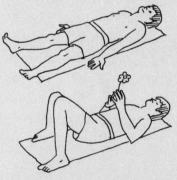

This yoga workout can be found on the *YOU: Being Beautiful Workout* DVD.

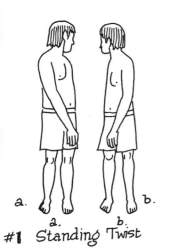

a.   b.

#1 Standing Twist

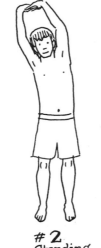

#2 Standing Leaning Stretch

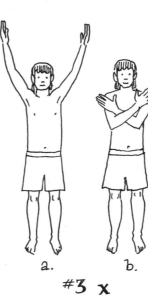

a.   b.

#3 x

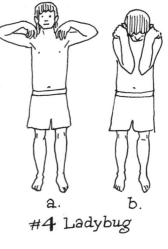

a.   b.

#4 Ladybug

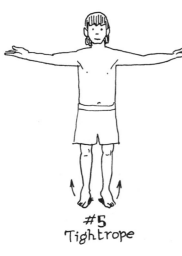

#5 Tightrope

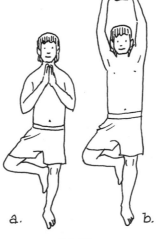

a.   b.

#6 Tree

#7 Stork

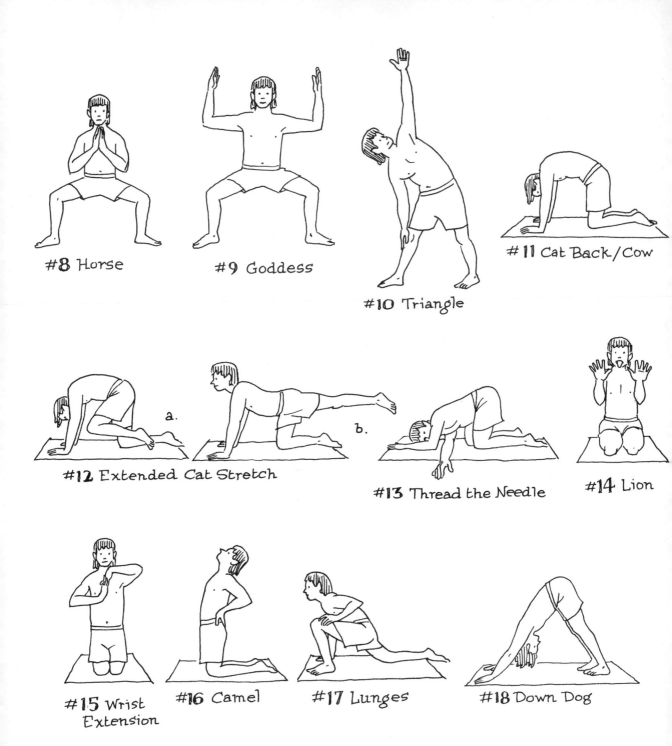

#8 Horse

#9 Goddess

#10 Triangle

#11 Cat Back/Cow

#12 Extended Cat Stretch

a.

b.

#13 Thread the Needle

#14 Lion

#15 Wrist Extension

#16 Camel

#17 Lunges

#18 Down Dog

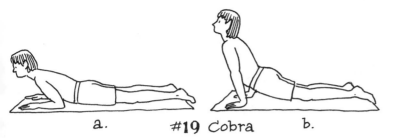

a.   #19 Cobra   b.

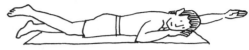

#20 Diagonal Reach

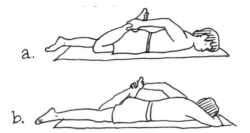

#21   Half Frog

#22 Down Dog One Leg

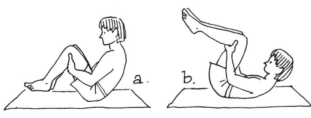

#23 Roll and Massage Back

#24 Little Boat

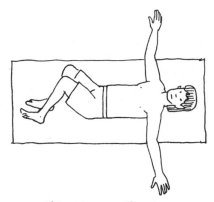

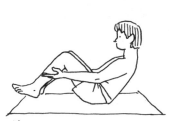

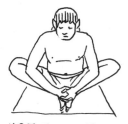

#25 Little Boat
Twist

#26 Half Boat

#27 Butterfly

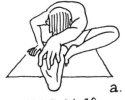

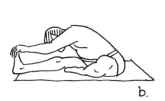

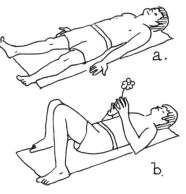

#28 Half
Butterfly

#29 Corpse

YOU Tool: The Perfect Gym Bag

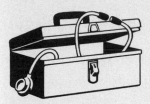

Gym bags of yesterday carried two things—a pair of sneakers and a stench that resembled bad bologna. If you do your workout someplace other than your home, you can stock your gym bag with a few other items. These items will not only help make your workout more comfortable but can also make you healthier.

Clothes

- Shirt and socks that wick away moisture and keep you cool and comfortable (and shorts or warm-up pants, of course)
- Well-fitting shoes for sport of choice
- Flip-flops for the shower, to decrease your risk of being exposed to fungi
- Gloves for weight lifting (so you avoid small cuts and calluses from lifting, and also to lessen the chance of passing along germs when you shake hands or picking up germs from the equipment)
- A towel (even if the gym provides one, bring your own, because gyms tend not to use enough detergent at a high enough temperature to kill MRSA, methicillin-resistant *Staphylococcus aureui*)

Equipment

- Heart-rate monitor (keep heart rate at 80 percent of max, which is 220 minus your age, for most of the time you're on a cardio machine, and push to maximum heart rate for last minute of every ten, with doc's approval)
- Earphones and audio player (but keep volume level under 85 decibels; that's about a 6–7 on most handheld audio players)
- Elastic bandages for tight wrapping (RICE protocol) if you twist an ankle
- Ice containers (plastic bags) into which you can place ice for injuries

Goop

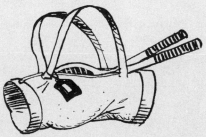

- A pocket-size bottle of antibacterial gel if your gym doesn't have some (use after your workout since you have been gripping sweaty objects)
- Alcohol spritzer to wipe off sweaty machines (if the bozo ahead of you didn't wipe them down himself)

YOU Tool: Health Utensils

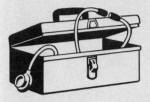 While much of this book focuses on beauty issues that have big health implications, we want to address a few more health-related issues, because, after all, there's nothing that looks or feels beautiful when you're sick and run-down.

STAY STOCKED: YOUR MEDICINE CABINET

You've likely snooped in enough medicine cabinets to know that they tend to be not only full of used medicine but also a breeding ground for makeup, Allen wrenches, and bills from 1975. Do yourself a favor and clean out your collection of nastiness and stock your medicine cabinet full of things that can make you feel good—even when times are tough.

Tools

Dental floss

Soft-bristle toothbrush (don't brush as you brush a toilet, and change every two months);
    a sonic brush is even better

Mouth mask (if you get the flu, to avoid spreading it to your family)

Home blood pressure–testing device

Self-heating wraps that don't burn skin (for muscle soreness)

Nail clipper

Cleaners

Healthy toothpaste; if you have frequent mouth ulcers, avoid sodium laurel sulfate (foaming agent)
    or whitening agents

Soap without antibacterial properties (which encourage resistant bacteria) or fragrances (which are
    allergens)

Skin exfoliant (removes dead cells and reduces adult acne)

Deodorant (without an antiperspirant, so you can let the natural process of sweating happen)

Pain Relievers and Medicines

Topical muscle reliever, such as Bengay, Tiger Balm, capsaicin cream, or arnica

General first aid kit

Butterfly tape strips (to close little cuts)

Band-Aid Liquid Bandage (cyanoacrylate Dermabond for home for blisters and small cracks—
same as doc's Dermabond)

Petroleum-based Vaseline, Neosporin, or bacitracin cream (to keep wounds moist)

Tea tree oil (for pilonidal cysts and feet)

Burt's Bees beeswax lip balm

Glyoxide (soothes canker sores)

Pepto-Bismol (for traveler's diarrhea)

Antacids (OTC Prilosec)

Epsom salts (use in bath for soreness)

Elastic bandages for tight wrapping (RICE protocol)

Ipecac to induce vomiting (we hope you won't need this)

Benadryl tablets for minor allergic reactions

Think Twice About

Tamiflu (may be overkill, plus can cause psychotic reactions)

Imodium (generally, when you have the runs, you want the bacteria or virus to come out, not stay
stuck inside)

Cough medicines with pseudoephedrine, which will jack up your blood pressure (and absolutely
avoid these if you're on any medicine or supplement for blood pressure)

Old, expired drugs, particularly liquids, which can grow bacteria and change chemically

KEEP CLEAN: HOME HYGIENE

Whether your home is clean and organized or whether it looks as though the familial tornado has just made its way through every room of the house, your home is packed with places where germs can breed and spread. Let's take a tour and figure out how you can keep the contamination to a minimum.

Kitchen

Garbage disposal. A veritable whirlwind of bacteria sprays up every time the disposal is turned on, leaving a germ-heavy mist hanging over the kitchen. Make sure the disposal opening is properly covered before you flip the switch.

Sponges and dishrags. These are fertile bacteria breeding grounds, containing more than 100,000 germs per square inch. Microwave wet sponges (dry ones can catch fire) for two minutes on high when they're particularly dirty (preferably each day) to kill bacteria, or get rid of them and just use dishrags cleaned in a dilute bleach (aka Clorox) solution.

Cutting board. Despite what you may have heard, wooden cutting boards are safer than plastic ones. In one study, the bacteria on the wooden board died off in three minutes. On the plastic board, the bacteria remained and actually multiplied overnight. It seems that wood has a natural bacteria-killing property that plastic and glass don't.

Countertops. You're never going to control the bacteria in your house, so don't go ballistic over this. Antibacterial countertops are useless. Clean off your counters with water after preparing food. If your food is contaminated with bacteria, as all chicken and hamburger is, kill those germs with Lysol, bleach, or a green alternative such as vinegar. Ditto for your refrigerator and freezer.

Bathroom

Toilet. Toilets contain a bacterial line just below the water level called a biofilm. The bacterial biofilm is very difficult to remove even with household cleaners. Once airborne, these microdroplets land on everything within the flush zone: drinking cups, toys, toothbrushes used by children, etc. Some of these pathogens live for a week on surfaces. Every toilet flush creates an unseen mist detectable at head height that can travel up to 15 feet away from the toilet bowl—known as the

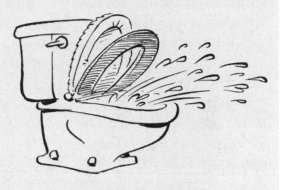

aerosol effect. Always put the toilet seat down before you flush the toilet, as it will prevent some of the fecal particles from floating up and landing on every other bathroom surface, and keep your toothbrush covered.

Cleaning solutions. All bathroom surfaces should be cleaned regularly. These include the door handle, faucets, toilet, sink, floor, and shower/bathtub. Clean inside the toilet at least twice a week with a disinfectant or disinfectant toilet bowl cleaner. Clean the toilet and sink with separate cloths to avoid transferring germs.

Showerheads. Occasionally remove your showerheads and soak them overnight in vinegar or a commercial cleanser. This removes the mineral residue and mold that clog the head and contaminate shower water.

Bedroom

Mattress. We all sweat during the night, excreting up to half a pint of moisture, and that goes somewhere—into the mattress—and forms an ideal environment for dust mites. Add to that the fact that we shed skin as we sleep, around nine pounds per person per year, which gives the mites something to eat. These little buggers can irritate your skin and cause swelling. The scary statistic is that an average bed is home to about 10,000 dust mites, which can cause hay fever and asthma, among other things. Turn the mattress every six months, replace it every ten years, and vacuum it monthly. Use a latex cover or a 1-micron filter sheet cover.

Pillow. Every night you're inhaling the waste of the dust mites that live in the pillow. Use a latex cover or a 1-micron filter pillow cover.

INFECTION PROTECTION

Let's face it. Nobody feels all that beautiful when they're facedown in the toilet trying to expel the toxic remains of last night's dinner. Ugly scene, ugly feeling, ugly cleanup duty. While many people assume that their so-called bug comes from a virus, the truth is that a lot of intestinal tumult comes from something even scarier—food poisoning. Though we don't advocate that you be so germphobic that you hole up in your house and restrict yourself to unseasoned rice, we do think that you should be aware of the kinds of toxins that can send you scurrying for the closest porcelain basin. When it comes to food poisoning, here's a fact that will scare the sashimi right out of you: The Center for Disease Control says that for every reported case of food poisoning, there are anywhere from 20 to 100 that go unreported. Why? People often blame the heaves on a 24-hour bug. Another reason: It often takes from 24 to 72 hours for food-borne illnesses to take effect, so you don't associate a potentially bad food with sickness; salmonella can take three days for symptoms to appear, while *E. coli* can take up to eight days. Adding to the problem is that people have various misconceptions about food poisoning—for example, that bad smell and taste will tip off whether a food is spoiled (germs and toxins often don't change the taste), or that home food is safer than restaurant food (also not true). There are 2,500 deaths and 50,000 to 2.5 million severe cases of food poisoning a year. This wide range of estimates reflects how poorly reported this condition really is. The only real protection is proper storage and preparation of food.

If you see an unsavory practice in a restaurant—such as a worker not washing his hands between mopping the floor and making your pizza—let the management and the board of health know it. If your waiter has conjunctivitis, or if the chef sneezes in your pasta primavera, open your mouth (and not to swallow the food). You're not being a snitch; you're saving yourself and others from food poisoning.

Another serious health risk is nosocomial infections—that is, infections spread in the hospital. As you know (or can imagine), hospitals are breeding grounds for such germs because of all the sick people and the constant contact from person to person and from person to thing. Many hospitals are doing a lot to reduce the risk of spreading infections, but it's a tough task—and it's a problem you should be aware of if you're admitted to or are visiting a hospital. You won't be offending your doctor or nurse if you ask them to wash their hands; ask them if they used soap and water or alcohol (tell them you're taking a poll). They'll get the message. Sometimes they get sloppy, and you must protect yourself.

By the way, there are several theories as to why we get sick in the winter. It might be because we huddle in confined areas to avoid the cold or that we become vitamin D deficient from lack of sun so our immune systems are compromised. It also may be that microbes survive a lot longer in cold weather and low humidity, so they can hang out longer before infecting us.

The real secret of preventing infection is making sure you keep your hands clean. In fact, it's the single best way to stop the spread of illness-causing germs. While you may think that washing hands is as instinctual as blinking, there is a correct method and form to reduce the germs.

Correct hand-washing method (an alternate is using an alcohol gel sanitizer, but doing both is better, and alcohol gel alone misses many bad bacteria):

Use very warm running water and soap.

Scrub both sides of the hands for about 20 or 30 seconds.

Pay close attention to under the fingernails and around the hair follicles on the fingers and on the backs of the hands.

Rinse well with very warm, running water.

Dry hands with a disposable paper towel.

Hands should be washed after:

Using the toilet

Changing diapers (wash the hands of the diapered child, too)

Helping a child at the toilet

Your hands come in contact with any bodily fluid, e.g., vomit, saliva, a runny nose, etc.

Fixing or eating food (and before also)

Touching raw meat, poultry, fish, or eggs

Shaking hands

Coughing, sneezing, or blowing your nose (though you can change your sneeze habits, so that you sneeze into the crook of your elbow)

Handling money

Riding public transportation

And at any point where you feel your hands might be at risk: When in doubt, wash 'em out.

YOU Tool: Your Eyes

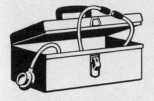

If the eyes are the windows to the soul, we sure have a lot of options for curtains. We can dress up our eyes and improve our vision with things that nobody can notice (like LASIK) or with things that can make pretty bold fashion statements (nice monocle, Dad!). Research shows that people who wear glasses are perceived to be more intelligent than those who don't (half of people say they would put glasses on just to be thought of as smarter on a date or job interview). That means you'll want to think carefully about how you dress up your eyes. Here are a few options:

GLASSES
Types of Lenses

You're nearsighted if you can see better near and farsighted if you can see better far. And when you hit 40, that inability to see near—called presbyopia—becomes a bigger problem, meaning that you may need bifocals, or different lenses for seeing close *and* far. (By the way, some people say that eye exercises can eliminate the need for glasses; this is as yet unproven, but remember that traditional Inuits never needed glasses for distance vision because they were looking to the horizon all the time.) Progressive lenses eliminate the bifocal lines on the lens that may make you seem older than you feel.

If your eye is squished on one side, called an astigmatism, your lenses should compensate for that. (Astigmatism will make you a little harder to fit for contact lenses, because the curve of your cornea will be different on the top and bottom.)

Both the lens in the front of the eye and the retina in the back of the eye can be damaged by ultraviolet A- and B-spectrum radiation. Caps and visors alone are not enough because much of the light is reflected from the road or water. Some clear eyeglass lenses need to be treated to protect your eyes from UV light, but ones made of polycarbonate don't need extra coatings. Lenses should have a label indicating that they block over 90 percent of UVA and 95 percent of UVB. (Sunglasses are usually made to this standard.) While it may be counter to fashion, the larger the lenses, the more protection they will provide.

YOUR SHAPE OF FACE	IDEAL SHAPE OF GLASSES
Oval	Any type of frame
Long, thin	Round frame to make face seem shorter
Square, with strong jawline	Round or oval frames
Round	Rectangular to make face look longer and thinner
Heart (wide at forehead, thin at chin)	Wider at bottom and low on the temples to balance the wide forehead
Neanderthal	Just smile a lot

Types of Frames

You should pick a frame based not only on what looks best but also on comfort and how it'll function with your particular lifestyle.

Plastic: Lightweight but breaks easily

Titanium: Strong, expensive; will resist bending if you're active; just get it

Beryllium: Resists corrosion; good for people who work around water

Stainless steel, aluminum: Strong, light, good all-around frames

CONTACT LENSES

Sitting directly on your cornea, contacts are made of various materials and can be hard or soft, reusable or disposable. They have plenty of advantages—no glare from glasses and no worrying about losing or breaking your specs. But they have their risks (1 in 20 users have complications). Corneal abrasions are a constant risk, not only from placement of the lens but from the lens rubbing on the cornea with each blink. Conjunctivitis, as well as allergies to either the lenses or the cleaning solutions, are common and are related to the type of lens and whether you wear them overnight. Bacteria can invade your eyes if they're irritated by contacts, causing severe corneal infections that can endanger your vision. Disposable lenses do not reduce the chance of infection, as the lens-cleaning solution may be the source of bacteria. You should write the date on the bottle when you open a lens-wetting or -cleaning solution and throw it out after a month. Lenses can rob your cornea of oxygen, causing your body to grow blood vessels into the normally clear cornea and impairing your vision. So make sure you take them out every night unless they're specifically marked as continuous wear. Follow the manufacturer's guidelines carefully to avoid corneal damage.

LASIK

Five million people in the United States have thrown away their eyeglasses *and* contacts, opting to have their eyeballs reshaped by a laser. LASIK (laser-assisted in-situ keratomileusis) is a high-tech method of altering the shape of your eye to improve your vision. The goal of LASIK is 20/20 vision. This means that at 20 feet, you'll see the 20 line on the eye chart; this is the level of acuity that is considered to be acceptable by most people. Some people want the best possible vision for the average person, shooting for 20/12. Because of the way the light-sensing cones in the retina and the neurons in the brain process light and space, the best vision any human can have is 20/10.

While LASIK sounds great, it's still an imperfect procedure. LASIK relies on lasers to cut the cornea, and that's where problems can occur. As with any surgical procedure, about 3 to 5 percent of people have complications. Though eyeballs have even been perforated, most problems are just nuisances that leave you with irregular vision and halos around light, particularly at night. Your eyes might feel dry afterward, and you might need saline drops. If this happens, be careful if you plan on having cosmetic eyelid surgery in the future, and make sure to tell your doc about your problem. LASIK is irreversible and can't treat some shapes of eyeballs. Occasionally, blood vessels can grow into the cornea after the procedure, harming vision. Newer techniques are being developed in the hope of solving these problems. LASIK is a great procedure and one that we expect to improve with newer generations of computerized lasers, but if your job depends on perfect vision, such as flying an airplane or performing surgery, you might want to wait a few more years before considering LASIK.

YOU Tool: The Biophysical Battery: Energy Blood Tests

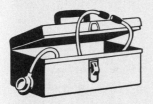

If you don't have enough energy, you can ask your doc to explain your results on the following tests. The complete test is available through Biophysical at www.biophysicalcorp.com. But your doc can also order routine blood tests to measure many of these functions. Remember, we still believe that your history is the key to diagnosis, but these can aid your doctor.

THYROID FUNCTION TESTS: These tests look to see if you have hypo- or hyperthyroidism, both of which are often associated with lack of energy (yes, hyper- causes you to feel hyper before you feel fatigued).

- **TSH LEVEL:** The thyroid gland is regulated by a pituitary hormone called thyroid-stimulating hormone (TSH). TSH is one of the best indicators of how your thyroid gland is functioning. Hyperthyroidism usually results in a decreased TSH level, while hypothyroidism usually results in an elevated TSH level. Subclinical hyperthyroidism typically occurs when you have a low or borderline low TSH level and normal levels of triiodothyronine (T3) or thyroxine (T4). Subclinical hypothyroidism, on the other hand, typically occurs when an individual has a high or borderline high TSH level and normal T3 and T4 levels. Subclinical hypothyroidism is more common in people over 60.
- **FREE T4 LEVEL.** This is the less active hormone from the thyroid that is converted to the more active T3 to regulate metabolism. Too much T4 leads to excessive energy and a profound feeling of the jitters— not to mention weight loss. This is hyperthyroidism. Too little T4 leads to reduced energy and a profound feeling of the blahs—and of course weight gain.
- **FREE T3 LEVEL.** This is the most active thyroid hormone, and it regulates metabolism in much the same way as T4. Both of these hormones influence the pituitary's secretion of TSH. If there is too little T3 or T4 in circulation, TSH goes up. If there is too much T3 and T4 in circulation, the TSH goes down. This seesaw between pituitary hormone and the active hormone of the gland is known as a feedback relationship.
- **THYROGLOBULIN AB AND THYROID MICROSOMAL AB** are autoantibodies to the thyroid gland. This means that some people make antibodies against their own thyroid rather than an intruder bacteria or virus, which is what our antibodies are designed to do. People who have thyroid autoantibodies and an elevated level of TSH progress to overt hypothyroidism at a rate of 3 to 5 percent per year. These are the two most common thyroid autoantibodies seen in people with hypothyroidism.

ANEMIA OR HEMOCHROMATOSIS LEVELS: These tests look to see if you have abnormal blood cell amounts that are commonly associated with fatigue. By the way, if you have anemia as a cause of fatigue, you need more tests to determine the cause of your anemia.

- **HGB LEVEL:** Hemoglobin is an iron-containing protein that enables red blood cells to carry oxygen from the lungs to body tissues. All of our tissues need oxygen. This is an essential energy source. Without enough hemoglobin, the tissues lack oxygen and the heart and lungs must work harder to try to compensate. Low levels of hemoglobin may indicate anemia, excessive bleeding, nutritional deficiencies, destruction of cells because of a transfusion reaction or mechanical heart valve, or abnormally formed hemoglobin such as is found in sickle-cell anemia.
- **FERRITIN:** Ferritin is a protein that stores iron in the blood. The ferritin level is a sensitive indicator of the body's iron stores. Serum ferritin levels are very helpful in the evaluation of blood disorders such as iron-deficiency anemia. In this variety of anemia, the hemoglobin is low because there is not enough iron in the body. Usually this is the case because of very gradual blood loss from menstrual periods or from the stomach (ulcers) or colon (polyps). Hemochromatosis is a condition in which the ferritin level is elevated and therefore the body's iron stores are quite high. If you have it, too much iron can build up and hurt vital organs such as the liver and the pancreas. This condition is uncommon and affects 1 in 600 people.

INFLAMMATION: These tests look to see if you have high levels of inflammation in your body—these, or what is causing the inflammation, can cause fatigue. Your doctor may follow up with more specific tests (such as for rheumatoid factors or lupus or other less common diseases if these screening tests for inflammation indicate that your fatigue may be due to these causes).

- **C-REACTIVE PROTEIN (CRP)** is produced in the liver, and its levels rise dramatically in the presence of inflammation or infection. Although not a telltale diagnostic sign of any one condition, CRP may be measured to check for rheumatoid arthritis or to measure a patient's response to treatment. As a marker of inflammation, CRP has also been established as an important predictor of cardiovascular risk. CRP levels between 3 and 10 ug/mL are suggestive of the inflammatory process caused by the formation of plaque within arteries or atherosclerosis. Most docs think the evidence to treat such elevations with a statin drug after a search for other causes warrants that such treatment be recommended to patients. Levels greater than 10 ug/mL suggest other types of inflammation that can occur with such conditions as arthritis or infection.
- **ERYTHROCYTE SEDIMENTATION RATE.** This is another way to measure inflammation in the body.
- **IL-6, IL-8, AND/OR TNF ALPHA:** These are special chemicals or biomarkers in the blood that are released by one group of inflammatory cells to tell the others that there is a site of inflammation within the body and that more help (more inflammatory cells) is needed to respond to the problem. These biomarkers may signal a greater intensity of inflammation.
- **VASCULAR ENDOTHELIAL GROWTH FACTOR (VEGF):** This is a very interesting biomarker that is often associated with inflammation. Since it stimulates the growth of tiny blood vessels, it can be elevated in healing wounds or nasal polyps. Perhaps related to inflammation in general, many people with sleep apnea have an elevation of VEGF.

DIABETES AND IMPAIRED GLUCOSE METABOLISM: Diabetes mellitus is a disease in which the body cannot make or respond to insulin, allowing glucose to build up in the bloodstream. Insulin is a hormone produced by the pancreas that helps the body's cells to take in glucose and convert it to energy. When the pancreas does not make enough insulin or the body is resistant to the insulin that is present, excess glucose builds up in the bloodstream, setting the stage for diabetes. Diabetes is a growing health concern, affecting about 8 percent of the U.S. population. It plays a major role in strokes and cardiac and vascular disease, and can cause injury to the kidneys, eyes, and other parts of the body. Diabetes is divided into two types: type 1 (also called juvenile or insulin-dependent diabetes) and type 2 (also called adult-onset or non-insulin-dependent diabetes). In addition, there is a form of prediabetes called impaired glucose metabolism (IGM). IGM is often observed in individuals with an increased waist size and increases one's risk of developing type 2 diabetes and heart disease.

- **FASTING BLOOD GLUCOSE LEVEL:** A level from 79 to 99 mg/dL indicates normal glucose metabolism. A level from 100 to 125 mg/dL indicates impaired glucose metabolism, while a level above 125 mg/dL on two separate occasions indicates the presence of diabetes.
- **HEMOGLOBIN A1C (HbA1c):** This biomarker level is an indication of the average amount of glucose in your blood over time, as HbA1c levels are not influenced by daily fluctuations in the blood glucose concentration. An insulin measurement helps determine whether a high blood glucose reading is the result of insufficient insulin or poor use of insulin. Individuals with type 2 diabetes mellitus may have elevated levels of insulin.

KIDNEY FUNCTION: Kidneys are the beanlike organs that are essential for micro-managing your blood chemicals and often the first organ injured by chronic disease.

- **CREATININE.** Creatinine is a protein waste product generated by muscle metabolism and is eliminated by the kidneys. Because creatinine is released at a constant rate (depending on muscle mass), its serum level is a good indicator of kidney function. Creatinine levels can increase temporarily as a result of muscle injury.
- **BUN:** Measures the amount of urea nitrogen in the blood. Urea is the major breakdown product of bodily protein and contains nitrogen. Urea and other nitrogen-rich waste products are normally eliminated from the bloodstream by the kidneys, so an increased BUN level may indicate impaired renal (kidney) function. However, many conditions other than renal disease can cause BUN alterations. An elevated BUN level may also be caused by dehydration.

LIVER DISEASE: The liver is the body's filter for toxins and is the main metabolic engine for creating new proteins.

- **AST:** Aspartate aminotransferase (AST) is an enzyme found in liver, muscle, and heart tissues. Increased levels of AST can be seen with liver diseases (e.g., hepatitis), and injury or disease to the muscles. The

AST test is often done to determine liver function in conjunction with other tests, including alanine aminotransferase (ALT) and alkaline phosphatase (ALP).

- **BILIRUBIN:** Bilirubin is a breakdown product from the hemoglobin released from dying red blood cells and is elevated if the liver or gallbladder are too congested to process this waste product.

HEART FAILURE: The heart cannot pump enough blood to the body; it's not hard to understand why fatigue occurs.

- **B-TYPE NATRIURETIC PEPTIDE (BNP):** It's produced only in the ventricles of the heart. Increased levels may indicate heart failure. There is strong correlation between the degree of heart failure and the BNP level. Studies suggest that the BNP may have important prognostic significance in people with acute coronary syndrome (ACS). If your BNP is significantly elevated, heart disease may be the cause of your fatigue.

VITAMIN INADEQUACIES: Specific vitamin levels.

- **VITAMIN B12** is important for metabolism, the formation of the red blood cells, and the maintenance of the central nervous system. A deficiency of vitamin B12 may occur as a result of an inability to absorb the vitamin from food. It can also occur in strict vegetarians who do not consume any animal foods. Some individuals who develop a vitamin B12 deficiency have an underlying stomach or intestinal disorder that limits the absorption of vitamin B12.
- **VITAMIN D** is essential for enabling the digestive system to absorb calcium and phosphate. It also causes the release of calcium from bone into the bloodstream. Vitamin D is also required for normal development of teeth and bones, and it's important for normal immune and cardiovascular functioning. The body acquires and activates vitamin D from particular food sources and exposure to ultraviolet radiation or sunlight.

BOWEL DISEASES: Chronic bowel problems and parasitic diseases can also rob you of energy and cause fatigue.

- **TISSUE TRANSGLUTAMINASE (tTG):** Certain antibodies can signal inflammation within the small intestine. tTG is an antibody that indicates gluten (wheat, barley, rye, oat) intolerance, also known as celiac disease. Some people with celiac disease do not absorb important nutrients well and as a result may become chronically fatigued.
- Antibodies for gluten (wheat, barley, rye, oat) intolerance.
- Stool for ova and parasites.
- You may also use your history to help confirm or help with management.

OBESITY AND METABOLIC SYNDROME: Over a third of obese individuals have a condition known as metabolic syndrome. This syndrome combines five parameters: high blood pressure, high glucose, high triglycerides, low HDL (the good cholesterol), and a bulging waistline. Most of these people have a resistance to insulin and may be on the road to adult diabetes.

- **INSULIN:** This important hormone allows glucose (sugar) to enter cells. Obese people may be resistant to insulin so that their glucose is elevated as well as their insulin. This problem improves a great deal with weight loss.
- **LEPTIN:** This is a hormone made by fat cells. In normal people it helps curb the appetite so that we don't gain too much weight. This mechanism may not work as efficiently in obese people.
- **ADIPONECTIN:** This is another fat hormone, but this one decreases with weight gain. Higher levels of adiponectin are desirable because it protects us from heart attacks. Adiponectin increases as we lose weight.
- **MYOGLOBIN:** This is an important muscle enzyme. Petite people with very little muscle have lower levels of myoglobin.

HORMONES

- **DHEA-S LEVEL:** Dihydroepiandrosterone sulfate (DHEA-S) is a steroid hormone produced by the adrenal glands, testes, and brain. It is a precursor hormone, meaning that other steroid hormones, such as estrogen and testosterone, are made from DHEA-S. Research has shown that as men age, their levels of DHEA-S tend to decrease.
- **TESTOSTERONE** for men, especially if shaving frequency has changed or libido is decreased, or for women over 45 or if leg-shaving frequency has changed.
- **SEX HORMONE BINDING GLOBULIN (SHBG):** This is the flatbed truck for our sex hormones. SHBG is a protein that transports testosterone and estrogen from one place to another in our bloodstream. During transport sex hormones are so tightly bound to SHBG that they are temporarily unavailable.
- **ALBUMIN:** This is one of the most important proteins in our bloodstream. It too transports sex hormones but binds to them less tightly so that they are more active and available.
- **BIOAVAILABLE TESTOSTERONE (CALCULATED):** The testosterone in the bloodstream that is available for biological activity is called the bioavailable testosterone. This calculation can help determine if someone has enough testosterone to get the job done.
- **IGF-1 LEVEL:** This hormone is made by the liver and is directly related to growth hormone. Insulin-like growth factor (also called somatomedin) is a protein hormone similar in structure and function to insulin, but with much higher growth-promoting activity than insulin. It stimulates the proliferation of various types of cells, including muscle, bone, and cartilage. Factors that are known to cause variation in the levels of growth hormone (GH) and IGF-1 in serum include genetic makeup, amount of sleep, time of day, age, gender, exercise status, stress levels, nutrition level, waist size, disease state, race, and estrogen status.

If it is in the purview of chronic fatigue (lasting longer than six months) . . .

INFECTIOUS CAUSES

- **CYTOMEGALOVIRUS ANTIBODIES:** CMV is a common virus that may cause a mononucleosis-like illness in healthy individuals or more severe disease in immunosuppressed persons. The presence of CMV antibody indicates recent infection or exposure. CMV infections in humans are widespread: 60 to 90 percent of adults have had CMV infection. Infection of healthy children and adults usually results in asymptomatic disease but can cause hepatitis or mononucleosis and in rare cases may result in chronic fatigue.
- **EPSTEIN-BARR VIRUS ANTIBODIES:** EBV is a virus that causes infectious mononucleosis. Infection with EBV is common and occurs most frequently in late adolescence or early adulthood. Once infected with EBV, individuals develop virus-specific antibodies. Some infected individuals develop chronic fatigue syndrome.
- **TOXOPLASMOSIS TITERS:** Toxoplasmosis is a common infectious disease caused by the *Toxoplasma gondii* parasite. You can become infected with toxoplasmosis if you accidentally touch your hands to your mouth after gardening, cleaning a cat's litter box, or handling undercooked meat. In healthy individuals, it causes only mild symptoms of fatigue.
- **LYME DISEASE:** Lyme disease is a bacterial infection carried by ticks that often causes an expanding target-like skin rash, which is followed by arthritis, fatigue, malaise, nervous system problems, and heart rhythm disturbances several months later. Sometimes people with untreated Lyme disease develop persistent fatigue associated with aching muscles and joints, mood swings, and memory problems, so learning if you have been infected by measuring whether your antibodies have responded to the bacteria is worthwhile.

APPENDIX:
HEALING WITH STEEL

Finding the Right Plastic Surgery for You

If you've gotten this far, then surely you know that the point of the book is that beauty equals health, not supermodel looks. While we've given you tips and tricks for helping you look, feel, and be as beautiful as you can, we also know the reality: some people will never feel happy with the body or face that genetics (or life) has dealt them. Because of that, we believe that a variety of cosmetic options *may* be right for you. With nearly 2 million cosmetic surgeries a year, 10 million minimally invasive procedures, and nearly as many reality shows detailing them, it's clear that our culture has embraced these beauty-enhancement options. Here's a quick guide to some of the most popular procedures—and what you should know before you decide to nip, tuck, pull, vacuum, and/or lift. And those of you who are are up all night Googling plastic surgery can check out *Straight Talk About Cosmetic Surgery* by our coauthor Dr. Arthur W. Perry. It's your toolbox to stay on the safe side of the scalpel.

BREAST IMPLANTS: Jockeying back and forth each year with liposuction as the most popular plastic surgical procedure, breast augmentations, euphemistically called "breast enhancement," have skyrocketed in popularity since silicone gel was allowed back on the market in 2006 after a 14-year absence. Now women can sit down with their plastic surgeons and choose from a bewildering array of gel, saline, smooth, textured, or shaped implants.

These outpatient procedures (best done with general anesthesia) are the biggest "wow" technique in plastic surgery (go into the operating room with an A cup and come out with a stage job

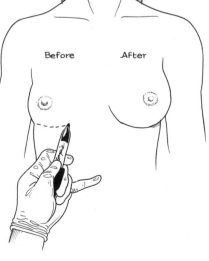

Before   After

at the Risqué Room). Implants are placed either in front of or behind your pectoralis muscle in this two-hour surgery. The newest technique, in which the muscle is actually cut through to let the implant hang more naturally, makes it harder for women to flex their pecs. Unless you're headed for the Olympics, this won't hurt your athletic performance. The main problem with breast augmentations is that implants distort X-ray mammograms, meaning you'll require MRIs to check yearly for breast cancer. We're not in favor of anything that will hurt your health, so if you decide to make your breasts larger, stay safe by having MRIs along with your mammograms.

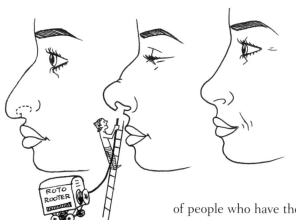

RHINOPLASTY: It sounds like a procedure performed on zoo animals, but nose jobs are serious business. This two- to three-hour procedure can be done with you either awake or asleep ("just a little tapping now"). The doc will sculpt the cartilage and bones in your nose, making you look like . . . yourself, but hopefully without that hump. The noses of today are much more conservative than your mother's rhinoplasty, but even so, 15 percent of people who have their noses operated on have to go under the knife for a touch-up. Don't expect your insurance to cover rhinoplasty; it's usually cosmetic.

LIPOSUCTION: Liposuction is more than just fodder for a great doctor T-shirt (Fat Sucks, So We Suck Fat). Liposuction has been the most popular procedure in plastic surgery for almost two decades, and the 457,000 procedures performed annually make it nine times as popular as in 1992.

While women most often have fat suctioned from their thighs, men have it removed from their "love handles." Liposuction is safest when less than ten pounds is removed. More than that, and you could wind up on the wrong end of a complication. Don't do it to lose weight; do it when you're near your ideal weight but still want to change your shape. Choose your surgeon wisely—make sure she has privileges to do liposuction in a hospital and make sure that your doc doesn't inject too much of the anesthetic lidocaine—if you're asleep for the procedure, you won't need any. It's the lidocaine that makes the procedure more dangerous. You can check out the surgeon with a second opin-

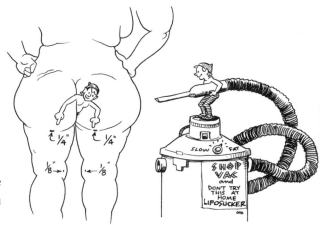

ion (see *YOU: The Smart Patient*). Checking docs' backgrounds and their use of lidocaine will make you able to celebrate the results.

EYE PROCEDURES: The eyes are the first part of the face that hints at aging, because those little crinkles in your lower eyelids can be accompanied by extra skin on the upper lids, giving you an 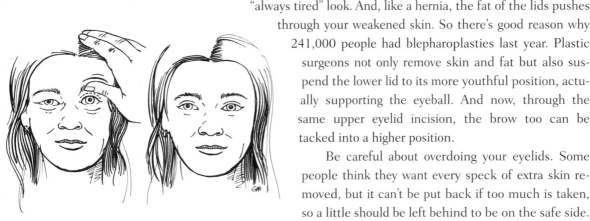 "always tired" look. And, like a hernia, the fat of the lids pushes through your weakened skin. So there's good reason why 241,000 people had blepharoplasties last year. Plastic surgeons not only remove skin and fat but also suspend the lower lid to its more youthful position, actually supporting the eyeball. And now, through the same upper eyelid incision, the brow too can be tacked into a higher position.

Be careful about overdoing your eyelids. Some people think they want every speck of extra skin removed, but it can't be put back if too much is taken, so a little should be left behind to be on the safe side. And leaving a little skin will leave you looking more natural. Most blephs are done with you awake but groggy. Afterward, you'll look as if you went three rounds with Ali. It takes nearly two weeks to look good again, but then your eyes should sparkle.

If you have dry eyes or very loose lower lids, you're at high risk for the complication called an ectropion if you have your lids lifted, leaving you resembling a basset hound. To avoid this complication, your lower lids might need a tightening procedure called a canthopexy (no clever marketing surgeon has come up with a catchy name for this one) along with skin and fat removal. There is a 4 in 10,000 chance of blindness from blephs, but a good surgeon who also properly evaluates your medical issues should be able to steer you clear of problems.

TUMMY TUCKS: The fastest-growing cosmetic procedure and among the most popular ones is the abdominoplasty. Baby boomers have had their kids, and tummy tucks reverse the damage those little tykes did while inside. While someone was camping out in your uterus, your abdominal muscles relaxed and thinned so your belly wouldn't crush your baby.

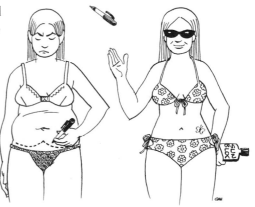

A tummy tuck tightens the rectus muscles in the abdomen and also pulls in the obliques (muscles on the sides of the abdomen) to improve their tone. You'll stand up straighter, and your lower-back pain may be relieved.

Liposuction of the flanks is usually done along with the tummy tuck, and the extra skin and fat of the lower belly is tossed into medical waste. What's left behind is tightened so much that you won't stand up straight for two weeks. Sounds terrible, but when it's all done, your tummy will be flatter. But choose your doctor wisely; tummy tucks are the most dangerous of all cosmetic surgery, with bleeding, blood clots in the legs, and even deaths occurring. Do it in a hospital, and don't fall for that "mommy makeover" marketing stuff; most careful plastic surgeons will not do any procedures other than the hip liposuction along with a tummy tuck to reduce the complication rate.

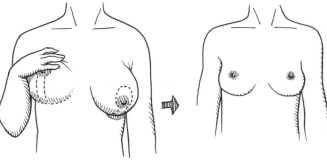

BREAST REDUCTIONS: No, no, no, men say. Don't do it. But if you have an extra five pounds of breast dragging on your neck and shoulders, what a relief it is to lighten the load. So breast reductions are useful for both functional and cosmetic reasons. And men themselves are not immune to growing large breasts (it's called gyneco-mastia). Almost half of men have some degree of breast growth around puberty, although most settle down by the time they're 20. This problem is rising because so many of our drugs, such as blood pressure medicines and steroids, can cause breast tissue to grow. Breast reductions in men and women are usually outpatient procedures with a high satisfaction rate.

Face Fixers: Minimally Invasive Procedures

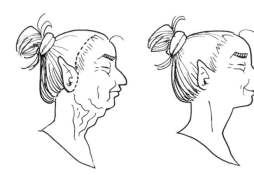

FACE-LIFTS: While the face-lift may be declining in popularity, don't count it out yet. More than 138,000 people couldn't be wrong, or could they? The docs who were proficient on their sewing machines lift and shape aging faces through smaller and smaller incisions. Most plastic surgeons don't just pull on the skin—they lift the jowls in a separate layer, suck fat, and tie those two turkey gobbler bands together. There are a lot of overpulled cheeks, so choose your artist-surgeon wisely to make sure you don't wind up looking as if you're driving through a wind tunnel. We recommend putting off that lift until there are no other options. New techniques of Botoxing, peeling, filling, and less invasive lifting techniques can keep your face looking younger longer.

The New Numb

WHAT IT IS: Pliaglis—the newest helper for cosmetic procedures—helps take the sting out of Botox and wrinkle filler injections, mole removal, and laser procedures. It is similar to EMLA cream but easier to apply correctly. Studies have shown that Pliaglis decreases pain by about 50 percent. Pliaglis is a combination of 7 percent lidocaine and 7 percent tetracaine, mixed together in a cream that forms a mask on your skin.

HOW TO USE IT: As directed by your doc, Pliaglis is spread on your skin 30 minutes before the procedure. (It should not be left on your skin for more than two hours.) It is to be spread out thinly (about the thickness of a dime) with a tongue depressor or a dull butter knife. You may feel comfortable applying Pliaglis over your whole face, missing the eyes, nostrils, and lips. Then leave it in place (a doc or nurse will remove it before the procedure).

FINE PRINT: The numbing from Pliaglis lasts 11 hours, so you can put it on your skin and expect pain relief for a long time. Don't use it if you're allergic to lidocaine or tetracaine or are pregnant or nursing, and don't use it if you use tocainide or mexiletine. Pliaglis may have a hard time catching on because of draconian marketing philosophy—the company is selling it to the docs, who then sell it to you (usually for a profit). We can't figure out why they're bypassing pharmacies.

BOTOX. Almost one and a half million people knowingly had poison injected into their bodies last year. And that makes Botox the most popular of all cosmetic procedures. Like a smart bomb in search of a target, Botox locks onto your nerves and destroys them within days. This leaves your muscles unable to move. Great if you want to get rid of those scowl lines between the brows or your crow's feet, bad if too much is injected into your upper lip. Can you say "drool"? (Not if you had too much Botox, you can't.) So that's why most plastic surgeons won't inject those smile lines. It's too difficult to balance the smile and get rid of lines. Botox is as much of an art form as rhinoplasty is (over-Botoxing can leave you expressionless). So make sure a real doctor injects your Botox (and don't do it if you're pregnant or you have any sort of neurologic disease).

And make sure you get Botox from the real manufacturer, not the industrial-strength research-grade varieties, which have been associated with all types of complications. You might have heard about a dozen or so deaths from Botox over the last decade. These problems were seen in patients with complex neck muscle problems using doses 100 to 1,000 times above the normal cosmetic doses. There have been other reports of non-life-threatening complications in cosmetically treating wrinkles around the eyes, but these are rare. Botox injections need to be repeated every two to six months.

PEELS: Peels have been popular for two decades; more than a million people had them in the last year alone. They range from "lunch-hour" peels that have subtle effects at best all the way to laser peels that vaporize your skin, leaving you looking like someone in a Schwarzenegger movie. All peels wound the skin. The deeper the wound, the more profound the effect. Peels take advantage of your body's response to injury—your skin heals by shrinking and tightening. Peels will remove anything from the dead superficial layers of cells (glycolic acid) to the mid-dermis (phenol).

The appeal of the glycolic peel is not to peel (whew!). Your doc will gradually increase the concentration of the glycolic acid and the time it is applied to your skin. This lets your skin acclimate to the chemical. By the time you're on the fourth monthly peel, your new superskin will be able to handle much higher concentrations—and that's when you'll start looking like you're ready for your close-up. Your skin will look refreshed, and its tone will improve. Acne often improves, and your skin's collagen may actually thicken. The advantage of the lunch-hour peels, of course, is that you won't miss more than an hour of work. But many people give up because the effects are so subtle and take months to be seen. One midlevel peel using the chemical TCA (trichloroacetic acid, for you budding chemists) will give you the results of at least six consecutive monthly glycolic peels. The effects of TCA peels are striking, particularly if you are troubled by splotchy brown pigmentation. You need to prepare your skin with vitamin A creams and pigment reducers to thin the layer of dead cells and turn off pigment production before this peel, and get ready for some pain. This half hour is not for the faint of heart or, for that matter, for anyone with heart problems.

If your face looks like a moonscape or a desert with ripples, don't waste your money on those pansy peels. You need industrial-strength peeling—a laser or a phenol peel. These procedures blast off the epidermis and part of the dermis, leaving you looking like a weeping pumpkin. Order up two weeks worth of DVDs and a lot of popcorn made with olive oil. But as your weeping face gradually heals, those wrinkles will shrink-wrap away, leaving your face looking years, sometimes decades, younger. Along with your wrinkles, invisible early skin cancers can also be blasted into oblivion.

Any peel can cause scarring, and the deeper the peel, the more likely scarring is. If you have a tendency to scar, you shouldn't have peels deeper than the TCA peel. And the deeper peels can cause lightening of the skin, so if you have darker skin, there's danger in peels deeper than those that use glycolic acid. Make sure that a doctor performs any peel using anything stronger than 10 percent glycolic acid—especially to properly analyze skin and treat the occasional complications. And as for those "no downtime" lasers, those plastic surgeons haven't quite figured out which of those lighter "nonablative" lasers really do the trick. So stay tuned; we're sure the evening news will follow this story.

MICRODERMABRASION: We actually exfoliate every time we wash our skin. We do it more aggressively with a loofah pad or washcloth. We can do it chemically with glycolic acid, or we can do it mechanically with microdermabrasion. Let's make this perfectly clear: Microdermabrasion cleans your skin (that's a good thing). But don't do it if you believe those signs in the windows of salons that say it removes wrinkles and scars. It can't because it simply exfoliates and sucks out the oils and dirt from your pores. (It's a facial without the soft music and aromatherapy.) Micro-dermabrasion either blasts the skin with salt or sand particles or rubs the skin with diamond crystals. A vacuum then cleans your pores. Your skin feels smoother and cleaner. Acne, blackheads, and whiteheads are reduced. Do it every two to four weeks to keep your face as clean as possible. *Micro*dermabrasion is harmless unless the operator goes too deep, creating *macro*dermabrasion. *That's* the procedure that plastic surgeons use to smooth wrinkles and scars, and that's a surgical procedure, whereas microdermabrasion can be safely performed by trained aestheticians or nurses.

WRINKLE FILLERS: The most popular wrinkle fillers are made of hyaluronic acid, a normal constituent of your skin. This is one of the few procedures that reliably give a "wow" reaction even before leaving the office. Wrinkle fillers are done with the aid of cream anesthetics or lidocaine injected into facial nerves. While current forms of hyaluronic acid last about a year, scientists are hard at work to improve their longevity. For deeper folds such as those between the nose and mouth, fillers containing calcium hydroxylapatite last nearly two years. This generation of fillers is helping cut the number of face-lifts.

Hyaluronic acid can be injected into lips for that Angelina Jolie look and can even lessen the appearance of jowls when injected between the jowl and chin. Why not permanent fillers like silicone or plastic? We've learned from the mistakes of the 1960s that any substance that doesn't dissolve eventually needs to be removable in the event of infection or if it drifts to an unwanted position. Permanent fillers can't be removed, and so if they become infected, the entire piece of skin needs to be cut out. Now, that ain't pretty, is it? Gel or cream fillers treat the wrinkles below the midnose level. They work best around the mouth and cheeks and chin. Deeper fillers can smooth out jowls and fill dents in the nose. Many docs feel they're too dangerous to inject around or between the eyes, however. They can cause blisters, blindness, or even strokes in these areas. A little too much pain for the gain.

ACKNOWLEDGMENTS

Ted Spiker continues to amaze the entire YOU docs team. Besides being one of the sharpest people we have ever met (which is acknowledged by his own University of Florida, which wisely awarded him a tenured position in journalism), Ted magically keeps all of our balls in the air without fail. He coalesces our insights into an accessible and humorous work that has attitude but is never condescending.

Gary Hallgren has perfected the medical cartoon and helps the readers (especially the males) chortle as they enjoy his humor. His cartoons dot our YOU books with crucial insights that bring alive the text. We just hope to hold off the onslaught of *MAD* magazine customers who want him full-time.

Craig Wynett and his son Ryan brought remarkable clarity to the extraordinarily opaque topic of beauty. Craig has the broadest-thinking mind we know and identifies trends in science better than any physician we know. Craig transforms us and you with his profound insights, which form the foundation of the text.

Dr. Arthur Perry is our good friend and great ally in the battle to clarify cosmetic medicine. His own remarkable book, *Straight Talk About Cosmetic Surgery*, educated us, and he served as a sage adviser throughout the book on topics ranging quite far from his specialty of plastic surgery. His meticulous attention to detail improved the quality of the final work.

Lisa Oz's honest and insightful editorial advice keeps us on our toes. Marrying her is the luckiest thing that ever happened to one of us.

Dr. Mark Rudberg was instrumental in bringing together thoughts about several of our early chapters. Dr. Art Markman is one of the world's leaders in happiness research and created the fundamental aspects of the YOU-Q test. Besides being a pleasure to work with, he helped us combine decades of research into a succinct quiz that will fascinate our readers.

Adam Snavely worked tirelessly to fact-check and research many of the questions created whenever scientists are researching a book. He was helped by Jeff Roizen and Jeff Oestricher, who labored hardily to root out answers to even the esoteric questions. We thank Joel Harper for his remarkable effort to make the *YOU: Being Beautiful Workout* the perfect tool for us to get procrastinators to exercise. Joel also supervised the great culinary video of Joel Odhner. Linda Kahn continued to provide profound and valuable criticisms of our work and helped us revise the text into the wonderful final result. She reminds us that "no pain, no gain" applies to books as well. Without Linda, we would have a far inferior product. Finally, our agent Candice Fuhrman's honest commentary and tough advice allowed this book to mature into the manuscript America deserves. While the hours of conference calls, research, and writing were often exhausting, this powerful group functioned seamlessly to resolve style and content conflicts.

We also want to thank the people at Free Press (Simon & Schuster) who so enthusiastically supported this material and who have dedicated themselves to bringing our ideas to the world. Martha Levin leads a wonderful team with the strong support of Jill Siegel, Carisa Hays, Susan Donahue, Linda Dingler, Nancy Singer, Nancy Inglis, and Alex Noya. Thanks especially to our visionary editor, Dominick Anfuso, and his assistant, Leah Miller.

We are indebted to our close partners at RealAge.com, including Charlie Silver, Rich Benci, and Val Weaver. We appreciate the continued support of Discovery Health, including Carol Tomko, Alon Orstein, Wayne Barbin, and John Whyte. And as always, thanks to Billy Campbell for being such an honorable lifelong friend.

We have become very close with our friends at the *Oprah Show* and will list a few colleagues only to symbolize how much we treasure the relationships. Jack Mori deserves an honorary medical degree and should soon be joined in practice by Terry Goulder. Jill Van Lokeren (and sometimes Jill Barancik) harnesses this dynamic duo with a down-to-earth sensibility. Sheri Salata and Lisa Erspamer lead a powerful team, including Lisa Morin, Chris Martin, Leslie Grisanti, Joanna Moel, Stacey Stazis, Anne Rovak, Rick Segall, and Ann Lofgren and many more supremely talented colleagues.

Thanks to the Harpo strategy whizzes Harriet Seitler and Ellen Rakieten and for the inspired leadership of Tim Bennett and Doug Pattison. Thanks to Lisa Halliday and Don Halcombe for keeping me safe.

The web team Robyn Miller, Josh London, and Jenn Horton have kept us digital. The XM radio team of John St. Augustine, John Gehron, Laurie Cantillo, Katherine Kelly, Megan Robertson, Theresa Rodriguez, and Tracy Square have kept the airwaves hopping.

And of course thanks to the continuing mentorship of Ms. Oprah Winfrey, who really is the fairest woman of them all.

Our books contain so broad a range of topics that we are compelled to ask advice from many world experts who selflessly share their insights in the true academic tradition. We list them all here without details of their contributions in order to save space for the actual book, but we deeply appreciate your dedication to your specialities and willingness to sacrifice your time to help craft the most scientifically accurate book possible. We thank Ivan Kronenfeld, Jon Lapook, Paul Rosenberg, Nancy Roizen, Jennifer Ashton, Dac Benasillo, Alphonse Gallizia, Ridwan Shapsig, Francis Levin, Robin Golan, Julide Tok, Evan Johnson, Scott Forman, Marty Becker, Arthur Agaston, Manny Alvarez, Daniel Amen, Theresa Dews, Gary Ginsberg, Lillian Gonsalves, Mac Lee, Harriet Imrey, Leo Kapural, Eric Klein, John LaPuma, Nagy MeKail, Stephen Post, Keith Roach, Marc Sharfman, Jason Theodosakis, Jim Zins, Laura Shenkar, Bill Levine, Jonathon

Levine, Erin Olivo, Rowe Jones, Mary Matsui, Irvin Schorsh, George Rodgers, James Zacny, John Ellis, Marsha Lowry, Paula Begoun, Bruce Ames, Glenn Copeland, Alfonse Gallizia, Mary Carmen Gasco-Buisson, Dean Ornish, and especially Jacob Teitlebaum, for teaching us about beauty and reviewing our work.

From Mehmet Oz

Dr. Oz thanks his colleagues in cardiothoracic surgery for their tireless support in and out of the operating rooms. Dr. Craig Smith, Dr. Yoshifuma Naka, Dr. Mike Argenziano, Dr. Henry Spotnitz, Dr. Allan Stewart, Dr. Mat Williams, Dr. Eric Rose, and the other superb surgeons on our team all chipped in. The physician assistants, especially Laura Altman, the nurses in the OR and on the floor, and our spectacular ICU team always care meticulously for my patients. My clinical office manager, Lidia Nieves, and her remarkable memory keep my patients safe. My administrative coordinators, Michelle Washburn and Celia Taylor, kept me on time and on target. Thanks to Melanie Fernandi for pitching in whenever we were in need. Finally, as on our other books, our Divisional Administrator, Diane Amato, was on target with her witty criticisms and courageous commentary. Thanks to the dedicated public affairs group at New York–Presbyterian, including Bryan Dotson, Alicia Park, and Myrna Manners, who have taught me to stay on message.

My parents, Mustafa and Suna Oz, taught me that success was working hard for a goal no matter the outcome. My parents-in-law, Gerald and Emily Jane Lemole, created a loving and supportive environment that fosters harmony. Besides being our coauthor, the love of my life, Lisa, brought our four children, Daphne, Arabella, Zoe, and Oliver, into the world, and we have enjoyed their every moment in our lives.

From Michael Roizen

Dr. Roizen wants to thank his administrative associates Candy Lawrence and especially Beth Grubb, who made this work possible. And to thank many of the staff at the Cleveland Clinic and physicians elsewhere who answered numerous questions. Many of the clinic's Wellness Institute staff and associates made scientific contributions and constructive criticisms, and allowed the time to complete this work. Cleveland Clinic CEO Toby Cosgrove has said that while the clinic will continue to be one of, if not the best, in illness care, wellness and fostering being beautiful is what the clinic will do for every employee and person we touch. I am fortunate to work with such a talented and creative group as Nabil Gabriel, Dr. Beth Ricanati, Dr. Martin Harris, Dr. Brigette Duffy, David Strand, Scott McFarland, Cindy Hundorfean, Chris Ayers, Dennis Kenny, Bill Peacock, Gene Lazuta, and many nutritionists and exercise physiologists, chef Jim Perko, Drs. Rich Lang, Tanya Edwards, Rene Seballos, Steve Nissen, Jim Young, David Bronson, Glen Copeland

(and many more), and clinicians and leaders who span the gamut from inner-city schoolteachers to executive coaches.

Our family was fully engaged, with Jeff as our M.D./Ph.D. research associate and Jennifer and Nancy as critical readers, joined at times by the "enlarged family" of the Katzes, Unobskeys, Wattels, and Campodonicos. I also want to thank Sukie Miller, Diane Reverend, Eileen Sheil, Erinne Dyer, Erica Foreman, Susan Petre, John Maudlin, Zack Wasserman, and others for encouraging and critiquing the concepts and the RealAge team, especially founding partners Charlie Silver and Martin Rom, and Rich Benci, Val Weaver and Drs. Keith Roach, Mark Rudberg, Carl Peck, and Axel Goetz, who validate and verify content. Dirk Wales and the leadership (and membership) of the American Association of Nurse Anesthetists encouraged the study of choices that are associated with inner beauty and happiness.

Having a great partner to ablate stress daily is clearly a magnificent way to help you feel and be more beautiful—thank you, Nancy.

From Ted Spiker

Thank you to my colleagues and students at the University of Florida, to the magazine editors and writers I've worked with and learned from (especially from *Men's Health* and *Women's Health* magazines), and the entire YOU team for embracing the concept that the most potent literary medicine should include humor as an active ingredient. And to my wife, Liz, kids, Alex and Thad, and the rest of my family and friends: Thank you for being beautiful in so many ways.

From Craig Wynett

To all the beautiful women in my life. My grandmother Ann Staples, my mother, Priscilla Wynett, my aunt Sallie Burke, and my wife, Denise, have all led by example on how to be authentically beautiful. I just took notes.

From Arthur Perry

For a doctor, to be called to duty by the esteemed physicians Drs. Michael Roizen and Mehmet Oz is like a politician being summoned to work in a presidential administration. The opportunity to watch these two minds churn away was too tempting and just couldn't be passed up, no matter how many weekends and evenings would be sacrificed. And so Mike and Mehmet, along with Craig and Ted, challenged my knowledge and pushed me to think broader than with the scalpel. But it was my wife, Bedonna, who supported and nurtured my writing and endured all those Sunday conference calls. And my son and aspiring filmmaker, Benjamin, and my daughters, Meredith and Julia, who are just beginning their careers, keep me in check every day, reminding me that my most important job is to be their dad. I am indebted to my parents, Michael Perry, D.D.S., and Harriet, still inspiring and guiding as octogenarians. And special thanks to my nurse, Pam Mayers, R.N., for organizing my clinical life. Many thanks to Dr. Robert Grant at Cornell/Columbia for his insight and reviews. And to all who have contributed to my thought-provoking approach to plastic surgery: At Robert Wood Johnson University Hospital, it was the In the OR staff who endured my nascent theories and daily rants; at WOR radio it was Noah Fleishman and Jen Buckley who pushed me to expand my horizons; and at New Vitality, it was Jonathan Greenhut who gave me the pulpit to design skin "dream creams."

From Gary Hallgren

Praise be for Ted Spiker, who thought there was a place for a chuckle in this YOU series. And thanks to Mehmet and Michael, and to my beautiful wife, Michelle, who sometimes laugh out loud at my corny jokes.

INDEX

abdominal muscles, 145, 184, 185, 186, 190, 345
acetyl-L-carnitine, 222
aches. *See* pain/aches; *type of ache*
achilles tendonitis, 206
acid reflux, 219
ACL strains and tears, 206
acne, 44, 56, 58, 84
ACTH hormone, 258
"active ingredients," 47, 48
activity level, 158, 169, 171, 186, 191–92, 202, 346. *See also* exercise; *specific exercise*
acupressure, 210
acupuncture, 179, 218, 326
addiction, 6, 74, 131, 238–41, 243, 244–45, 246–51. *See also specific addiction*
adrenal gland, 36, 160, 164, 167, 258, 259, 260
aerobic exercise, 216
African Americans, skin color of, 45
age, 37, 39–41, 71, 113, 114, 231, 291
age spots, 40, 50, 54, 124–25
agreeableness, 237
alcohol, 53, 165, 212, 220, 231, 239, 243, 344
allergies, 40, 41, 45–46, 47, 64
aloe, 51
alpha-hydroxy acid, 49, 58, 339
alternative medicine, 178, 324
androgens, 72, 108, 142
anemia, 74, 388
anger, 23, 34, 89, 231, 246, 255, 306, 317, 321, 344
animals. *See* pets; Safari Secrets

ankles, 200–201, 205
antibacterials, 92
antibiotics, 45, 50, 96–97, 100, 220
antidepressants, 160, 222, 235, 241, 242
antifungals, 218, 220
antioxidants, 47, 49–50, 56, 60, 174, 198, 242, 340. *See also specific antioxidant*
anxiety, 225, 227, 231, 235, 241, 246, 248, 256, 258, 293
appearance
  automatic reactions to, 154
  and first impressions, 24
  as instant message to others, 3
  and self-image, 29
  and standards of beauty, 23–24, 26–29, 130
  YOU-Q for, 10–12
Arm Circle, 355, 359
arms/shoulders, exercise for, 144–45, 195, 355, 359
arnica, 178
aromatherapy, 51, 348
arrhythmias, 230
arthritis, 47, 178, 182, 201, 202, 204, 216
aspirin, 52–53, 124, 167, 191, 196, 204, 215, 341
ASU (avocado-soybean-unsaponifiables), 203
athlete's foot, 120
ATP, 157, 158, 163, 164, 170
attraction
  biology of, 285–88
  and biology of sex, 297
  evolution of, 300
  and phi, 24, 26

and relationships, 285–88, 297, 300, 303, 308
attractiveness, 2, 4, 5, 68, 130, 131, 136, 139, 268. *See also* outer beauty
authenticity, 4, 8, 9, 318–20, 330
awe, 312

back brace, 182, 345
back pain, 6, 176–77, 179, 180–93, 218, 258
bacteria, 122, 123, 157. *See also* antibacterials
bad breath, 91, 98, 105, 340
baldness, 69, 71, 72, 73, 74, 79–80
bananas, 242, 296
band workout, 243, 345–46, 351–60
baths
  foot, 51
  olive oil, 52
Be-YOU-tiful Plan, 337–48
beautiful day, ultimate, 6, 338–48
beauty
  advantages of, 22
  authentic, 8, 9
  biology of, 3
  cliches about, 2
  detectors of, 5–6, 24
  formula, 24, 25, 26
  as full-circle concept, 281
  importance of, 1
  kinds of, 3–4
  as managing stress, 256
  markers for, 88, 89–97
  money equated with, 268
  perceptions of, 22–24
  as serious business, 5

beauty (*cont.*)
  standards, 2, 23–24, 26–29, 130
  See also specific topic
beauty industry, 4–5
beauty reflex, 23–24
Begoun, Paula, 64
being, levels of, 318, 319, 320
being beautiful
  and feeling good about yourself, 5
  overview about, 280–81
  and YOU-Q, 14–17
  See also authenticity; happiness; relationships
beliefs, 330–31
biking, 201, 216
biofeedback, 212
biology
  of attraction, 285–88
  of beauty, 3
  of decision making, 273
  and energy, 156
  and feeling beautiful, 152–54
  of headaches, 208
  of love, 288–91
  and relationships, 285–301
  of sex, 291–301
  of stress, 258, 260
biomechanical stimulation, 161
biotin, 50, 111, 343
bipolar disorder, 229
birth control pills, 218
bisphenol, 333
blackheads, 42
blindness, 286
blisters, 37
blood flow, 158–59, 290, 294, 310
blood pressure, 172, 175, 211, 258, 300, 310
blood sugar, 160, 173, 222, 258
blood tests, 164, 166, 167, 235, 387–92
body art, 61–63
body dysmorphic disorder, 131
body hair, 75, 80
body language, 27, 305–6
bone-on-bone grinding, 197, 199
borage, 217
Boswellia (olibanum), 178, 204
botox, 32, 53–54, 124, 213, 397
botulism, 54

bowel diseases, blood tests for, 390
brain
  and addiction, 239, 240, 241
  building a better, 331
  and decision making, 272
  and depression, 232, 233, 235
  and emotions, 153, 154, 227, 228, 242, 244–45
  and energy, 158, 162, 164, 165, 320
  and evolution, 154
  and feeling beautiful, 152–54
  and happiness, 313, 315, 316, 317–18, 320, 321–24
  and headaches, 208, 211
  and health, 33, 264
  and helping others, 256
  importance of, 23
  and instincts, 268, 269
  and irritable bowel syndrome, 219
  networks of, 270
  and pain, 154, 175, 177, 179
  and relationships, 286–91, 293–94, 296, 297, 298, 300, 310
  and satisfaction index, 147
  and sex, 293–94, 296, 297, 298, 310
  and shape, 133–40, 146, 147
  and spirituality, 322–24, 331
  and standards of beauty, 23–24, 26–27
  and stress, 259, 260, 331
  and thyroid, 75
  and vitamins and supplements, 174, 341
  See also biology
bras, 147–48
breakfast, 340
breasts, 131, 136, 148, 217, 294, 393–94, 396
breath, smell of, 91, 98, 105, 340
breathe-free program, 246–51
breathing, deep, 212, 243, 246–51, 330, 341, 361
Buddhism, 317
buddies, 247, 250, 251, 275, 280, 284, 292, 345
bunions, 117, 118, 119, 125
bupropion, 250, 251, 293–94. *See also* Wellbutrin
burnout, 255

burns, 36–37, 51–52
Butt Blaster, 356, 360
butt/thighs, exercises for, 143–44, 356, 360
Butterfly, 370, 374

C-reactive protein (CRP), 230, 388
caffeine, 79, 124, 165, 174, 215, 217, 220, 239, 275, 341
calcium, 146, 172, 204, 217, 341, 345
calluses, 119, 124, 125
calories, 141, 142, 146
Camel, 366, 372
cancer, 35, 37, 41–42, 64, 92, 105, 174, 186, 231, 333
canine smile, 96
canker sores, 92
cannabinoids, 137, 138
capsaicin, 178
carbonated drinks, 220
cardiovascular system, 146, 190, 230, 344
carotenoids, 50
cars, efficient, 336
cartilage, 47, 198–99, 201, 202, 203, 204
Cat Back/Cow, 365, 372
cellulite, 142
ceramides, 39–40
charity, 313–14, 329, 332. *See also* helping others
chemotherapy, 221
cherries, 204
Chest Opener, 352, 358
chia, 172–73
Chicken Wing, 353, 358
childhood traumas, 293
children, 303, 346
chiropractic treatment, 189
chlorine, 79, 343
chocolate, 160, 212, 215, 309
cholesterol, 52, 100, 166, 167, 258, 260
chondroitin, 198, 203
chronic fatigue, 159, 161, 162, 166, 168, 172, 391, 392
cigarettes. *See* smoking
cleaners, ingredients in, 42
Clock Lunge, 143–44
cloning, 74
clothes/fashion, 147–50
cluster headaches, 213–14

Cobra, 367, 373
coenzyme Q10, 49, 53, 208
coffee, 212, 215, 242
cognitive behavioral therapy, 212, 242
cognitive-control network, 270
cold packs, 190–91
cold sores, 92
collagen, 32, 35–39, 49, 51–53, 56, 106, 186, 196, 203
community, sense of, 329–30
complementary medicine, 324
compression, and RICE, 201–2
conscientiousness, 237
contact lenses, 384–85
coping strategies, 242, 327
corns, 117, 125
Corpse, 370, 374
cortisol, 33, 232, 258
cortisone, 192
cosmetics, 47, 48, 64, 113
cramps, 217–18
cravings, 160, 244, 260, 290, 293–94, 317
CRH hormone, 258
Cross Leg Drop, 356, 360
Cross-Legged Lift, 357, 360
Cross-Legged Twist, 357, 360
crying, 230
cryotherapy, 125
CT scans, 188, 216
curling irons, 78, 339
cuticle, 111, 112, 122, 123, 339
cysts, 97, 217

dandruff, 78, 80–81
day, Ultimate Beautiful, 6, 338–48
Dead Bug, 145
decision making, 264–65, 267, 268–72, 273, 274, 305
deep breathing, 212, 243, 246–51, 330, 341, 361
delusions, 244, 317
dementia, 231
deodorants, 340
depression
    and addiction, 246
    and brain, 232, 233, 235
    characteristics of, 225, 232, 234
    as chemical disease, 229
    clinical, 229, 231
    diagnosis of, 226

and drugs/medications, 231, 235–36, 241, 242–43
and energy, 232
and exercise, 242–43, 244
Factoids about, 229, 230, 234
and gender, 229, 231
and goal of feeling beautiful, 154
and hormones, 233
and irritable bowel syndrome, 219
kinds/categories of, 231–32
major, 231–32, 242–43
and menstruation, 160
myths about, 229
and pain, 179, 184
recurrent episodes of, 235
and relationships, 280
situational, 232
and skin, 33
and stress, 258
and supplements, 241
survival benefit of, 234
symptoms of, 231–32, 234, 235
testing for, 235
vascular, 232
YOU Test for, 223, 226
YOU Tips for, 242, 244
and YOU-Q, 15, 17
dermabrasion, 125
dermatitis, 41, 42, 50, 64, 75
dermis, 32, 34, 36, 39, 52
Devil's claw, 178
DHA, 146, 161, 169, 184, 189, 202, 203, 217, 221, 241, 309, 341
DHEA, 167, 241, 391
DHT (dihydrotestosterone), 74, 79, 80
diabetes, 39, 221, 222, 231, 310, 333, 389
Diagonal Reach, 368, 373
diet
    and back pain, 188–89
    and energy, 157, 158, 172–74
    and female pains, 217
    and hair, 50, 69, 79, 80
    and headaches, 212, 215
    and infections, 174
    and irritable bowel syndrome, 220
    and nails, 50, 111
    and portion size, 147

and shape, 139, 143, 146
and skin, 44, 50–51, 52, 59
and teeth, 99
and tics, 215
and weight, 343
digit-length ratio, 108, 115
disconnection, 321–22
discs, and back pain, 182–84, 186, 188, 189, 191
disease. See type of disease
disuse atrophy, 186
divorce, 227, 263, 274
DMAE, 42
DNA, 34, 35, 39, 177
dopamine, 231, 239, 240, 256, 269, 288, 289, 290, 302, 308
Down Dog, 367, 372
Down Dog One Leg, 368, 373
drugs/medications
    and addiction, 247
    for back pain, 183, 184, 191
    and bipolar disorder, 229
    and depression, 231, 235–36, 241, 242–43
    and emotional disorders, 236
    for fungal infections, 115–16
    and hair, 84
    and headaches, 211, 212, 215–16
    and joint pain, 205, 213
    and neuropathies, 222
    over-the-counter, 215
    and sex, 300, 310
    and shape, 140, 142
    side effects of, 91
    for thyroid, 165, 166, 167
    and tics, 215
    and weight, 140
    withdrawal from, 215–16
    See also specific drug/ medication

ears, pressure points near, 210
eczema, 45–46, 56
elasticity, 40
elastin, 32, 36, 38, 39, 49, 51, 52, 56
electrocautery, 46
electrolysis, 67
emergency accounts, 273
emotional intelligence, 270–72
emotional stability, as personality type, 237

emotions
 and action, 331
 and brain, 153, 154, 228, 242,
  244–45
 and decision making, 274
 embracing, 321–22
 and environment, 242
 and evolution, 154
 and exercise, 242–43
 facilitating, 271
 and finances, 265
 and goal of feeling beautiful,
  152, 154
 and happiness, 321–22
 and hormones, 230
 ID-ing, 270
 importance of, 6
 influence of, 154
 managing, 272
 observing, 321
 and spirituality, 243
 and stress, 270, 313
 thinking with, 321
 understanding, 271
 YOU Tools for, 246–51
 See also addiction; depression;
  emotional intelligence;
  mood; personality; specific
  emotion
empathy, 314–18, 330
Empty Can, 145
endorphins, 212–13, 216, 242
energy
 and activity level/exercise, 158,
  169, 171
 and adrenals, 167
 and biology, 156
 and brain, 158, 162, 164, 165,
  320
 in crisis, 157–59, 161–68
 and depression, 232
 and diet, 157, 158, 172–74
 Factoids about, 159, 165
 and feeling beautiful, 4, 152,
  154, 156
 and hormones, 161–64,
  167–68
 and how it works, 157–59,
  161–68
 and infections, 157, 158,
  159–61, 174
 and insulin resistance, 159
 management of, 275, 277,
  342

 and muscles, 161, 162, 163,
  168, 169
 and pain, 161, 162, 163, 166,
  167, 168, 171, 176
 saving, 335
 and sex, 167–68, 309
 and sleep, 157, 158, 159, 161,
  171–72
 and spirituality, 325–26
 and stress, 157, 159, 164
 and sugar, 157, 160, 164, 165,
  169, 170, 172
 and thyroid, 164, 165–67, 387
 as warning signal, 168
 YOU Test for, 155, 160, 166
 YOU Tips for, 169, 171–74
 and YOU-Q, 13, 14
"energy" drinks, 165
environment
 and emotions, 236–37, 242
 and Ultimate Beautiful Day,
  342, 344
 work, 276–77, 342
Environmental Protection Agency
 (EPA), 42
epidermis, 34, 51, 52, 69
epigamic hair, 71
epileptics, 322–23
estrogen, 40, 132, 140, 167, 212,
 215, 217, 230, 310
evening primrose, 217
evolution
 of attraction, 300
 and biology of sex, 292–93,
  294, 295, 297
 and brain, 154
 and decision making, 265, 267
 and emotions, 154
 and gender, 263
 and genetic differences, 26
 and relationships, 291,
  292–93, 294, 295, 297, 300
 and shape, 132
 and worry, 256
exercise
 for abs/core muscles, 145, 190
 and addiction, 250, 251
 for arms/shoulders, 144–45
 and back pain, 180, 182, 190,
  192, 193
 for butt/thighs, 143–44
 cardiovascular, 146, 190
 and depression, 242–43, 244
 and emotions, 242–43

 and energy, 171
 facial, 32, 96
 and female pains, 218
 and headaches, 216
 intensity of, 146
 for joints, 195, 199, 200–201,
  202, 205, 206
 and neuropathies, 222
 and pain, 184
 and sex, 310
 and shape, 131, 139, 143–46
 and skin, 32, 47, 52
 See also Band Workout;
  walking; yoga; type of exercise
exfoliation, 41, 57–59, 60, 347
expectations, 326, 327
exposure therapy, 236
Extended Cat Stretch, 365, 372
extroversion, 227, 237
eyelashes, 34, 66, 68
eyelids, swelling of, 40
eyes, 46, 53–54, 64, 210, 230,
  300, 339, 383–85, 395

face
 exercise for, 32, 96
 exfoliation of, 347
 expressions on, 27, 94, 306
 as means of communication,
  27
 moisturizer for, 339, 340, 347
 plastic surgery for, 60, 396–99
 professional care of, 60
 and relationships, 306
 symmetry/shape of, 27–29,
  384
 tingling, 221–22
 and Ultimate Beautiful Day,
  339, 340, 347
 and YOU-Q, 11, 12
 See also eyes; mouth; smile;
  wrinkles
Factoid
 about addiction, 241
 about back pain, 180, 182,
  184, 188, 189
 about depression, 229, 230,
  234
 about energy, 159, 165
 about female pains, 217
 about finances, 256, 261,
  269
 about hair, 66, 68, 69, 71, 72,
  74, 75, 76, 77, 84, 85

about hands and feet, 108, 115, 121, 127
about headaches, 208, 211, 212
about joints, 198
about lips, 104, 105
about mouth, 96, 99
about nails, 109, 111, 113
about nose, 100
about pain, 179
about personality, 227
about relationships, 290, 291, 293, 297, 309
about sex, 293, 297
about shape, 133, 137, 139, 142
about shoes, 125
about skin, 32, 34, 36, 40, 45, 46, 59
about splinters, 120
about teeth, 91, 93, 99, 100
fat
    and energy, 164
    and irritable bowel syndrome, 220
    and shape, 132, 141, 143, 146
fatigue
    and biomechanical stimulation, 161
    and blood tests, 387, 388, 390, 391, 392
    chronic, 159, 161, 162, 166, 168, 172, 391, 392
    as degree of energy, 156
    and depression, 230
    and energy in crisis, 159, 161, 162, 166, 168
    and feeling beautiful, 4
    and menstruation, 167
    misunderstandings about, 162
    and pain, 159
    and thyroid, 165, 166
    as warning, 168
    and yeast overgrowth, 160
    YOU Tips about, 169, 172
fats, 52–53, 202–3. *See also type of fats*
fatty acids, 39–40, 45, 217. *See also* omega-3 fatty acids
fear, 177–78, 225, 227, 236
feedback, 169, 171, 298, 299

feeling beautiful
    energy as heart of, 156
    and feeling good about yourself, 5
    goal of, 152–54
    and happiness, 313
    importance of, 4
    and looking beautiful, 33
    overview about, 152–54
    YOU-Q for, 13–14
    See also emotions; energy; finances; pain; work
feeling good. *See* happiness
feet
    Factoids about, 108, 121, 127
    function of, 108
    moisturing of, 124
    and neuropathies, 222
    pain in, 205
    problems with, 109, 116–21, 122–25
    and sex, 6, 108, 126
    shape of, 121
    size of, 108
    smell of, 123–24
    swelling of, 158
    as symbol of fertility, 127
    tingling in, 221–22
    views about, 108
    YOU Tips about, 122–25
    YOU Tool for, 126–27
    See also nails; toenails
female pain, 217–18
Fibonacci sequence, 6, 24
fibroblasts, 34, 39
fibromyalgia, 161, 162, 163, 168, 172, 178
finances, 152, 256, 257, 260–70, 272, 273–78, 345
finasteride, 79, 80
fingernail polish, 42
fingernails, 109–12
fingers, size of, 108
first impressions, 24
fish oil, 169, 184, 202–3
flexibility, 190, 194, 195, 201
flossing, 102–3, 174
fluoride, 100
folate, 80, 92
folic acid, 222, 309
food, 136, 296, 308–9, 310, 340, 343, 344, 380. *See also* diet; *specific food*

Food and Drug Administration (FDA), 48, 53, 64, 80
foot baths, 51
foot rubs, 126
foreplay, 6
fragrances, 42, 47, 64
full denture smile, 96
fungal infections, 113–16, 120, 122–23, 157

G-spot, 296, 298, 307
gastrointestinal problems, 258
gate-control theory, 179
gender
    and biology of sex, 291–300
    and crying, 230
    and depression, 229, 231
    and evolution, 263
    and finances, 263–64
    and personality, 227
    and relationships, 291–300
gene therapy, 74
generosity, 313–14, 329, 332. *See also* helping others
genetics, 26, 69, 71–72, 133, 227, 229, 236, 239, 286, 322
genital warts, 120
ghrelin, 135, 137–40
ginger, 178
gingivitis, 99, 100, 105, 157
ginkgo biloba, 290, 310
ginseng, 290, 310
giving. *See* charity; generosity; helping others
glasses, 383–84
glucosamine, 198, 203
glycation, 39, 56, 125
glycolic acid, 49, 58
glycosaminoglycans, 39
Goddess, 364, 372
Going to Jail, 355, 359
golden ratio, 24, 25, 26, 28, 29, 115
gossip, 309
gout, 198
gratitude, 330, 345
green algae, 178
"green" cosmetics, 64
green living, YOU Tool for, 333–36
green tea, 50, 79, 82, 174, 341
grief, 244
Groin Pull, 206

growth hormone, 140, 171, 339
guided imagery, 212, 243
gums, 88, 95, 99–101, 102, 103, 105, 174, 213
gym bag, 375

hair
    and aging, 71
    and attractiveness, 68
    big, 76
    care of, 83–85
    coloring/bleaching of, 76–77, 78, 80–81, 85
    combing/brushing, 84, 85, 339
    destruction/abuse of, 68–71, 76–77, 83–85
    and diet, 50, 69, 79, 80
    and drugs, 84
    drying, 78, 83, 84, 339
    Factoids about, 66, 68, 69, 71, 72, 74, 75, 76, 77, 84, 85
    functions of, 66, 68, 75, 78
    and genetics, 69, 71–72
    graying, 73
    growth cycle for, 72, 74, 79
    and health, 68, 69
    and hormones, 69, 72, 74, 75–76, 79
    length of, 68
    loss of, 67, 68–76, 79–80, 84
    and menopause, 67, 72
    oily, 85
    pubic, 72
    pulling on, 74
    removal of, 67, 77
    replacement, 69
    Safari Secrets about, 71
    saving your, 65–85
    and sex, 71, 75, 79, 85
    structure of, 68–71
    teasing, 84
    and thyroid, 166
    transplants, 68
    and Ultimate Beautiful Day, 339
    unwanted, 67
    and vitamins and supplements, 49, 71, 80
    washing, 76, 78–79, 81–82
    and weight, 67
    YOU Test for, 65
    YOU Tips for, 78–82
    YOU Tools for, 83–85
    and YOU-Q, 11, 12

Half Boat, 369, 374
Half Butterfly, 370, 374
Half Frog Pose, 368, 373
hallucinations, 244
hammertoes, 125
Hamstring Pull, 206
hands, 59, 108–12, 115, 121, 122–25, 126–27, 199, 210, 221–22, 381. See also nails
handshakes, 306
hangnails, 112, 123
happiness
    and being beautiful, 4, 313
    and brain, 313, 315, 316, 317–18, 320, 321–24
    contributors to, 284
    and emotions, 321–22
    and feeling beautiful, 313
    and health, 2, 327
    importance of, 314
    and inflammation, 326
    and looking beautiful, 313
    and love, 332
    overview about, 280–81
    paths to, 312, 313–28
    and relationships, 280, 281, 284, 320, 328
    secret of finding, 312–13
    and sex, 292, 295
    and spirituality, 312–13, 322
    and stress, 326
    and survival, 327
    and understanding unhappiness, 326–28
    YOU Tips about, 329–32
    YOU Tool for, 333–36
    and YOU-Q, 8, 11, 14–15
hatred, 317
headaches
    biology of, 208
    control of, 179
    drugs/medications for, 211, 212, 215–16
    and exercise, 216
    Factoids about, 208, 211, 212
    kinds and causes of, 98, 99, 208–14, 215, 216
    prevalence of, 176–77
    rebound, 215–16
    and stress, 258
    YOU Tips for, 215–22
healing, 33

health
    beauty as, 1, 2
    and brain, 33
    and finances, 263–64
    and hair, 68, 69
    and happiness, 2, 327
    and nails, 107, 117
    and pets, 292
    and relationships, 284, 292
    and shape, 131–32
    and spirituality, 325, 329
    and teeth, 88, 97–101
health utensils, 377–81
heart, 100, 231, 232, 257, 258, 292, 329, 333, 340, 341, 390
heels, 205
helping others, 256, 281, 302, 314, 316, 329, 330, 347
hemochromatosis levels, 388
hepatitis, 61, 123
herpes infections, 92, 97
hips, 195. See also waist-to-hip ratio
HIV/AIDS, 61, 123
holistic medicine, 220
home
    green living at, 334–35
    health utensils for hygiene in, 378–80
    safety in, 343
home ownership, 276
homeopathy, 326
hormones
    blood tests for, 391
    and depression, 232, 233
    and emotions, 230
    and energy, 158, 161, 164–65, 167, 171
    and female pains, 217
    and hair, 69, 72, 74, 75–76, 79
    and headaches, 212
    imbalances of, 161–64
    and joints, 206
    and sex, 294, 299, 300, 309
    and shape, 137, 140
    and spirituality, 324
    and stress, 233, 258, 259
    and weight, 140
    See also specific hormone
Horse, 364, 372
hospitals, infections in, 380
humor, 277

hyaluronic acid (HA), 49, 53, 58–59, 106, 203, 399
hydrocortisone, 45
hypersensitivity, 232, 234
hypochondriacs, 234
hypothalamic-pituitary-adrenal (HPA) axis, 258, 259

illusions, 244
imidazolidinyl urea, 42
immune system, 29, 50, 81, 100, 161, 219, 230, 258, 260, 324–25, 329
impulsiveness, 270, 272
infant formulas, 241
infections
  and aromatherapy, 51
  and back pain, 184
  blood tests for, 392
  and depression, 230
  and diet, 174
  and energy, 157, 158, 159–61, 174
  and headaches, 211
  health utensils for, 380–81
  home remedies for, 122–23
  in hospitals, 380
  and irritable bowel syndrome, 219–20
  and neuropathies, 221, 222
  nosocomial, 380
  and skin, 51–52, 56, 61, 63
  and sleep, 174
  and sugar, 174
  See also specific infection
inflammation
  and back pain, 184, 186, 188–89, 190–91, 192
  blood tests for, 388
  and chia, 172
  and depression, 230
  and energy, 174
  and female pains, 218
  of gums, 88, 99, 100, 174
  and hair, 75, 81
  and happiness, 326
  and headaches, 208, 211
  and irritable bowel syndrome, 221
  of joints, 198, 199, 201, 203, 204, 205, 206
  in leg, 188
  markers for, 230
ingrown toenails, 112

inner beauty, 2, 6, 17, 29. See also happiness; spirituality
inspiration, 361
instincts, 24, 268–72, 318, 320, 331
insulin, 137, 140, 159, 164, 390, 391
insurance plans, 250
iron, 74, 92
irritable bowel syndrome, 219–21

jaw/jawbones, 97–99, 100–101, 103, 159, 213
joints, 176–77, 194–207, 213, 361. See also specific joint
journals, 244

Kegel exercises, 218, 307, 309, 341
keratin, 109, 111
kidneys, blood tests for, 389
kissing, 104
knees, 199, 200–201, 206. See also menisci
kyphoplasty, 186

L-arginine, 310
L-lysine, 80
labels, 48, 60, 80, 340
lactic acid, 45
Ladybug, 363, 371
laser therapy, 67, 125
lasik, 385
Lateral Circle, 353, 358
Lateral Hold, 354, 359
Lateral Pull-Down, 353, 359
Lateral Raise, 352, 358
lavender, 51, 52
lead, in cosmetics, 64
leg, 158, 188, 192
lemon, 51
leptin, 135, 137–40
Lewis, C. S., 332
licorice, 49
life
  changes in, 232, 234
  purpose in, 5, 281, 313, 314, 322
  satisfaction with, 15–16, 17
ligaments, 196, 198, 205, 206
light, 244, 276, 334. See also sun; ultraviolet light
Lion, 366, 372
lipoic acid, 222

liposuction, 394–95
lips, 37, 53, 91–92, 94–96, 103–6, 172, 294, 399
lipsticks, lead in, 64
lists, 278, 342
Little Boat Pose, 369, 373
Little Boat Twist, 369, 374
liver disease, blood tests for, 389–90
locus of control, 269–70, 342
Locust, 144
longevity, 280, 292, 314, 347
loofahs, 58
looking beautiful
  and feeling beautiful, 33
  and feeling good about yourself, 5
  and happiness, 313
  importance of, 3
  and relationships, 285
  YOU-Q for, 10–12
  See also feet; hair; hands; mouth; nails; shape; skin
love, 285, 288–91, 332
lunch, 343
Lunges, 190, 192, 367, 372
lycopene, 51
lymphatic system, 36, 361
lymphoma, 80

maca, 173
magnesium, 172, 204, 208, 217, 341, 345
makeup, 52, 58, 60
malaria, 66
manicures, 123
Markman, Art, 9
mascara, 64
massage, 6, 51, 126, 142, 191, 192, 193, 210, 348
mattresses, 180
medications. See drugs/medications
medicine cabinet, health utensils for, 377–78
meditation, 47, 191, 212, 216, 313, 317, 321–25, 330, 339, 346, 348, 361
melanin, 36–37, 45, 46
melatonin, 291
menisci, 197, 198, 199, 203, 204
menopause, 67, 72, 74
menstruation, 160, 166, 167, 206, 211, 212, 217–18, 291

mental accounting, 267–68
mental problems
    biology of, 227
    See also addiction; depression;
        emotions; personality
metabolism, 140, 146, 343,
    390–91
metal, in hair, 72
microdermabrasion, 60, 398–99
migraine headaches, 211, 212,
    215
minerals, 203–4, 208. *See also*
    specific mineral
minoxidil, 79, 80
moisturizing, 40–41, 45, 57, 112,
    123, 124, 172, 339, 340,
    347
money. *See* finances
mood
    YOU Tips about, 242–45
    YOU Tool for, 246–51
    See also addiction; depression;
        emotions; personality
mouth
    anatomy of, 91–97
    as beauty marker, 89–97
    bleeding in, 105
    cancer of, 92
    Factoids about, 96, 99
    function of, 89
    infections in, 92, 96
    muscles in, 93, 94, 95, 96
    shape and size of, 89–90
    sleeping with open, 99
    sores in, 92
    YOU Tips for, 102–6
    See also jaw/jawbones; lips;
        smile; teeth
MRI tests, 188, 288, 317
MSM (methylsulfonylmethane),
    203
muffins, chia, 173
muscles
    aching, 178
    and back pain, 182, 184–86,
        188, 189, 190, 191, 192,
        345
    and Band Workout, 345
    and botox, 53–54
    categories of, 184
    and energy, 161, 162, 163,
        168, 169
    function of, 140, 141, 142
    and headaches, 212

psoas, 189
    and shape, 140–42, 143
    and skin, 32
    spasms of, 188
    and yoga, 361
    See also specific muscles
music, 244, 329
mustache, 67
myelin, 178–79, 186–88, 189

nails, 47, 49, 50, 107, 109, 110,
    111, 112, 113–17, 120,
    122–23
naps, 172, 344
neck, 179, 195, 216
Neck Stretch, 352, 358
nerves/nervous system
    and addiction, 248
    and back pain, 186–88, 192
    and crying, 230
    and depression, 230
    and headaches, 208, 209, 211
    and irritable bowel syndrome,
        219
    and pain, 177–78
    and relationships, 286–87,
        297, 298
    and sex, 297, 298
    and spirituality, 323
    and stress, 258
    tingling, 221–22
neuroticism, 227
niacin. *See* vitamin B3
nicotine, 124, 239, 310. *See also*
    smoking
noise, 257, 262
nose, 77, 100, 285–87, 288, 294.
    See also smell

obesity, 182, 258, 390–91. *See*
    also weight
obsessions, 131, 234
obsessive-compulsive disorder,
    236, 238
olive oil, 52, 146, 203
omega-3 fatty acids, 44, 50, 79,
    146, 169, 172, 189, 217,
    221, 222, 241, 309, 341
omega-6 fats, 44
openness, 237–38, 330–31
optimism. *See* positive, being
osteoarthritis, 178, 199, 201,
    204
osteoporosis, 186

outer beauty, 1–2, 3, 6, 17, 29.
    See also attractiveness
overeating, 134, 220. *See also*
    satiety centers
oxytocin, 33, 126, 242, 289, 290,
    294, 299, 302, 309

pain threshold, 211
pain/aches
    acute, 179
    alternative therapies for, 178
    and brain, 154, 175, 177, 179
    chronic, 14, 176, 179, 185,
        192
    cycle of, 179
    and depression, 179, 184
    effects of, 176
    and empathy, 315
    and energy, 161, 162, 163,
        166, 167, 168, 171, 176
    Factoid about, 179
    fear as remembered, 177–78
    and feeling beautiful, 4, 152,
        154
    female, 217–18
    gate-control theory of, 179
    getting used to, 179
    and nervous system, 177–78
    physical versus emotional, 177
    response to, 154
    sensing of, 178–79
    and sex, 292, 294, 309
    and shoes, 205
    and skin, 179
    and sleep, 161
    and spirituality, 329
    and Ultimate Beautiful Day,
        339
    as warning signal, 168
    what is, 177–79
    YOU Test for, 175–76
    YOU Tips for, 243
    and YOU-Q, 13, 14
    See also specific type of pain or
        ache
Palms Out, 354, 359
pantothenic acid. *See* vitamin B5
pedicures, 123
peels, 398
Penguin, 355, 359
pepper, 80
peppermint, 51, 52, 220
periodontal disease, 99, 102,
    340

personality, 2, 224, 225, 227, 237–38, 244, 252–54. *See also specific disorder*
perspiration, 42. *See also* sweat
pets, 292
pheromones, 72, 286, 287, 288, 309
phi, 24, 26
piercings, 63
Pilates, 190
pineal gland, 291
pituitary gland, 258, 259
plantar fasciitis, 205
plastic, 333
plastic surgery, 131, 393–99
Pliaglis, 397
PMS, 217–18
polycystic ovarian disease (PCOS), 140
polyphenols, 174, 203, 343
polyunsaturated fats, 146
positive, being, 313–14, 329, 331
postpartum depression, 231
posture, 103, 108, 112, 159, 186, 189, 191–92, 213, 341
prayer, 323, 324–25, 326, 329, 330
predispositions, 322
pregnancy, 131, 132, 161, 210, 212, 298
pressure points, 210
probiotics, 174, 220–21
progesterone, 167, 206, 217
prolactin, 230
proprioception, 205
prostate gland, 298, 300, 307
protein, 111, 146, 147, 160, 172, 203, 230, 326, 340, 344
Prozac, 235
psoriasis, 46–47, 82, 116
pubic hair, 72
pulsed electromagnetic fields, 326
Punching Bag Crunches, 145

recycling, 334
reflexology, 126
Reiki, 326
relationships
    and attraction, 285–88, 297, 300, 303, 308
    and authenticity, 320
    and biology, 285–301, 310
    of blind people, 286

and buddies, 280, 284, 292
conflicts in, 293
and decision making, 305
decline in, 290
and depression, 280
and evolution, 291, 292–93, 294, 295, 297, 300
Factoids about, 290, 291, 293, 309
and gender, 291–300
and genetics, 286
and happiness, 280, 281, 284, 320, 328
and health, 284, 292
overview about, 280–81, 284–85
with pets, 292
reinventing, 302
Safari Secrets about, 288
and smell, 285–86, 287, 288, 294, 309
and spirituality, 312
and stress, 256, 284, 300
and survival, 291
and talking, 290, 298, 299, 302, 304–6, 309, 310
and teeth, 98
and togetherness, 289, 304
and touch, 286
and Ultimate Beautiful Day, 342, 344, 345, 347, 348
YOU Test for, 283
YOU Tips for, 302–6, 307–10
YOU Tool for, 307–10
See also love; sex
relaxation therapies, 313
religion, 313, 322–23
Remeron, 235
reproduction, and shape, 130, 131, 133, 136
resistance training, 47, 142, 143, 200–201
rest, and RICE, 201–2
restaurants, food in, 380
retinoids, 48, 57
retirement, 278
revitalization. *See* energy
rhinoplasty, 394
Rhodiola rosea, 173–74
ribose, 157, 169, 170
RICE, 201–2, 205
risk-taking, 264, 270, 274, 290, 293
rituals, 329–30, 347

role playing, 249
Rolfing, 189
roll around massage, 193
Roll and Massage Back, 368, 373
rosacea, 45, 50
rotator cuff, 202, 207
running exercises, 201

Safari Secrets, 26, 33, 44, 71, 93, 97, 288, 294
Saint John's wort, 241
SAMe, 178, 241
satiety, 133–37, 139, 146
satisfaction index, 147
saturated fats, 44, 52, 53, 146, 157, 172, 174, 217, 310
saw palmetto, 80
seabuchthorn oil, 45
seasonal affective disorder, 231, 244
sebaceous glands, 34, 36, 52
sebum, 34, 36, 50, 71, 85
second opinions, 204
Seidman, Daniel, 246
selenium, 309
self-esteem, 5, 16, 17, 230, 236–37
self-image, 29
self-love, 280
self-worth, 262
serotonin, 160, 175, 211, 212–13, 219, 231, 235, 242, 290, 309
sex
    and back pain, 180, 184
    biology of, 291–301
    and blind people, 286
    and brain, 136, 293, 294, 296, 297, 298, 310
    and depression, 230, 235
    and drugs/medications, 310
    and energy, 309
    and exercise, 310
    Factoid about, 297
    and feet, 6, 108, 126
    and female pains, 218
    and food, 296, 308–9, 310
    and hair, 71, 75, 79, 85
    and happiness, 292, 295
    and headaches, 212
    and hormones, 309
    and Kegel exercises, 341
    money equated with, 268
    and pain, 292, 294, 309

sex (*cont.*)
purpose and function of, 291, 292
and relationships, 285, 288, 290, 291–300
Safari Secrets about, 294
and smell, 309
and talking, 310
and Ultimate Beautiful Day, 348
and vitamins and supplements, 341
and weight, 310
YOU Tips for, 307–10
sex hormones, 132, 167–68, 391. *See also specific hormone*
shampoo, 6, 42, 66, 76, 78–79, 80, 81–82, 83, 84, 85, 339
shape
apple, 132
and attractiveness, 130, 131, 136
and brain, 133–40, 146, 147
and clothes/fashion, 147–50
and diet, 139, 143, 146
and drugs, 140, 142
and exercise, 131, 139, 143–46
Factoids about, 133, 137, 139, 142
and genetics, 133
and ghrelin and leptin, 137–40
and health, 131–32
and hormones, 137, 140
how to change, 133–42
ideal, 130
and muscles, 140–42, 143
pear, 131, 132
and sleep, 136, 137, 140
and waist-to-hip ratio, 129, 130, 131, 132–33, 136, 139
and weight, 131, 140, 146
YOU Test about, 129
YOU Tips for, 143–48
YOU Tool for, 149–50
YOU-Q for, 10–11, 12
shoes, 117, 118, 120, 125, 200, 205, 206, 343
Shoulder Height, 354, 359
The Shoulder Matrix, 144
shoulders
exercises for, 195
See also rotator cuff
Side Curl, 355, 359
Side Tricep Extension, 354, 359

simplicity, 332
sinuses, 100, 211, 340
sinusitis, 157, 160, 220
sitting, 186, 191–92
situational depression, 232
skin
aging of, 37, 39–41
and alcohol, 53
and allergies, 40, 41, 45, 47
body art for, 61–63
and burns, 51–52
cancer, 35, 37, 41–42
characteristics of healthy, beautiful, 39
color of, 39, 45, 59
as communicator, 33
composition of, 33–36
and cosmetics, 47, 48, 64
and diet, 44, 50–51, 52, 59
dirty, 52, 60
and exercise, 32, 47, 52
exfoliation of, 57–59, 60
near eyes, 46
Factoids about, 32, 34, 36, 40, 45, 46, 59
and fats, 52–53
function of, 33–34
glycation of, 125
and healing, 33
heaviness of, 33
and how it works, 36–41
and immune system, 50
and infections, 51–52, 56, 61, 63
and makeup, 58, 60
marks and blemishes on, 54–55
moisturizers for, 40–41, 45, 57
and muscles, 32
myths about, 39
and oil, 52
and pain, 179
problems with, 41–47
puffy, 40, 41, 53
Safari Secrets about, 33, 44
sagging, 37, 38, 40
and sleep, 40, 46, 52, 53
and stress, 37, 44
and sun, 38, 40, 44, 45, 50, 51, 52, 54, 56, 59–60
thinning, 38, 40, 46
and thyroid, 166
type of, 43

and Ultimate Beautiful Day, 339
and ultraviolet light, 34, 35, 39, 44, 45, 46, 48, 49, 50, 52, 59, 340, 343
and vitamins and supplements, 48–50, 54, 56, 59, 60, 341
washing and cleansing, 56–60
YOU Test for, 31, 43
YOU Tips for, 48–55
YOU Tools for, 56–60
YOU-Q for, 11, 12
See also skin care products; wrinkles
skin care products, 42, 46, 47, 48–49, 54, 57, 125
sleep
and addiction, 246
and brain, 136
and depression, 230, 232
and energy, 157, 158, 159, 161, 171–72
and eyes, 46
and infections, 174
with mouth open, 99
and naps, 172
and pain, 161
pills for, 231
problems with, 161
and shape, 136, 137, 140
and skin, 40, 46, 52, 53
and stress, 258
supplements for, 172
and Ultimate Beautiful Day, 339, 347, 348
smell, 285–86, 287, 288, 294, 309, 340
smile, 6, 88, 90, 93, 95–96, 306, 313, 342
smoking
addiction to, 239, 241, 246–51
and female pains, 217
and hair, 66
and happiness, 327
and neuropathies, 222
quitting, 327
as risk factor for back pain, 182
and secondhand smoke, 222
and skin, 37, 38, 53
and tongue, 96
and wrinkles, 53
See also nicotine
snacks, 343, 344

soap, 41, 42, 56
socioemotional network, 270
socks/stockings, 158
spastic colon, 160, 219–20
specialists, 168, 216
Spinal Twist, 357, 360
spine, 182–84, 186, 188, 191,
    192, 199, 221
spirituality
    and brain, 322–24, 331
    definition of, 6
    and emotions, 243
    and energy, 325–26
    exploring, 322–26
    and genetics, 322
    and happiness, 312–13, 322
    and health, 325, 329
    learning, 323
    overview about, 312–13
    and relationships, 312
    and stress, 329
    as tool, 330
    and Ultimate Beautiful Day,
        345, 347
    YOU Test for, 311
    YOU Tips about, 329–32
    and YOU-Q, 15, 16, 17
splinters, 112, 120
squats, 144, 190, 192, 356, 360
Squeeze Squats, 144
stamina training, 146
Standing Chest Press, 351, 358
Standing Chest Pull, 352, 358
Standing Leaning Stretch, 362,
    371
Standing Twist, 362, 371
steroids, 36, 45, 116, 184, 192,
    231
Stork, 364, 371
strength
    and shape, 130
    See also muscles
strength training/exercises, 142,
    182, 201, 205, 216, 309
stress
    acute, 260, 262
    and aromatherapy, 51
    beauty as managing, 256
    benefits of, 257, 260
    biology of, 258, 260
    and brain, 259, 260, 331
    chronic, 260, 262
    control of, 270–72
    and depression, 233

effects of, 258
    and emotional intelligence,
        270–72
    and emotions, 243, 270, 313
    and energy, 157, 159, 164
    and exercise, 216
    and gratitude, 330
    and hair, 74
    and happiness, 326
    and headaches, 212
    and healing, 33
    and hormones, 233, 259
    and irritable bowel syndrome,
        219
    and joint pain, 213
    as lack of control, 256
    and locus of control, 269
    management of, 331
    and personality, 237
    and relationships, 284, 300
    and sex, 300
    and skin, 37, 44
    and spirituality, 329
    and sugar, 160
    and teeth, 97, 99, 101, 103
    and Ultimate Beautiful Day,
        342, 344, 345
    See also worry; type of stress
stretch marks, 36, 49, 55
stretching exercises, 143, 191,
    216, 339
strokes, 211, 231, 232, 292
substance P, 175, 178
sugar
    craving for, 160
    and energy, 157, 160, 164,
        165, 169, 170, 172
    and headaches, 215
    and infections, 174
    and sex, 310
    and shape, 137
    simple, 146, 172, 174
    and yeast overgrowth, 220
    See also blood sugar; type of
        sugar
suicide, 229, 232
sun
    and hair, 75
    and hands, 59
    and lips, 105
    screens, 59–60, 64
    and skin, 38, 40, 44, 45, 50,
        51, 52, 54, 56, 59–60,
        343

and wrinkling, 50
    See also ultraviolet light
superficiality, 320, 328
supplements, 48–49, 80, 172,
    217, 241, 341, 345. See also
    minerals; vitamins; specific
    supplement
support groups, 236, 276
surgery, 119, 143, 186, 204, 206,
    222, 232. See also laser
    therapy; plastic surgery
survival, 5, 264, 291, 317, 327
sweat, 34, 36, 72, 114, 124, 215,
    294, 340
swimming, 202, 216
symmetry, 27–29
synovial fluid, 196, 198, 199, 203

talking, 225, 242, 244, 276, 290,
    298, 299, 302, 304–6, 309,
    310
tanning, 36–37
tantric sex, 307–8
tattoos, 61–63
teeth
    and anatomy of mouth, 92–93
    appearance of, 98
    brushing of, 102, 105, 340,
        347
    and diet, 99
    discoloration of, 100, 104–5
    Factoids about, 91, 93, 99, 100
    fillings for, 93
    flossing of, 102–3, 340
    function of, 88
    grinding of, 87, 88, 89, 98,
        100–101
    and health, 88, 97–101
    and jaw pain, 213
    Safari Secrets about, 93, 97
    shape of, 93
    and smile, 90, 95, 96
    and stress, 97, 99, 101
    and tics, 215
    and Ultimate Beautiful Day,
        340, 347
    whitening of, 103–4, 105
    wisdom, 91
    YOU Test about, 87, 89
    YOU Tips about, 102–6
temporomandibular joint (TMJ),
    159, 211, 213
tendons, 196, 207
tennis balls, massage with, 6, 193

tension headaches, 212–13, 216
testosterone, 72, 73, 74, 79, 132, 167, 288, 310, 391
    and, 140
tests. *See type of test*
thank you. *See gratitude*
Thatcher, Margaret, image of, 149, 150
therapy. *See type of therapy*
thinking, too much, 331
Thread the Needle, 356, 360, 366, 372
thrush, 97
thyroid, 75–76, 79, 140, 164, 165–67, 220, 231, 235, 387
tics, 215
Tiger Balm, 188
Tightrope, 363, 371
tocopherol, 50
toenails, 113–21
togetherness, 289, 304
toluene, 42
tongue, 91, 96–97, 98, 340
toothpaste, 92, 100, 102, 104
topical ointments, 196
touching, and healing, 33, 286, 306
trans fats, 44, 52, 146, 172, 217, 310
transplants, hair, 68
Tree, 363, 371
Triangle, 365, 372
triglycerides, 52, 167, 258
TSH levels, 75, 165, 387
tummy tucks, 395–96
Turkish Getup, 145

ulcers, 97
Ultimate Beautiful Day, 338–48
ultraviolet light
    and emotions, 244
    and nails, 113
    and skin, 34, 35, 39, 44, 45, 47, 48, 49, 50, 52, 59, 340, 343
uric acid, 198

vagina, pain in, 218
vaginitis, 157, 174
vagus nerve, 33
varicose veins, 55, 158
vascular depression, 232
vertebrae, 182–84, 189

vertebroplasty, 186
Viagra, 235, 290
viruses, 157, 159–61, 174. *See also specific virus*
vitamins
    and cancer, 174
    and hair, 49, 71, 80
    and headaches, 208
    and immune system, 50
    and joints, 203–4
    and nails, 49
    and skin, 48–50, 56, 59
    and Ultimate Beautiful Day, 341, 345
    See also specific vitamin
vitamin A, 40–41, 48, 49, 50, 54, 57, 347
vitamin B, 80, 111, 157, 174, 189
vitamin B3 (niacin), 45, 48, 49, 52, 56, 125, 339
vitamin B4, 157
vitamin B5 (pantothenic acid), 48, 49, 56, 339
vitamin B6, 217, 222
vitamin B12, 92, 174, 222, 235, 390
vitamin C, 45, 49–50, 54, 56, 203–4, 309, 347
vitamin D, 45, 59, 174, 341, 343, 390
vitamin D3, 203, 204, 221
vitamin E, 40–41, 49, 50, 56, 71, 203–4, 309, 339

waist-to-hip ratio, 129, 130, 131, 132–33, 136, 139, 300
walking, 139, 146, 171, 216, 244, 250, 251, 292, 342, 343
warts, 119–20, 123
water, 136, 146, 172, 220, 334, 341, 343, 347
waxing, 67
weight
    and addiction, 247
    causes of gain in, 140
    and depression, 230
    and diet, 343
    and energy, 162, 171
    and hair, 67
    and joints, 200–201, 202
    and sex, 310
    and shape, 131, 140, 146
    and thyroid, 166

and Ultimate Beautiful Day, 343
    See also obesity
weight bells, 182
weight-bearing exercises, 200, 201
Wellbutrin, 235, 250. *See also* bupropion
willow bark, 178, 191, 204
work, 257, 258–62, 266, 269–70, 273–78, 342
worry
    and instincts, 268–72
    overview about, 256–57
    purpose of, 256
    types of, 256
    YOU Test about, 255
    YOU Tips about, 273–78
    See also finances; stress; work
wrinkles, 32, 33, 37–38, 40, 42, 50, 53–54, 56, 341, 399
Wrist Extensions, 366, 372

X, 362, 371
xanthomas, 52

yeast, 97, 160, 220
yoga, 143, 189, 190, 201, 216, 243, 339, 345, 361–74
yohimbine, 290
YOU Test
    for back pain, 181
    for depression, 223, 226
    for energy, 155, 160, 166
    for finances, 261, 266
    for hair, 65
    for joints, 195
    for nails, 107
    for pain, 175–76
    purpose of, 6
    for relationships, 283
    for shape, 129
    for skin type, 43
    for spirituality, 311
    for sugar cravings, 160
    tape skin, 31
    for teeth, 87, 89
    for thyroid, 166
    for work, 266
    for worry, 255
YOU Tips
    for addiction, 244–45
    for back pain, 190–93
    for depression, 244

for energy, 169, 171–74
for feet, 122–25
for finances, 273–78
for hair, 78–82
for hands, 122–25
for happiness, 329–32
for headaches, 215–22
for joint pain, 200–204
for mood, 242–45
for mouth, 102–6
for pain, 243
purpose of, 6
for relationships, 302–6, 307–10
for sex, 307–10
for shape, 143–48
for skin care, 48–55
for spirituality, 329–32
for teeth, 102–6
for work, 273–78
for worry, 273–78
YOU Tools
for addiction, 246–51
band workout as, 351–60
body art as, 61–63
for emotions, 246–51
energy blood tests as, 387–92
for eyes, 383–85
for fashion, 149–50
for feet, 126–27
for green living, 333–36
for hair care, 83–85
for hands, 126–27
for happiness, 333–36
health utensils as, 377–81
for joint pain, 205–7
for mood, 246–51
perfect gym bag as, 375
for personality, 252–54
purpose of, 6
for relationships, 307–10
for shape, 149–50
for yoga workout, 361–74
YOU-Q Test, 6, 8–20, 280

zinc, 59, 309
Zoloft, 235